Biomedical Ethics

FUNDAMENTALS OF PHILOSOPHY SERIES

Series Editors
John Martin Fischer, University of California, Riverside
and
John Perry, Stanford University

Biomedical Ethics
Walter Glannon

Mind: A Brief Introduction
John R. Searle

Free Will
Robert Kane

Biomedical Ethics

WALTER GLANNON

New York ◆ Oxford
OXFORD UNIVERSITY PRESS
2005

Oxford University Press

Oxford   New York
Auckland   Bangkok   Buenos Aires   Cape Town   Chennai
Dar es Salaam   Delhi   Hong Kong   Istanbul   Karachi   Kolkata
Kuala Lumpur   Madrid   Melbourne   Mexico City   Mumbai   Nairobi
São Paulo   Shanghai   Taipei   Tokyo   Toronto

Published by Oxford University Press, Inc.
198 Madison Avenue, New York, New York, 10016
www.oup.com

Oxford is a registered trademark of Oxford University Press

Library of Congress Cataloging-in-Publication Data

Glannon, Walter.
  Biomedical ethics/by Walter Glannon.
    p. cm—(Fundamentals of philosophy)
  Includes bibliographical references and index.
  ISBN 978-0-19-514431-4 (pbk.)
    1. Medical ethics. I. Title. II. Series

R724.G58 2004
174.2—dc22   2004050092

Printed in the United States of America
on acid-free paper

For Yee-Wah

Contents

Preface

These are exciting times in medicine and biotechnology. Advances in these fields are occurring at a rapid pace and are having a profound influence on our lives. Mechanical ventilation can keep humans alive indefinitely in the absence of most brain functions. The participation of human subjects in medical research may lead to drugs that can control or cure the most debilitating and deadly diseases. Computed tomography (CT), magnetic resonance imaging (MRI), and positron emission tomography (PET) scans of the body and brain can reveal disorders before symptoms appear. Genetic testing of embryos can predict whether persons will have diseases earlier or later in life. Genes can be inserted into the body and brain to correct disorders and possibly improve physical and mental capacities. It may even become possible to clone human beings. But these and other developments raise important and controversial ethical questions.

The aim of this book is to engage readers in critically reflecting on and analyzing these questions. It is a philosophical introduction to the most important ethical positions and arguments in six areas of biomedicine: the patient-doctor relationship; medical research on humans; reproductive rights and technologies; genetics; medical decisions at the end of life; and allocation of scarce medical resources. The topics cover both perennial ethical issues in medicine, such as doctors' duties to patients, and recent and emerging ethical issues in scientific innovation, such as gene therapy and cloning. The scope of the book captures the historical, contemporary, and future-oriented flavor of these areas in a concise and accessible way. I do not merely describe arguments so that they are understood, but also use them to reach reasoned conclusions on controversial matters in Chapters 2 through 7. The general point of this method is to show that debates in biomedical ethics can be resolved in more than one reasonable way.

Strictly speaking, "ethics" and "morality" have distinct meanings. The first derives from the Greek and is concerned with individual character and the sorts of lives that are good or bad for persons to lead. The second derives from the Latin and emphasizes social expectation, taking into account the needs and interests of others when we act. In practice, though, most people use the two terms interchangeably, and I will follow that custom here.

I thank John Perry and John Martin Fischer, editors of the Fundamentals of Philosophy series, for inviting me to write this book. I am grateful to the four readers of the book proposal and the four readers of the manuscript commissioned by Oxford University Press, as well as to John Fischer, for many constructive suggestions. My editors at OUP, Robert Miller, Emily Voigt, and Celeste Alexander, were very helpful and supportive throughout the project. David Schmidtz gave me valuable comments on the first chapter that set the stage for the discussion in the subsequent chapters. David Benatar, Lainie Friedman Ross, and Teresa Yee-Wah Yu read the entire manuscript. Teresa's keen stylistic and substantive comments led to significant improvements. I am especially grateful to David B. and Lainie, each of whom generously provided many pages of insightful points and constructive criticisms on both medical issues and philosophical arguments that have been extremely helpful. The book is much better as a result of the thoughtful reading of all these people.

Biomedical Ethics

CHAPTER 1

History and Theories

Introduction

Biomedical ethics began in the fifth century B.C.E. in the School of Hippocrates. Upon graduation from medical school, many doctors still take the Hippocratic Oath: "I will use treatment to help the sick according to my ability and judgment, but never with a view to injury or wrongdoing." This is the basis of the central Latin maxim of medical practice: *Primum non nocere* ("First, do no harm"). How doctors should treat patients rests on general moral principles about how a person should treat other people. These principles in turn derive from the more fundamental question of ethics that Socrates raises in Plato's *Republic*: "How should one live?" Biomedical ethics is thus grounded in the study of moral philosophy.

The Hippocratic tradition was carried on through the centuries by, among others, the Jewish philosopher and physician Moses Maimonides (1135–1204). But it was the English physician Thomas Percival who first used the term "medical ethics" when he published a book with this title in 1803. Percival expanded the Hippocratic focus on the doctor-patient relationship to a broader social ethic of medicine, emphasizing the professional responsibility of the physician. This idea was incorporated into the first version of the American Medical Association's *Code of Medical Ethics* in 1849, which was subsequently revised in 1903 under the new title, *Principles of Medical Ethics*. After many transformations, the 1946 version of the Code embodied a set of principles that, in the spirit of Percival, emphasized not only *nonmaleficence* (not harming) and *beneficence* (benefiting) toward patients, but also doctors' responsibility to the medical profession and to society at large. In 1971, Van Rensselaer Potter described "bioethics" as "a new discipline that combines biological knowledge with knowledge of human value systems." One year later, Warren Reich, editor of the *Encyclopedia of Bioethics*, drew from the ideas of Potter and Andre Helligers in defining bioethics as "the study of the ethical dimensions of medicine and the biological sciences." By this time, biomedical ethics had become a discipline in its own right, a discipline emerging at the intersection of science, medicine, and ethics.

Developments in medical practice and research over the second half of the twentieth century led to ethical principles in addition to nonmaleficence and beneficence. Before this time, the interpretation and application of these two principles were excessively paternalistic. The physician alone determined what was in the best interests of the patient. Experimentation on human subjects in Nazi Germany and the United States in the twentieth century was a perverse extension of the authoritarian aspect of paternalism. Humans were entered into medical experiments without consent and without any consideration of the risk of harm to them. The abuses committed in these experiments, and the recognition that patients were the best judges of their own interests, led to a gradual shift in decisional authority from doctor to patient. This turned the Hippocratic tradition on its head. As a result, the patient-based principle of *autonomy* came to complement the physician-based principles of nonmaleficence and beneficence.

Autonomy (from the Greek *auto* = "self" + *nomos* = "law") means having the capacity and the right to self-determination, to formulate and follow a life plan of one's own making. Individuals with the capacity for autonomy have the right to exercise that capacity. This includes the right to accept or refuse medical treatment in accord with one's interests, which may not be limited to medical considerations alone. Respect for autonomy derives from two fundamental principles from two distinct traditions of moral theory. The first is Immanuel Kant's principle of respect for persons as autonomous ends-in-themselves. We are autonomous in the sense that we have the capacity for reason and can apply the moral law to ourselves. Kant's principle is at the core of the deontological tradition. The second is John Stuart Mill's principle of liberty, which says that a person is sovereign over his or her own body and mind. It specifies that an individual's freedom can be restricted only when its exercise would harm others. Mill's principle is at the core of the liberal tradition. We will discuss the theories of these and other philosophers in more detail throughout this chapter.

Advances in medical technology over the years have had significant ethical implications. In the 1960s, the availability of dialysis for people in chronic kidney failure made it possible to purify the blood of patients who otherwise would have died. But dialysis was expensive and not accessible on a large scale, which meant that not all people who needed it could receive it. This marked one of the first instances of the need to allocate a scarce medical resource. The feasibility of organ transplantation was another example of a life-saving technology; but it involved the same problem of demand exceeding supply. The main issue was how a scarce medical resource could be distributed fairly among people with equal needs when its scarcity meant that not everyone's needs could be met. Because justice is usually defined in terms of fairness, *justice* emerged as the fourth main principle in medical ethics.

The introduction of the respirator in the late 1960s and early 1970s made it possible to maintain breathing and heartbeat when patients were no longer able to do these on their own. Before this life-sustaining technology became available, patients died when they stopped breathing and their hearts stopped beating. The ability to artificially sustain life forced a revision of the definition of death, shifting the focus from the heart and lungs to the brain. On this view, death occurs when all brain functions permanently cease. This view has had significant medical and ethical implications for decisions at both the beginning and end of human life. The respirator and related technology enable us to sustain the lives of low-weight babies born at the margin of viability, with immature lungs and other organs. These tools also enable us to indefinitely sustain the lives of patients with no higher-brain function but only a functioning brain stem. Debate continues on whether the benefits of these and other life-sustaining interventions outweigh the burdens to the patients who receive them.

In the area of genetics, presymptomatic testing for individuals at risk of late-onset genetic diseases such as Huntington's is now available. Embryos and fetuses can also be tested for mutations that can result in severe disease and disability for the people who develop from them. Genetic testing raises questions about how genetic information should be used and how it might benefit or harm people. In addition, the use of human subjects in clinical trials raises questions about informed consent, equal access, and the ratio of risks to benefits for those who participate in these trials.

These developments force us to consider ethical questions such as the following: How can scarce organs for transplantation be allocated fairly and efficiently to those who need them? When is it permissible to withhold or withdraw life-sustaining medical treatment? Should doctors be prohibited from assisting terminally ill patients in committing suicide? Can suspected carriers of a genetic mutation be obligated to undergo genetic testing and inform their siblings or children of the results? Should embryo selection on the basis of genetic status be prohibited? Is it permissible to allow human subjects to participate in clinical trials when it puts them at risk and offers them no direct benefit?

The Need for Theories

To respond to these questions, we need to appeal to ethical theories in giving reasons and arguments to justify a particular action or policy. Ethical theories provide a framework that enables us to critically reflect on and refine the intuitions generated by issues and cases. This process will enable us to give reasons for or against a position. An argument can be understood as a consistent set of reasons logically leading to a conclusion. The stronger the reasons one gives for an action or policy, the more convincing will be the argument and the stronger the justification for doing or implementing it. In most cases, the reasons one gives will be motivated by one of the four ethical principles we have mentioned. And these principles will be shorthand for different ethical theories. Before we examine these theories, some additional definitions are in order.

In the process of justification, reasons determine which actions or policies are obligated, prohibited, or permitted. An action or policy is *obligated* if it is supported by an ethically decisive reason. That is, the reason outweighs any opposing reason for not acting or not implementing a policy. An action or policy is *prohibited* if there is an ethically decisive reason against it. And an action or policy is *permitted* if there is no ethically decisive reason against it. What makes the action or policy permissible is the absence of a reason for not doing or not implementing it. Whether a reason is decisive will depend to some extent on the particular context in which it is cited. For example, if one claims that it is morally permissible to withhold or withdraw treatment from a patient, then this claim implies that there is no ethically decisive reason for initiating or continuing that treatment. The treatment has no clear therapeutic benefit and is not in the patient's best interests. On the other hand, the claim that a patient with symptoms of a late-onset genetic disease is obligated to undergo genetic testing and share the result with siblings or children implies that there is an ethically decisive reason for testing. In this second case, the reason applies not only to the patient with the symptoms, but also to his family. The information can prevent harm to and benefit those who are at risk of inheriting the disease by enabling them to plan their lives accordingly. Also, the claim that withholding or withdrawing treatment from a newborn with multiple medical conditions should be prohibited implies that there is an ethically decisive reason against these actions. The reason is based on a presumption to treat the infant, unless his or her condition is terminal or the treatment is of no benefit.

Biomedical ethics is a species of practical normative ethics. It is the study of what one is obligated or permitted to do, or prohibited from doing, in different contexts of biotechnology, medical practice, and medical research. *Normative ethics* is concerned with how people ought to act, what sort of person one ought to be, or what sorts of polices ought to be implemented. It is "normative" in the sense that it specifies norms or standards of right and wrong action and behavior. We employ principles and theories of normative ethics to motivate and justify actions and policies in biomedicine. In contrast, *descriptive ethics* is concerned with how people do in fact behave, not how they ought to behave. Evolutionary theories of morality are descriptive in the sense that they claim that morality serves an adaptive purpose, enhancing human survival through social cooperation. Similarly, sociological and anthropological accounts of morality are descriptive in the way they focus on behavioral patterns among people in different cultures. The two types of ethical theory we have just outlined are to be distinguished from *metaethics*. While normative ethics deals with the substantive question of which actions are right or wrong, good or bad, metaethics deals with the formal question of the point of ethics. It focuses on the meaning of terms like "right," "wrong," "good," and "bad," and on the form of arguments used to justify actions. Metaethics is concerned with whether there are ethical facts independent of our normative judgments and social conventions, facts that ground these judgments and conventions. Put another way, whereas normative ethics focuses on the *content* of morality, metaethics focuses on the *nature* of morality.

Most normative ethical theories have two criteria in common: (1) *objectivity*, where the right course of action is based on the best reasons for doing it, and where these reasons can be recognized universally by anyone and therefore cannot be reduced to any particular point of view; and (2) *impartiality*, where reasons for action assume that each person's needs and interests are equally important, and that the claims of all people are given equal weight. Together, these two criteria are safeguards against arbitrariness and personal or group bias in justifying behavior.

Although biomedical ethics is a practical normative enterprise, it cannot be divorced from metaethics. For, in citing reasons to justify an action or policy, these reasons presuppose an implicit understanding of the meaning of such terms as "right," "wrong," "required," "prohibited," and "permitted." Moreover, the form of argument one uses in citing these reasons will be crucial to the justification. Metaethics is also concerned with the question of whether the two criteria of normative ethical theories cited in the previous paragraph can be met. These points are especially important in the light of the challenge that cultural relativism poses to the presumed objectivity and impartiality of ethical theories. On the view that there are no universally valid judgments about what constitutes right or wrong action, these judgments will always be relative to different belief systems in different cultures. As we will see later in this chapter and in Chapter 2, cultural relativism calls into question the value and meaning of practices and terms central to Western medicine. Among other things, the challenge of cultural relativism shows that the formal and substantive aspects of ethical theory are interconnected.

Consequentialism and Deontology

Consequentialism and deontology are the two ethical theories most frequently cited to defend different positions in biomedicine. The four ethical principles that we have mentioned are representative of these two theories. Nonmaleficence and beneficence are consequentialist principles concerned with benefiting and not harming patients in bringing about the best outcome of a treatment. Autonomy is a deontological principle concerned with such things as a patient's rights, dignity, and value, as well as the doctor's corresponding duty to respect them. This does not mean that consequentialists completely ignore autonomy. Nor do deontologists completely ignore consequences. Each group gives greater weight to one of these two general principles and lesser weight to the other. Justice may be characterized as either a deontological or consequentialist principle. It is concerned with what is due or owed to persons in terms of the distribution of benefits and burdens among them. In biomedical ethics, justice is especially pertinent to research involving human subjects and the allocation of scarce medical resources such as organs for transplantation.

Respect for autonomy protects a competent patient's right to refuse medical treatment. A doctor would be obligated to respect a competent adult Jehovah's Witness' refusal of a blood transfusion for severe anemia resulting from chemotherapy to treat leukemia. This means that the doctor would be prohibited from giving the transfusion, even if not giving it led to the patient's death. The patient's refusal is motivated by the idea that accepting blood or blood products violates his or her religious beliefs, which fall under the patient's autonomy. In a different instance, an individual who happens to be a good tissue match for a stranger in need of a kidney transplant would not be obligated to give up the needed organ. In each of these two cases, the person is exercising the right to noninterference in accord with personal interests, values, and beliefs. On the other hand, blood and tissue matches between organ donors and potential organ recipients mean that some recipients will have better outcomes with a transplant than others. With the newer immunosuppressive drugs, these matches have become less important. Still, the long-term outcomes of transplants where blood and tissue do not match are unknown. It would be unwise to ignore these biological factors altogether and give each person in need of a transplant an equal chance to receive one. Here considerations of fairness in giving equal weight to people's claims of need may be overridden by the goal of bringing about the best outcome. This is merely one example of the fact that different issues and cases in biomedical ethics require careful analysis of the relative weights of conflicting ethical principles and theories.

Ethical principles are not absolute, but prima facie, an idea that is traceable to the twentieth-century philosopher W. D. Ross. A prima facie moral obligation is one that is binding unless it is overridden or outweighed by a competing moral obligation. The four principles at hand are prima facie in the sense that each has considerable weight in serving to justify a given position. But each can be overridden if the weight of a different principle for a competing position is greater. In the majority of cases, the most defensible position will be arrived at only after carefully weighing the force of each principle against one or more of the other three. Rarely can a position be defended by consideration of one principle alone.

Consequentialism defines the rightness or wrongness of an action in terms of its consequences. Actions are justified by the amount of good they bring about. The most familiar form of consequentialism is utilitarianism, which says that one should act to promote the greatest good for the greatest number. It generates an obligation to increase happiness and diminish suffering in securing a net overall benefit. Many philosophers use "consequentialism" and "utilitarianism" interchangeably. There are differences between these two theories, however. Noting that the intensity of a good may vary across people, consequentialists are more concerned with the greatest good than with the good of the greatest number. Moreover, ethically relevant outcomes in different areas of biomedicine include but are not limited to happiness and suffering. Hence, we will use the more general term "consequentialism" in the remainder of this chapter and in subsequent chapters.

Deontology (from the Greek *deon* = "duty") defines the rightness or wrongness of an action in terms of a duty or obligation to respect the rights and values of persons. It specifies constraints on what we can or cannot do to others, constraints that can prohibit actions that bring about good consequences. A modified version of deontology, nonconsequentialism, says that consequences can matter; but they are not the main motivation for action. We are permitted not to maximize overall best consequences, and there may be constraints on promoting these consequences. The focus remains on rights, duties, and the person as an end-in-itself.

Despite their differences, consequentialism and deontology both prescribe principles telling us what we should do. In this sense, they specify moral obligations. In consequentialism, the obligation is to promote good outcomes. In deontology, the obligation is to respect persons as ends-in-themselves. It will be helpful to further elaborate the defining features of these two theories and assess their comparative strengths and weaknesses.

Consequentialism says that what makes an action or policy right is that it brings about better consequences than any alternatives. We have noted that utilitarianism is the most well-known version of consequentialism. Jeremy Bentham (1748–1832) articulated the principle of utility, or the Greatest Happiness Principle. This says that actions are right if they promote happiness, and wrong if they promote suffering. John Stuart Mill (1806–1873) refined this principle and added to it a condition of equality. This means that, in applying the principle of utility, we should act in such a way that each person counts for one, and nobody counts for more than one. It is important to distinguish the principle of utility from Mill's principle of liberty, which, together with Kant's idea of respect for persons, forms the basis of personal autonomy.

There are two types of consequentialism: act-consequentialism and rule-consequentialism. These correspond to two types of utilitarianism: act- and rule-utilitarianism. Act-consequentialism says that an act is obligatory if it promotes better consequences than any of its alternatives. An act is permissible if it promotes consequences that are at least as good as any of its alternatives. Consider an intensive care unit (ICU). When the number of patients needing care exceeds the number of available beds, doctors have to decide to admit some patients but not others. Giving highest priority to admitting the patient with the highest likelihood of being restored to normal functioning, and lowest priority to the patient with the lowest likelihood of surviving, can be justified on act-consequentialist grounds. The act of selecting one patient over the other is permissible, if not obligatory, because it brings about a better consequence than giving each of the patients an equal chance for treatment.

In other cases, adherence to act-consequentialism can be short-sighted and result in more harm than good. Suppose that one of a doctor's patients shows symptoms of a neurodegenerative disease and tests positive for the genetic mutation that causes Huntington's disease. This mutation has virtual 100 percent penetrance, which means that anyone who has it will develop the disease. The patient has several children, each of whom has a 50 percent chance of having the mutation and developing the disease later in life. The doctor asks the patient to tell his children that he has the disease and to explain the risk to them; but he refuses. Intending to prevent potential harm to the children in not knowing their genetic status and not being able to plan for their future, the doctor breaches confidentiality and informs them of their father's genetic status without his consent. While this act might be justified if it prevented harmful consequences to the children, it could lead to more harmful consequences in the long term. If breaching confidentiality were practiced on a broad scale, then many people might distrust the medical profession and be discouraged from seeing doctors for prevention and treatment of diseases.

Rule-consequentialism is often invoked to avoid this problem with act-consequentialism. Whereas the latter asks, "Which action will promote the best consequences in this particular situation?" the former asks "Which general rules will promote the best consequences in the long term, assuming that everyone accepts and complies with them?" Following the guidance implicit in this second question, doctors should try to persuade their patients with heritable disorders that they should inform their children, spouses, or siblings of their genetic status. Their patients may refuse. But unless the probability of harm to these relatives is high, by upholding confidentiality doctors will promote public trust in the medical profession, better relations between patients and doctors, and thus better consequences for patients overall.

The most serious objection to consequentialism (in both "act" and "rule" forms) is that doing whatever promotes the best consequences may violate individuals' interests and rights. This was evident in the example of the physician who disclosed genetic information about the Huntington's patient without his consent. A second objection is that consequentialism fails to take seriously the separateness of persons. It is an impersonal theory concerned more with the aggregative question of *how much* of some good there should be than with the distributive question of *who* should have it. Consequentialism may at first blush appear to be superior to deontology in determining how a scarce resource should be allocated to maximize overall benefits and minimize overall burdens. But it does not pay sufficient attention to the claims of each person who stands to benefit or be burdened by these decisions or policies. Only deontology can adequately respect the force of these claims.

The most well-known deontologist is Immanuel Kant (1724–1804). Kant held that there is one fundamental principle of morality, the categorical imperative. This principle is based on reason alone, specifically on the idea that humans are defined essentially in terms of the capacity for reason. Emotions should play no role in the motivation for action because they are too unstable to serve as a basis for moral behavior. The categorical imperative consists of two formulations: (1) act only on that maxim by which you can at the same time will that it should become a universal law; and (2) act so that you treat humanity, whether in your own person or in that of any other, always as an end and never as a means only. This imperative is "categorical" in the sense that it is unconditional and therefore allows no exceptions. It applies to all humans regardless of personal desires, plans, or interests. And it is based on reason alone, which tells us which action is right in every situation. This is distinct from a hypothetical imperative, which is conditional in the sense that it is based on particular desires and the conditions that will satisfy them. A hypothetical imperative states: "If you want x, then do y." A categorical imperative states: "Do not kill!", "Always keep your promises!", or "Always tell the truth!" An action is right when it aligns with the moral law, which embodies the categorical imperative and is self-legislated by rational human beings.

For Kant, the nature of moral judgment rests on maxims. A maxim is a subjective rule that guides one's actions. It is not actions such as suicide or killing that Kant judges as wrong, but killing oneself or others on the basis of a particular maxim. To be universalizable, a maxim must be both conceived and willed as a universal law. Regarding the maxim to keep one's promises, for example, one would have to pass the following test: "What if everyone, without exception, acted on the principle that, when I am in need, I shall make promises I have no intention of keeping?" Kant's general point is not about the consequences of lying. Rather, if it were universally willed, lying would be inconsistent with what is essential to the will of every self-interested agent. It would be inconsistent with our rational humanity.

The second formulation of the categorical imperative is more germane to biomedical ethics. It specifies constraints on what we can do to others, prohibiting even actions that would maximize overall net benefit. Consider a patient who is comatose and in respiratory distress following an automobile accident. Although he is put on a respirator, doctors treating him believe that he will regain consciousness and recover. Other than the areas of his body affected by the accident, his organs are functioning well. A transplant surgeon would like to disconnect the respirator keeping him alive and immediately procure his organs for transplantation. By doing this, he could save the lives of several other patients needing transplants. But the act of disconnecting life-support in this case would amount to wrongfully killing the patient. If the patient still has the capacity for consciousness and still has an interest in and right to continue living, then the doctor would be violating the patient's interest and right. He would be harming and wronging the patient, treating him merely as a means and not also as an end-in-itself. There would be a decisive reason against the doctor's action and thus it would be prohibited. Deontology prescribes an absolute prohibition against killing in such a case, no matter how good the consequences of the action might be. Deontology does not prohibit all forms of killing, though. Self-defense and just wars are two examples of morally justified killing on deontological grounds.

A more common example of a deontological constraint in medical practice is when a patient refuses chemotherapy for a form of cancer that can be treated and controlled. The oncologist is obligated to try to persuade the patient to accept the treatment. But if the patient is competent enough to understand his or her diagnosis, prognosis, and the consequences of refusing the treatment, then the oncologist is obligated to uphold the patient's decision. The doctor is obligated to respect the patient's autonomy in exercising the right to refuse treatment in accord with his or her best interests. By not overriding that decision, the doctor is treating the patient as an end-in-itself.

Perhaps the most instructive application of the second formulation of the categorical imperative to biomedical ethics is in research involving human subjects. The goal of medical research is to gain scientific knowledge about drugs, surgery, or other interventions that can benefit future patients. When recruiting subjects for clinical trials to achieve this goal, researchers effectively are using subjects as means. Yet, provided that subjects give informed consent to participate in and understand the potential reasonable risks and benefits of the trials, they are respected as autonomous decision-makers. The subjects *are* being used as means, though not *only* as means but *also* as ends-in-themselves. In this regard, using human subjects for medical research can be justified on deontological grounds. There are problems with informed consent in medical research, however, as we will see in Chapter 3.

Deontology has shortcomings regarding the allocation of scarce resources. The main objection to this theory is that it does not adequately consider the number of people who stand to benefit or be harmed by an action or policy. Nor does it consider the probability and magnitude of benefit and harm. Deontology does not offer much guidance about how to best meet the claims of need of many people in maximizing benefit and minimizing harm. By ignoring or not paying sufficient attention to outcomes, it cannot always provide a justification for action. Indeed, deontology can be untenable if it is strictly adhered to in situations of scarcity, as we saw earlier in the example of deciding which patients to admit into an ICU. If we simply give each patient in urgent need of care an equal chance regardless of the probable outcome of treatment, then we may end up benefiting none and harming many people.

Some will not be satisfied with consequentialism or deontology. They will claim that basing ethics on principles that specify obligations leaves other important dimensions of motivation and behavior out of the picture. Neither theory, nor their representative principles, can satisfactorily explain or justify every action. Let's explore some alternatives to principle-based ethics.

Virtue Ethics and Feminist Ethics

Virtue ethics is often seen as an antidote to the principle-based ethical theories of consequentialism and deontology. Instead of duties and obligations, virtue ethics focuses on such aretaic (*arête* = virtue, excellence) properties as "admirable," "reprehensible," "praiseworthy," and "blameworthy." The ancient Greeks, especially Aristotle, conceived of ethics in this way. It has made a comeback in contemporary moral philosophy, in the wake of what philosophers Elizabeth Anscombe and Alasdair MacIntyre have called the "bankruptcy of modern moral philosophy." Virtue theory is especially relevant to the patient-physician relationship and emphasizes the more personal, humane aspects of medicine. Ideally, a physician should display such traits as conscientiousness, courtesy, empathy, and compassion toward patients. Correspondingly, patients should display such traits as self-control and moderation in their lifestyle and reasonableness toward their doctors in terms of what they expect from them. Together, these traits engender mutual trust in the relationship.

Virtue ethics is agent based rather than action based. It is concerned with a person's motivation for action, the disposition or character from which the action issues, instead of with features of the action itself. Actions are evaluated as expressions of the agent's disposition or character. If one performs a compassionate act, for example, it is because one has a compassionate disposition to act in that way. The disposition is fundamental; the action is derivative. Our moral evaluation of human agents and their actions follows in the same order. Unlike Kantian deontology, the idea that a physician has a duty to act virtuously is not part of his or her motivation for acting. A virtuous disposition motivates virtuous action. Acting from duty is not the mark of excellence. The distinguishing feature of the virtuous person is that he or she believes that it is intrinsically good to be virtuous, and the person's actions reflect this belief. The virtuous person does not feel compelled to act from a sense of duty or obligation.

For Aristotle, a virtue is a mean between the extremes of excess and deficiency. Courage, for example, is a mean between the extremes of cowardice and foolhardiness. It is cowardly to run away from all danger; but it is foolhardy to risk too much in the face of danger. Generosity is a virtue between the extremes of stinginess and extravagance. But what should we say about honesty? Kant would say that we have an absolute duty to always tell the truth. Others would consider truth-telling a virtue. Yet if there is an absolute duty to always tell the truth, then it would seem that truth-telling, or honesty, is not a mean between extremes and therefore is not a virtue.

Suppose that honesty is a virtue. Suppose further that tests indicate that a patient with a history of depression has cancer. The patient's doctor wants to be honest in telling him all the medical facts about his condition. At the same time, she wants to be compassionate toward him and not precipitate another episode of severe depression. What should she tell him? Honesty and compassion are both virtues. Yet they are not always compatible, and there is no principle in virtue ethics to which one can appeal to resolve this sort of conflict. We will explore whether such a conflict can be resolved in other ways in Chapter 2. A more general criticism of virtue ethics is that it may have only limited relevance to biomedical ethics beyond the patient-doctor relationship.

Feminist ethics is considered by some to be an extension of virtue ethics, in the sense that it emphasizes an ethics of care involving human connectedness and the importance of interpersonal relationships. Presumably, it focuses on virtuous dispositions such as sympathy rather than on impartial reason. Yet this is an oversimplified, if not misleading, description. Although there is no single definition of the enterprise, feminist ethics can be characterized as a concern for the rights and welfare of all women. It affirms the general right of women to control their own bodies and lives. This includes the right to refuse unwanted medical interventions, as well as the right to equal access to medical treatment and participation in research. These rights provide a corrective to the discrimination against and oppression and exclusion of women that have occurred in patriarchal societies and institutions. Traditional Western medicine has been one of these institutions. Feminist ethics seeks to redress the balance of power between women and men and put them on equal terms. It involves a model of care and respect that incorporates both men and women.

The first major gain in women's status in health care occurred in the area of reproduction. The U.S. Supreme Court *Roe v. Wade* decision in 1973 recognized a constitutional right of women to an abortion up to the time when the fetus became viable, or capable of surviving outside the womb. Since then, women have gained considerable autonomy over their bodies. This autonomy is not absolute, however, and does not always outweigh the rights of the fetus. Court-ordered cesarean sections performed for the sake of the fetus are one example of this fact. Feminist ethics has contributed to the correction of wrongs to women in other areas of health care as well. For years, women were underrepresented in clinical trials for such conditions as heart disease. This resulted in a reprehensible ignorance of the prevalence of the disease in postmenopausal women. As a matter of justice, arguments for the right of women to participate in clinical trials have promoted equal representation with men and equal access to potentially beneficial research. The research on women is still understudied, though. Improvements in the number of women participating in research have been due primarily to a few all-women studies. Much work remains to be done. Also, the doctor-patient relationship traditionally has been a patriarchal one in which the doctor was male. Physician paternalism was largely a function of a patriarchal way of thinking. The recent emphasis on patient autonomy, combined with the fact that there are now more women practicing medicine, has eroded much of the old paternalism. These developments have done much to give women equality with men in medical practice and medical research.

Communitarianism and Liberalism

Communitarianism derives from Aristotle's claim that humans are essentially social beings. It does not conceive of persons as a collection of isolated, self-interested individuals, each with his or her own conception of the good. Instead, communitarianism conceives of persons as members of communities with shared values, ideals, and goals. The ethical norms that govern our behavior are not found in the universal tenets of rationality, but in different historical and religious traditions. Communitarianism thus rejects liberal individualism, or simply liberalism, which focuses on the rights, interests, and reasoning of individual moral agents. Liberalism says that people should have the right to act and live in accord with their own conception of a good life, provided that it does not interfere with the rights of others to do the same. As Thomas Hobbes (1588–1679) noted, self-interested individuals acting in an unconstrained way would make life "nasty, brutish, and short." Hobbes maintained that, if individuals were to have decent lives, their actions must be regulated by social rules that everyone would accept, or contract for, on the assumption that doing so would be mutually advantageous. These limits on liberty move us beyond the state of nature and are consistent with Mill's later conception of liberty. Because liberalism accepts some limits on liberty, the social contract theory of morality can be characterized as a development out of liberalism. Communitarianism and liberalism are not necessarily rivals to the other theories we have discussed. They are often considered to focus more on political than on moral aspects of social interaction.

Hobbes's conception of morality is basically negative, focusing on the idea of enforcement to ensure compliance with rules, rather than on positive incentives. John Rawls (1921–2002) developed a positive version of liberalism and contractualism as the foundation for his theory of justice. Generally, justice concerns what people's rights are, what we owe to others, and the proper distribution of benefits and burdens. Unlike consequentialism and its emphasis on maximizing outcomes, for Rawls a deontological theory of justice emphasizes the process through which people's claims to social goods are evaluated. Principles of liberty and equality are agreed upon by rational, self-interested individuals for mutual benefit. These principles are the bases of economic, legal, and political institutions that ensure fair procedures for assessing people's reasonable expectations of different goods. Health care is one example of a social good. When applied to health care, Rawls's principles of justice require that all people have access to a basic set of medical benefits so that they will have an equal opportunity to enjoy other goods over the course of their lives. His theory of justice as fairness is especially pertinent to the allocation of scarce medical resources. We will discuss this issue in Chapter 7.

Liberalism differs from communitarianism as a normative theory in two main respects. First, it says that there should not be one conception of the good or one overarching moral value that all individuals live by and share. Second, it says that the rights and interests of individuals should not be sacrificed for the interests of the larger society. Because different individuals have different values and different conceptions of what constitutes a good life, it would be wrong to try to adopt a particular conception of the good for everyone. Society should remain neutral on these normative issues.

Communitarians reject this view because of their conviction that individual conceptions of the good cannot be divorced from the community in which individuals live. What is good for one person is a reflection of the common good. Because we are social beings, questions about right or wrong, good or bad, actions or policies should always be raised within a common social framework. What we should ask is "Which actions or policies will promote the kind of community in which we want to live?"

Communitarianism has become quite influential in recent debates about biomedical ethics. Daniel Callahan, for one, maintains that questions such as what the goals of medicine should be must be framed by the larger question of what kind of life our society wants. This general question will influence more specific questions such as whether, given limited resources, we should try to extend life or focus on dignified palliative care in the last stage of people's lives. To be fruitfully discussed and resolved, these issues require a shared understanding of goals and values. Questions about rights to medical services and responsibility for health outcomes should be raised and deliberated not individually but socially.

One objection to communitarianism is that it is difficult to arrive at a consensus on the goals of medical treatment at the end of life.

Some patients and their families believe in the sanctity of human life. For them, prolonging life is a benefit that cannot be overridden by considerations of dignity or quality of life. Palliation can relieve a patient's pain and suffering; but it might not be the most important goal for everyone. Others may want to preserve the patient's dignity and quality of life by refusing or deciding to withdraw life-sustaining interventions they consider nontherapeutic. Different people have different understandings of what constitutes "futile" treatment. The point here is that the values and wishes of patients and their families should be respected. And because not all patients and families have the same values and wishes about end-of-life care, liberalism seems to provide a more helpful ethical framework for addressing these issues than communitarianism. The latter theory may limit the freedom of individuals to act in line with their self-determined needs and interests, which may conflict with the principle of respect for autonomy. Rather than try to formulate one conception of the good for all people, we should adopt principles that encourage us to appreciate and respect the diversity of opinions of the good. These principles should accommodate different cultural and religious conceptions of a good life, as well as how health care fits in with these conceptions.

Nevertheless, as a society we will have to debate and agree upon such questions as the importance of health care compared to education, environmental protection, and other social goods. We will have to formulate health policies that determine how health services are distributed and who has access to these services. This is not likely to be done within a liberal or communitarian model alone, but will include elements of both.

The Rejection of Theories: Casuistry and Cultural Relativism

Those who are skeptical of ethical theories might adopt the method of casuistry, which focuses on practical decision making in particular cases. "Casuistry" comes from the Latin *casus*, or "case." It is traceable to the ancient discipline of rhetoric, as developed in Aristotle's *Rhetoric* and *Nicomachean Ethics*, as well as Cicero's *De Inventione*. A casuist will begin an ethical analysis by identifying particular features of a case, rather than by appealing to an abstract principle and applying it to the case. The casuist will move from cases to principles, rather than the other way around. Principles and theories divorced from actual circumstances will shed little, if any, light on the ethical issues at hand. Rejecting the primacy of principles, casuistry focuses on analogical reasoning, relying on precedents and existing paradigms to yield insight into and achieve shared agreement about new cases. There are parallels with law, where reasoning about new cases is done on the basis of legal precedent. For example, in deciding whether to respect a competent adolescent's refusal of life-saving treatment, we can look to similar cases in the past for guidance. As a descriptive ethical method, casuistry has many uses. Yet there are at least two grounds on which it can be questioned as a normative ethical method.

The same case may generate competing ethical intuitions in different people. Some people may pay attention to certain features of a case, while others may ignore them or judge them to be less important than other features. In this scenario, it is unclear how an appeal to a given paradigm or precedent could result in a decision or policy on which all parties could agree. There is no obvious mechanism in casuistry that could prevent or resolve a conflict of interpretations of a particular case. A consensus on the relevant ethical issues, or a resolution to a case involving an ethical conflict, cannot be assumed from the outset in a casuist model. This raises the more general question of how justification for an action can be given in casuistry. If principles are not objective, impartial standards outside of our intuitions, but only instruments on the way to a consensus, and if different parties have different intuitive judgments about a case, then it is unclear how anything about casuistry itself could adjudicate between these judgments.

Another criticism of casuistry is that, by relying on precedent and existing paradigms, it is not forward-looking enough to provide guidance in thinking about ethical issues in scientific innovation. For example, the method and aims of cloning human embryos are significantly different from those of existing forms of assisted reproduction. Casuistry does not offer much help in exploring the ethical implications of cloning and other new medical technologies. This point suggests that casuistry is more relevant to existing issues in clinical ethics than to emerging issues in the ethics of medical research and biotechnology.

Cultural relativism can also be viewed as a rejection of ethical theories. But its rationale is distinct from that of casuistry. It denies the criteria of objectivity and impartiality that define ethical theories. According to cultural relativism, there are no universal truths in ethics, only cultural codes that vary from one culture to another. No code has any special status. Each code is merely one among many, and each has its own sense of right and wrong. "Right" and "wrong" actions are determined by and within particular cultures. Cultural relativism pertains to both metaethics and normative ethics. It makes claims about the nature of ethical facts and the meaning of ethical terms, and from these claims draws the conclusion that there are no norms of behavior common to all cultures. It poses a challenge to the idea that there can be an objective basis on which to justify actions and policies. How persuasive is cultural relativism?

One can rebut the claims of cultural relativism on both formal and substantive grounds. Just because people from different cultures disagree about the motivation for or meaning of some type of behavior, it does not follow that there is no objective moral fact of the matter that justifies the behavior. To illustrate this formal point, James Rachels cites the example of infanticide among Eskimos as their way of surviving in a situation of scarce resources. Infanticide is practiced, not because infants have no rights or moral status, but because there is only enough food to support a certain number of people. In this situation, priority is given to adults because of their ability to gather and prepare food. Similarly, in the past the Japanese practice of *mabiki*, which means to "thin out," was the only way for the poor without an effective method of birth control to keep their families small enough to feed. A different interpretation of this concept is portrayed in the 1982 film *The Ballad of Narayama*, where people beyond a certain age in remote areas are expected to leave the family and allow themselves to die by exposure to the natural elements. The universal truth here is that, although their practices may differ, all cultures justify these practices by appeal to the notion of allocating a scarce resource in a way that achieves the best ratio of benefit to harm.

Moreover, most cultures have some moral rules in common because they are necessary for societies and cultures to exist and remain stable. Rules against lying and murder are just two examples. There are enough commonalities among people and cultures to support the claim that ethical facts are not relative to these cultures and that ethical truths are not merely social constructs. The examples cited here demonstrate that the principle used to justify allocation decisions in situations of scarcity is not itself a social construct. Underlying culturally relative interpretations of ethical principles are certain transcultural constants. The most basic of these is the right of all people to bodily noninterference. It is the basis of a competent patient's right to refuse medical treatment. Ethical universals like this right exist across all cultures, even if they are not always respected. But they are not equivalent to ethical absolutes. That is, the acceptance of a universal ethical truth such as the right to bodily noninterference does not commit one to ethical absolutism, the view that there is one theory or set of principles that applies to all cultures in the same way. We will elaborate on this in more detail in Chapter 2, when we discuss intercultural differences and the extent to which they depart from Western liberalism and influence the patient-doctor relationship.

This last point suggests a normative objection that gets at the heart of the problem with cultural relativism. It may involve accepting quite horrific practices. A particular culture may promote slavery or the sacrifice of children and have a way of defending these actions in its own descriptive terms. But no one could justify these practices in normative terms because they obviously violate the intrinsic dignity, worth, and rights of persons.

Conclusion

The principles and theories that have been laid out in this chapter provide a framework within which to test, refine, and systematize the ethical intuitions generated by the issues we will address in the next six chapters. The framework will give us the resources necessary to critically reflect on and assess different positions and arguments, as well as to see which actions or polices can be justified. Intuitions and theories should be mutually reinforcing, as we move back and forth between them in examining the issues. In this respect, we should adopt a model that is dynamic rather than static. We should aim at what Rawls called a "reflective equilibrium." The goal is to adjust our ethical intuitions so that they cohere with principles and theories. Yet because equilibrium is an ideal, intuitions constantly have to be readjusted and fine-tuned against principles and theories, and vice versa. Appeals to intuition alone or to theory alone will not yield a satisfactory analysis of or justification for a particular action or policy. Our intuitions feed and give substance to our theories. Our theories in turn shape and systematize our intuitions.

It is important to emphasize that none of the ethical principles outlined here alone is likely to adequately defend or justify every action or policy. Because they are not absolute but only prima facie, competing principles have to be weighed against each other. We must carefully assess their relative weights in analyzing different issues in biomedical ethics. No single ethical principle or theory will be endorsed because the issues we will be addressing raise different ethical questions, and the theories and principles we appeal to must be sensitive to these differences.

Selected Readings

Beauchamp, T., and Childress, J. *Principles of Biomedical Ethics*. 5th ed. New York: Oxford University Press, 2001.

Callahan, D. *Setting Limits: Medical Goals in an Aging Society*. New York: Simon & Schuster, 1987.

Jonsen, A. R. *The Birth of Bioethics*. New York: Oxford University Press, 1998.

Jonsen, A. R. *A Brief History of Bioethics*. New York: Oxford University Press, 2000.

Jonsen, A. R., Siegler, M., and Winslade, W. *Clinical Ethics: A Practical Approach to Ethical Decisions in Clinical Medicine*. 5th ed. New York: McGraw-Hill, 2002.

LaFollette, H., ed. *The Blackwell Guide to Ethical Theory*. Malden, Mass.: Blackwell, 2000.

McIntyre, A. *After Virtue*. 2d ed. Notre Dame, Ind.: University of Notre Dame Press, 1984.

Rachels, J. *The Elements of Moral Philosophy*. 4th ed. New York: McGraw-Hill, 2002.

Rawls, J. *A Theory of Justice*. Cambridge, Mass.: Belknap Harvard University Press, 1971.

Tong, R. *Feminist Approaches to Bioethics*. 2d ed. Boulder, Colo.: Westview Press, 1999.

CHAPTER 2

The Patient-Doctor Relationship

Introduction

The Hippocratic model of medicine was very much a paternalistic one. The good doctor determined what was in his patient's best interests, and the good patient was expected to follow the doctor's recommendations. But patient autonomy is now an established concept in medical practice. Doctors have a fiduciary responsibility to patients, one that rests on a trusting relationship between them. As part of this responsibility, there is a presumption to treat patients when it offers them some medical benefit. A patient's interests are not only physiological, however. Some treatments may conflict with a patient's religious beliefs. Other treatments may cause enough pain and suffering to outweigh any benefits to the patient. As an expression of their autonomy, patients have the right to refuse even medically beneficial treatments on these grounds. Decisional authority rests not with the doctor, but the patient.

Acknowledging the importance of respect for patient autonomy and of informed consent for any treatment, are there some instances in which a physician can justifiably override a patient's refusal and treat the person against his or her will? Can paternalistic intervention be justified at the expense of individual autonomy? Can a physician use a therapeutic privilege and not disclose potentially harmful medical information to a patient? Are there circumstances in which a doctor can disclose confidential medical information about a patient to a third party? When a Western-trained doctor treats a patient from a non-Western culture, and there is no initial shared understanding of medical practices and terms, can they arrive at a mutual agreement on the goals of treatment? Finally, what sort of doctors do patients want and need at different stages of their lives? We will discuss these and related questions in this chapter.

Informed Consent

Informed consent is a practical application of the principle of respect for patient autonomy. The notion of consent was first raised by Justice Cardozo in the 1914 legal case of *Schloendorff v. Society of New York Hospitals*. Cardozo stated that a patient must receive adequate medical information on which to make a decision about whether to accept or refuse treatment. To consent freely, a patient must be of sound mind and must not be subject to any coercion or undue influence. The term "informed consent" became firmly established in the law after the 1960 case of *Natanson v. Kline*.

The doctrine of informed consent consists of two components. The first component is the *doctor's disclosure* of medical information to the patient. This includes diagnosis, prognosis, available and alternative treatments, and the risks, benefits, and consequences of having or refusing treatment. The second component is the *competent patient*, who decides whether to accept or forego treatment on the basis of this information. A competent patient is one who understands the nature of his or her condition and the consequences of accepting or refusing an intervention for it. Ideally, informed consent serves as an ethical basis for a patient-doctor relationship characterized by mutual respect and shared decision making.

In an example from Chapter 1, a patient refuses chemotherapy for a form of cancer. The physician fulfills the duty of beneficence by exploring the patient's reasons for the refusal and by trying to persuade him that chemotherapy would be in his best medical interest. The patient explains that the burdens of the treatment outweigh the benefits. A few more years of life are not worth the pain and suffering he would experience with chemotherapy. By not overriding the patient's decision, the physician is respecting his autonomy and right to refuse such an intervention. Any potential conflict in this case is resolved by the determination that the patient's autonomy outweighs the doctor's duty of beneficence. For the doctor, the duty of beneficence is outweighed by the stronger duty to respect patient autonomy. Indeed, in one sense respecting patient autonomy is consistent with the doctor's duty of nonmaleficence. It prevents the adverse effects of chemotherapy from harming the patient.

Let's consider a more difficult case. A schizophrenic patient who has been living on the street and has been on and off antipsychotic medication admits himself to the hospital because of pain in his chest and arm. Coronary artery disease is suspected. An angiogram is performed to determine whether or to what extent there is an obstruction in the patient's arteries. This involves taking X-rays of the arteries after a dye has been injected into them. If there is an obstruction, then the next likely step would be angioplasty. In this procedure, the femoral artery in the leg is punctured with a large needle. From this opening, a catheter with a balloon attached to the tip is threaded into the diseased coronary artery. The catheter is positioned so that the balloon is at the level of the obstruction. The balloon is then inflated for several seconds and partially tears the inner layers of the arterial wall, thereby reducing the obstruction. Suppose that the patient has an obstruction but refuses to consent to angioplasty because it is an invasive procedure. He refuses angioplasty, despite the fact that he consented to the angiogram, which is also invasive, though perhaps to a lesser degree. While there is a slight risk of heart attack and death with angioplasty, the risk of not treating the obstruction is greater. The benefit of the angioplasty outweighs its risk, given the patient's condition.

Some might claim that the patient's psychiatric illness means that he is not competent to consent to the procedure. Therefore, the cardiologist would be justified in overriding his objection to treatment. The fact that the patient accepted the angiogram but refuses angioplasty suggests that he is inconsistent and thus irrational in his thinking. Yet he is not psychotic at the time of his admission and seems to have a sufficient degree of decisional capacity to understand at least the invasive nature of the procedure. Just because a person is irrational in assessing two related treatments does not imply that he lacks decisional capacity altogether. There is more of a conflict between beneficence and autonomy here than what might appear at first glance.

To resolve this sort of problem, some argue that the required level of competence to refuse a treatment should be on a sliding scale from low to high risk. The greater the level of risk in refusing a treatment, the higher the level of competence should be for the patient to make the decision. When a patient's decision to forego treatment entails a significant risk of harm to himself or others, the threshold of competence necessary to uphold patient autonomy should be high. If the patient in such a case fails to meet the threshold, then physician paternalism outweighs patient autonomy and an intervention can be justified. Generally, the less competent a patient is and the greater the risk in not intervening, the stronger reasons and justification there are for overriding a patient's refusal. On the other hand, the more competent the patient is and the lower the risk in foregoing treatment, the stronger reasons and justification there are for respecting autonomy and upholding the patient's decision. Still, some reject the idea of basing autonomy and consent on varying degrees of competence. They argue that minimal competence is enough for a patient to consent to or refuse a treatment. If the patient is competent enough to accept treatment, then he or she is competent enough to refuse it as well.

Yet there is a third dimension, in addition to competence and risk, that figures in the case at hand: the invasiveness of the procedure. Insofar as the schizophrenic patient knows what it means to have one's body invaded, and he objects to this, he is exercising his right to bodily noninterference. Suppose that this patient has enough decisional capacity to understand what is involved in a given procedure. If he objects to it because he believes that it is invasive, then more weight should be given to his autonomy and less weight to physician paternalism to override it. This point can be sustained despite the risk of harm to the patient in refusing the procedure. Because angioplasty is not related to the patient's psychiatric condition, his refusing it would not pose a risk of harm to others. If the blockage in his artery is not severe, then drug therapy might be an equally effective alternative to reduce the blockage. In the short term at least, this would be a more ethically desirable treatment because it would be less invasive. But if only angioplasty would be effective, then the patient's objection to it on grounds of its perceived invasiveness could be decisive. Only a minimal degree of competence would be necessary for his doctors to be obligated to respect and not override his decision. Does the same reasoning apply when patients want to be treated?

The right to refuse beneficial treatment does not imply a corresponding right to request any treatment. This is so for the following reason. Any right of a patient entails a corresponding obligation of a physician to respect that right. Doctors are obligated to provide treatment to patients, and patients have a right to it, only when it has some therapeutic benefit and thus falls within the goals of medicine. These goals include relieving pain and suffering and restoring patients to normal functioning. A patient with terminal lung cancer, for example, might request that cardiopulmonary resuscitation (CPR) be given to her in the event of cardiac arrest. But because the patient's condition is terminal, intervening with CPR cannot restore her to normal functioning or prolong her life and thus falls outside the goals of medicine. For this reason, the physician would not be obligated to give CPR, and the patient would have no right to it. Indeed, performing this action would violate the physician's professional integrity. Nor is a physician obligated to continue mechanical life-support on a patient if, in his or her professional judgment, it offers no therapeutic benefit. A brain-dead patient who is kept alive on a respirator is a case in point. This raises questions about futile treatment at the end of life, which we will take up in Chapter 6.

When a patient is not competent to make decisions about treatment, an appropriately designated *surrogate* can decide on the patient's behalf. A surrogate can act in either of two ways: (1) he or she can make decisions about treatment as the patient would make them if he were competent, thus exercising substituted judgment; or (2) the surrogate can decide on a course of action that he or she believes is in the patient's best interests. Alternatively, the patient's interests can be expressed in an *advance directive*, such as a living will. In this way, an autonomous patient can extend that autonomy to a time when he or she is no longer competent to make decisions. An advance directive can serve two goals: (1) it can express what the patient would want doctors to do (or not to do) to him or her; or (2) it can designate an individual to make decisions about treatment for the patient. The terms of the directive should be regularly updated so that they accord with the patient's interests at or near the time when a decision about an intervention must be made. In the absence of an advance directive, a surrogate can be chosen in the form of a court-ordered guardian. All of this indicates that it is not up to a physician to determine what is in a patient's best interests. But there are circumstances in which the issue of consent does not arise, as when critically ill patients are brought to the emergency room. Because of the urgency of the situation, there is a presumption to treat. Doctors need not consult with patients or their families in these cases.

Parents generally are the best judges of their children's best interests and make decisions about treatment on this basis. Yet their decisional authority can be overridden, as in instances of abuse or neglect. Parental refusal of treatment on religious grounds presents a unique problem. Recall the example in Chapter 1 of the Jehovah's Witness' refusal of a blood transfusion for severe anemia. The physician's decision not to challenge or override the patient's decision shows respect for the patient's autonomy and the determination of what is in his own best interests. Suppose that Jehovah's Witness parents of a child injured in an automobile accident refuse to allow a blood transfusion to be given to their child. Consistent with the principle that parents and physicians are obligated to act in the best interests of the child, a parental refusal of an intervention should be respected unless it causes direct and serious harm to the child. The child would die without the transfusion and so obviously would be harmed. Doctors have recourse to the legal system to obtain a court order to protect the welfare of those incapable of protecting themselves. In the case at hand, they would be justified in obtaining an order and overriding the parents' refusal of the transfusion.

Parents have considerable latitude in making decisions on behalf of their children. But state and local courts can intervene to protect children from risk to their health or life because of inaction due to their parents' religious beliefs. For those who cannot make decisions for themselves, the risk of serious physical harm and death outweighs the risk of eternal damnation. To borrow the words of Justice Oliver Wendell Holmes in his opinion on a child labor case: "Parents may make martyrs of themselves, but they are not free to make martyrs of their children."

When the individual in need of a transfusion is fourteen years old and legally determined by the courts to be a "mature minor," his or her refusal can be upheld. It is presumed that the patient fully understands his or her condition and the consequences of refusing a blood transfusion. The different judgment in this variant of the original example is that the patient is competent enough to know what is in his or her best interests and exercises personal autonomy in refusing the treatment. Provided that the patient has the requisite decisional capacity and is not unduly influenced or coerced by his or her parents, the decision is the patient's and should be respected. But if the patient is not legally considered to be a mature minor, then the parents may override the refusal.

The relationship between patients and physicians is more nuanced and complex than the examples we have discussed might suggest. Many cases involving difficult decisions about initiating, withholding, or withdrawing treatment cannot be analyzed adequately in terms of a simple conflict between physician paternalism and patient autonomy. Moreover, autonomy and beneficence, as well as the deontological and consequentialist theories on which they rest, may have been construed too narrowly thus far in our discussion. A patient who is confused about medical information presented in the form of a diagnosis and prognosis might ask the physician to make the decision, or at least suggest a course of action. In this respect, the patient would be transferring autonomy to the physician. But the voluntary request for help in making a decision could be described as an autonomous act.

Some argue that the importance given to autonomy has been exaggerated. For example, Edmund Pellegrino and David Thomasma (1988) say that "the patient autonomy model does not give sufficient attention to the impact of disease on the patient's capacity for autonomy. . . . Ill persons often become so anxious, guilty, unreasonable, fearful, or hostile that they make judgments they would not make in calmer times" (pp. 14–15). Illness, not a paternalistic physician, is the main obstacle to autonomy. In times of sickness, what some patients want is not so much the ability or opportunity to make their own decisions about treatment. Rather, such patients want a physician who, while respecting the patient's interests and values, takes control of the situation and acts on his or her best professional judgment, which the patient implicitly trusts. The patient's trust in the physician can be crucial to the patient's response to treatment. This can be accommodated only within a broader model of autonomy than a model in which a physician simply presents medical information to the patient, who then makes a decision about treatment. These considerations also suggest that beneficence should be more broadly construed to include trustworthiness, compassion, and other virtues that can work to the patient's benefit. Still, this is possible only if the physician respects the patient as an end-in-itself with interests of his or her own. If these interests are known, then paternalism should be distinguished from beneficence. Paternalism means that the doctor determines what is in the patient's best interests. Beneficence means that the doctor acts to promote the patient's best interests as determined by the patient.

Others argue that the idea of patients taking complete control over medical decision making is flawed because it depicts the physician as a competent but detached professional. Patient autonomy implies that the physician's role is simply to provide factual information to patients, who then make decisions on the basis of that information in accord with their values. Linda and Ezekiel Emanuel claim that this "informative model" perpetuates and accentuates the trend toward specialization and impersonality within the medical profession. It also suggests a misleading distinction between value-free information given by the physician and value-laden decisions made by the patient.

The Emanuels contrast the informative model with what they call the "paternalistic," "interpretive," and "deliberative" models of the patient-physician relationship. In the paternalistic model, the physician completely determines what is in the patient's best interests, with the patient playing a passive role in treatment decisions. In the informative model, the physician is obligated to provide all the available medical facts. On the basis of personal values, the patient then determines which treatments he or she will accept or refuse. There is a clear distinction between facts and values, which correspond to distinct roles of the physician and patient. In the interpretive model, the physician also provides the patient with information about the nature of his or her condition and the risks and benefits of different interventions. In addition, the interpretive physician helps the patient to elucidate his or her values, making them coherent so that the physician can choose a medical intervention that best realizes these values. In the deliberative model, the one the Emanuels defend, the physician is engaged in not only presenting medical information to the patient, but also in recommending treatment in line with the patient's health-related values and preferences. Unlike the other three models, in the deliberative model neither the patient nor the physician makes an exclusive decision about treatment. Rather, the decision follows from shared deliberation between physician and patient. Facts and values are intertwined in this deliberation. The physician tries to persuade the patient to have or forego a treatment, but steers clear of undue influence or coercion.

Yet because of physicians' authority, the persuasion they use on patients can influence them to the point where the presumed values behind a patient's decisions may not be really his or her own. An oncologist may strongly believe in the value of three additional life-years from chemotherapy, paying less attention to other health-related values such as the side effects of the treatment. More importantly, the deliberative model ignores the fact that the values that inform decisions about treatment are often not solely health related. An individual may decide to forego life-extending chemotherapy or radiation in order to take one last trip to a distant destination while his mental and physical capacities are still intact. Moreover, a surrogate making decisions for an unconscious patient whose death is imminent may ask that life-support be continued for a few days so that relatives can see the patient before she dies. The values that inform these sorts of decisions are not limited to considerations of health alone. This idea strengthens rather than weakens the concept of patient autonomy. The physician has a duty to engage the patient in deliberation about treatment. Ultimately, though, it is the patient who decides which treatment is in his or her own best interests and is consistent with his or her values. These interests and values go beyond the health-related values represented by the physician, and the physician should respect them.

Suppose that a patient has a serious disease and is confused about his options for treatment. He asks his doctor: "What would you do if you were me?" Consistent with both interpretive and deliberative models, the doctor should explore the patient's attitude toward sickness and the risks and benefits of different treatments. After giving a recommendation, the doctor would be obligated to say that it is all right if the patient does not agree, that he could seek a second opinion, and that it would not offend the doctor if the patient did so. Because the patient has explicitly asked the doctor for a recommendation, which suggests a trusting relationship between them, the deliberative model would be the most appropriate in this situation. On the other hand, when a patient wants the doctor's help in sorting out the relation between treatment options and his values, but wants to make the decision himself, the interpretive model would be more appropriate. It steers clear of an explicit recommendation and thus the potential for coercion, given the doctor's perceived authority. Which model is the most helpful guide for doctors in their professional relationship with patients depends on what patients reasonably expect from their doctors. It also depends on how strongly patients' values and interests influence their decisions about treatment.

Therapeutic Privilege

Physicians have an obligation to disclose relevant medical information to patients so that they can make informed decisions about treatment. This obligation is grounded in both deontological and consequentialist reasons. The disclosure of information shows respect for the patient's autonomy, and it enables the patient to make choices that will be beneficial and not harmful. Disclosure should include information about the patient's current medical condition, the likely progression if it is not treated, possible interventions, and the risks and benefits of these interventions. Disclosure is essential for informed consent.

But are there some cases where full disclosure of medical information would do more harm than good? Although it smacks of paternalism, are there some patients who would not want to know or could not handle the truth? Can "beneficent deception" ever be justified?

The idea that a doctor can withhold medical information when it is potentially harmful to a patient is known as "therapeutic privilege." Yet studies show that most patients would rather be told the truth, difficult though it may be to accept, than to be deceived for paternalistic reasons. Patients benefit from a trusting relationship with a physician, and honesty in disclosing information is more likely than deception to promote trust and to benefit patients in the long term. Robert Veatch cites two main objections to therapeutic privilege. First, doctors can exaggerate or otherwise make mistakes in assessing the benefits and harms of disclosure and nondisclosure. Second, and more importantly, withholding medical information fails to respect the autonomy of the patient and fails to fulfill the doctor's duties of honesty and fidelity. It is presumed that a competent patient can make informed, autonomous decisions about treatment. Disclosure of all relevant medical information is necessary to enable patients to make these decisions. Patients have the right of self-determination and access to all relevant information so that they can participate in decisions about their care. Therapeutic privilege violates this right. Therefore, there is no ethical justification for invoking therapeutic privilege. Given the importance of patient autonomy, a compelling argument is needed to support the claim that a reasonable person would not want medical information about his or her health.

Withholding medical information can be rejected on consequentialist grounds as well. Honesty is preferable to deception. Discovering that a physician is deceiving a patient by withholding information could undermine the patient's trust in the physician. It could discourage the patient from seeking needed treatment, or it could adversely affect how the patient responds to treatment. Either way, deception could result in more harm than benefit. On a broader scale, physicians who routinely deceive patients might risk losing public trust in the medical profession. Many patients might be reluctant to see doctors for necessary medical care and might be harmed by allowing disease to go untreated.

Still, is a physician obligated to disclose all medical information to a patient *all at once*? Recall the example from Chapter 1 of the patient with a history of depression who was diagnosed with cancer. The question of what his doctor should tell him was left unanswered. It seems that the most constructive approach for this sort of case is to adopt a strategy that falls between therapeutic privilege and Veatch's defense of full disclosure. The physician should give the medical information to the patient in a gradual, measured way so that he can have time to digest it and be able to rationally think through his treatment options. Initially, she should present the information to him in a positive, though not misleading, light. More specifically, if a course of chemotherapy has a 60 percent chance of extending the patient's life for three to five years, then it would be permissible to say at the first meeting that he has cancer but that it may be controlled (omitting "cured"). At a second meeting, at least several days after the first, the physician can discuss the prognosis in more direct terms. Separating discussion of diagnosis and prognosis may help the patient to accept the facts in a way that is not too disruptive to his fragile emotional state. The general point here is that *how much* information is disclosed to a patient and *how* it is disclosed are as important as the principle *that* it should be disclosed. Disclosure should be sensitive to the particular history and needs of each patient.

In other cases, once a diagnosis has been made, anything less than full disclosure of information amounts to maleficent deception. This can be especially serious regarding prognosis. A patient has been complaining of headaches, memory loss, confusion, and vomiting. A CT scan reveals a brain tumor. The neurosurgeon informs the patient and recommends that it be removed surgically. The patient then consents to the surgery. During the postoperative period, the neurosurgeon does not tell the patient which type of brain tumor she had or how much of it he removed. There are significant differences in prognosis, depending on whether the tumor is benign or malignant and whether it can be partially or completely removed. A *meningioma* is a tumor that develops from the meninges, the outer lining of the brain. Most of these tumors are benign, and most patients who have them recover completely once they are removed. In contrast, a *glioblastoma* is a malignant and rapidly growing tumor that develops from tissues surrounding and supporting nerve cells within the brain. Few people with these tumors are still living two years after diagnosis because they are aggressive and can metastasize. This makes it difficult to remove the tumor completely. Knowing the differences between these two types of brain tumor can be critical to an affected person's ability to make rational life choices in the light of the prognosis. Patients have a right to information necessary to rationally plan the rest of their lives, which is especially important when there is not much time left. In these cases, a physician has an obligation to disclose all relevant medical information once a diagnosis has been made.

We claimed in Chapter 1 that virtue ethics contained no principle that could adjudicate between competing virtues such as honesty and compassion. But this claim was too quick because the importance of how a physician discloses information to a patient suggests that these virtues are not necessarily competing and may be compatible. In many cases, physicians should not simply lay out a diagnosis and prognosis in a detached, clinically precise way. Instead, they should do it in a caring and respectful way, disclosing information in a gradual manner that is sensitive to the patient's feelings and emotions. To resolve any conflict between honesty and compassion, one needs to understand the first virtue in a broader sense. Gradual disclosure of medical information is not dishonest or deceptive. This is one respect in which the emphasis on absolute autonomy could be criticized. It fails to appreciate the importance of a caring physician, a doctor who respects the patient as a person with physical and emotional needs, not just as someone who processes information and always makes perfectly rational decisions. One's rational and emotional sides need to be attended to equally. This is not only because these mental faculties and the regions of the brain that generate and sustain them are interdependent. It is also because the pain caused by disease and the fear and suffering caused by pain or a grim prognosis involve emotional reactions. Medicine should be a healing art as much as a curative science. In order to realize these two goals, doctors should not only be competent, but empathetic and compassionate as well. We will discuss this point in more detail later in this chapter.

Confidentiality

Although doctors have a duty to disclose all relevant medical information to patients, they also have a corresponding duty *not* to disclose this information to a third party. This type of disclosure would violate the confidentiality that is essential to the patient-doctor relationship. Confidentiality is present in medicine when a doctor discloses medical information about a particular patient to that patient alone. The doctor pledges not to disclose the information to a third party without the patient's permission.

There are two arguments supporting physicians' obligation to uphold confidentiality with their patients. The first argument is deontological and involves respect for the patient's autonomy and privacy. Confidentiality is an extension of a patient's right to privacy, and disclosing information about the patient without consent is a violation of this right and fails to respect the patient's right to self-determination. The second argument is consequentialist. If physicians violate confidentiality by divulging information about their patients to third parties, then patients might lose trust in their physicians. They might become reluctant to seek medical care. Also, patients might not be forthcoming in providing an honest, accurate medical history. Without this information, physicians might not be able to make accurate diagnoses and prognoses or to recommend the best available course of treatment. As a result, doctors would not act in their patients' best interests.

But a different consequentialist argument supports breaching confidentiality when there is a significant risk of harm to others or to the patient. This was the opinion of the California Supreme Court in the 1976 case *Tarasoff v. Regents of the University of California*. A young male student, who had been treated at the University of California for violent and paranoid ideas, told his therapist that he intended to kill a particular female student. The therapist notified the campus police, who detained the male student but then released him. Shortly thereafter, he killed the female student. Her family sued the university and the therapist for failing to take appropriate action, which, they claimed, included warning them of the threat to their daughter. The court found in the family's favor. Recognizing the conflict between the duty to inform and the duty to uphold confidentiality, the court ruled that the protective privilege of confidentiality ends where public peril begins. The threat of harm was significant enough to infringe, or justifiably override, patient confidentiality and the deontological reason on which it was based. On purely consequentialist grounds, the direct risk of harm to the woman was significant enough to outweigh any indirect risk of harm to patients in general through the erosion of their trust in doctors. The act-consequentialist reason for preventing the direct risk of harm outweighed the rule-consequentialist reason for preventing the indirect risk of harm.

Let's test our intuitions further on this issue by considering another example. A patient is positive for HIV, the virus that causes AIDS. In discussing his health status and the risk of sexually transmitting the virus to his partner, his general practitioner recommends that the patient tell his partner. But the patient refuses to do this and adamantly insists that the doctor not tell his partner either. The doctor suspects that the patient is afraid that his partner will leave him if he knows that he is infected. He is obligated to try to persuade his patient to inform his partner of his HIV status and that doing so would be in their best interests. Still, the patient refuses. Would the doctor be justified in breaching confidentiality and telling his patient's partner directly?

Informing a third party that a patient is HIV positive without consent can be justified only when there is a significant risk of harm to an identified individual who could become infected and exposed to the health risks it entails. There are similarities between this case and *Tarasoff* in terms of the conflict between the doctor's duty to uphold patient privacy and confidentiality and the duty to prevent harm. Unlike *Tarasoff*, though, the patient in this example is not mentally impaired and could not lose his right to confidentiality for this reason. The probability of harm to the uninformed partner in becoming infected would appear to be significant enough to outweigh any probable harm to the patient by breaching confidentiality. Yet a complicating factor for the doctor is the possibility that overriding confidentiality may lead the patient to end his relationship with the doctor, who can give him the continuous care he needs.

There is another factor that distinguishes the HIV case from *Tarasoff*. In evaluating whether the partner of the HIV-positive patient should be notified, we should consider that the partner might already be infected. Indeed, the partner might have infected the patient. Even if his partner is infected, knowing his HIV status may nonetheless be beneficial in other ways. For instance, it may enable the partner to take steps to prevent the development of full-blown AIDS.

On balance, the risk of harm in this example is significant enough to justify overriding confidentiality and informing the patient's partner. Fear of abandonment notwithstanding, the fact that the patient refuses to allow his partner to know his HIV status indicates a disregard for his partner's welfare. This further supports breaching confidentiality. Yet breaching confidentiality could undermine public trust in doctors and result in the failure of patients to seek needed medical care. At the same time, doctors known to be concerned with preventing public harm could promote public trust in the medical profession. Doctors' primary responsibility is to individual patients. But their responsibility can extend to the social community if the risk of harm their patients pose to others is significant. In order to protect others from harm, there may be exceptions to the rule that confidentially must be protected unconditionally. The deontological constraint on breaching confidentiality may be overridden by this consequentialist line of reasoning.

Cross-Cultural Relations

In many of the cases we have discussed, ethical conflicts arise because patients and physicians disagree on the goals of treatment. The oncologist recommends chemotherapy because she believes that the goal should be extending life for a few years. The cancer patient refuses chemotherapy because he believes that the goal should be the quality of his remaining life. For patients from cultures distinct from that of the Western-trained physician, it can be difficult for them to agree with the physician on medical goals because they do not share the same vocabulary. Unlike intracultural conflicts, the meanings Western doctors and non-Western patients attach to terms such as "benefit" and "health" may be quite different. These divergent meanings may be reflections of different belief systems. And they may lead patients to ask for treatments that conflict with doctors' understanding of what is in their patients' best interests. Giving these treatments may violate the doctors' professional integrity as well.

These conflicts can often be prevented or resolved by relying on a broader understanding of concepts such as autonomy. In some cultures, it may be common for a competent adult to freely delegate decisional authority to another adult. Although this differs from our liberal understanding of individual autonomy and informed consent, it may be interpreted as a different expression of autonomy and consent. A member of the family may be designated as the decision maker for the entire family. This can be accommodated within a broad Western model of informed consent. Indeed, there are cases both in Western and non-Western cultures where the idea of family autonomy may be more important than individual autonomy. Decisions about treatment in such cases indicate that the interests of each family member cannot be separated from the interests of the family as a whole.

A Western-trained doctor is working in a Navajo community. One of his patients is a Navajo man who has not been taking his medication for hypertension. The doctor wants to make him more aware of his risk of stroke, kidney failure, and coronary artery disease, believing that this will motivate the patient to take the medication. But by focusing on the risks, the doctor may cause the patient to have a negative perception of treatment and discourage him from seeing the doctor. Too much emphasis on risk will conflict with his Navajo culture's concept of healing as a process of moving from a negative state of imbalance to a positive state of balance. By ignoring this concept, the doctor will be working against the aim of acting in his patient's best interests.

Confronted with this situation, the doctor shifts the emphasis from the idea of risk to the idea of balance. He tells his patient that taking the medication is the best way for him to regain this balance. The doctor thereby gives the patient a positive incentive to control his condition. By reframing his explanation of his patient's medical condition in terms of the meanings the patient attaches to "healing" and "harmony," the doctor can bring about a mutually agreeable plan of treatment. The doctor is not accepting a culturally relative interpretation of his ethical obligation to act in the best interests of his patient. Although the patient uses "harmony" and the doctor uses "health" to describe the goal of treatment, the goal is the same for both. Explaining the reasons for taking medication in culturally different terms is an alternative way of discharging the physician's duties of nonmaleficence and beneficence to patients. Moreover, by altering his discussion of the medical condition with the patient, the doctor is showing respect for the patient as an autonomous individual with the right to self-determination. There is nothing culturally relative about the underlying ethical norms in this case (Jecker, Carrese, and Pearlman 1995).

A different cross-cultural case is more problematic. A Navajo woman is brought to the emergency room of a hospital. She is confused, delirious, and has a fever. She has had these symptoms for several days, but has refused to go to the hospital or see a Western doctor. Given the woman's compromised decisional capacity, her daughters are her substitute decision makers. Despite admitting their mother to the hospital, they refuse to consent to a lumbar puncture to rule out meningitis as a possible cause of her symptoms. They claim that their mother would refuse any invasive procedure because it would violate her cultural beliefs in bodily integrity, harmony, and balance. She would also object to a CT scan to rule out a stroke on the ground that it too would disturb her integrity. The daughters discharge their mother from the hospital to participate in a healing ceremony conducted by the Navajo medicine man. The doctor knows that postponing or forgoing the lumbar puncture will prevent him from making an accurate diagnosis. He also knows that the woman's condition may worsen and become life-threatening without the proper treatment. Nevertheless, her daughters see the healing ceremony as the only way to restore the natural balance in their mother.

The doctor feels obligated to prevent harm to this patient. Allowing the patient to forego the lumbar puncture and treatment for the sake of the healing ceremony will be tantamount to allowing harm. This may violate the doctor's professional integrity. At the same time, the doctor has a duty to respect the patient's and her surrogates' autonomy. When a surrogate makes a decision about treatment, the doctor has a duty to respect the decision, provided that it is what the patient would have wanted or is in her best interests. Consistent with this respect, the doctor has a duty to be sensitive to the different values and beliefs informing the surrogates' decision. The doctor must be sensitive to the fact that "benefit" and "harm" have different meanings for them and for him, and that these meanings involve more than the physiological condition of the body. Mutual respect and openness between patient and doctor can lead to a cross-cultural reconciliation of value and meaning and a mutually agreeable course of treatment. But in this case the patient and her surrogates may believe that any invasive procedure (including the dye injected for the CT scan) would not benefit and only harm her. If the doctor believes that the only way to properly diagnose and treat the condition is through an invasive procedure, then it appears that the conflict between patient and doctor cannot be resolved. The doctor's only justifiable action is to respect the surrogates' decision to forego the conventional medical treatment and not treat the patient (Jecker, Carrese, and Pearlman 1995).

In some respects, this case is similar to that of the adult Jehovah's Witness who refuses a blood transfusion for severe anemia. In both cases, the doctor has a duty to respect patient autonomy and the right to refuse even life-saving treatment. Deontological considerations override consequentialist ones. The reasons for refusal as such are not decisive. What is decisive is that the reasons reflect a belief system that is part of the patient's right to self-determination. Because patients and their surrogates have this right, doctors have a corresponding duty to respect it.

Yet from the fact that a patient has a right to refuse any medical treatment, it does not follow that the patient has a right to receive any treatment. And if there is no such right, then a doctor has no obligation to grant a patient's request for a particular treatment. Put another way, *negative autonomy* does not imply *positive autonomy* for the patient. This asymmetry applies equally to intra- and cross-cultural situations. Doctors are permitted to perform procedures that put patients at some risk, as in transplanting kidneys from living donors. But they are prohibited from performing procedures or providing treatments known to harm patients. Although the duty of nonmaleficence is not absolute, it has considerable force and should not be ignored because of cultural differences between patient and doctor. If a patient asks a doctor to amputate a limb in order to drive evil spirits from his body, then the doctor would be prohibited from performing the amputation because of the obvious harm it entails. Although the patient could claim that there are religious reasons for the amputation, doctors are obligated to respect the wishes of competent patients on religious or cultural grounds only when patients *refuse* treatment, not when they *request* it.

Suppose that an African woman asks a Western doctor to perform a clitoridectomy, female genital mutilation. The woman may claim that this procedure is a part of her culture and that not having it would lead to her being shunned by her community. Yet it could be argued that this is a reflection of a patriarchal belief system that violates the right of women to bodily noninterference and perpetuates oppression against them. Clitoridectomies usually are performed because men want women to have them, not because women want them. A father will often request one for his daughter. When this occurs, a woman's request for the procedure is not truly autonomous. By refusing to perform female genital mutilation, Western doctors respect women's right to bodily noninterference. The universal truth here is the negative right not to be harmed. Even in a case where an autonomous adult woman requested such a procedure, she would not have a right to it. The doctor would have no obligation to do anything that would harm patients, and this procedure would cause obvious physical harm. It would be analogous to a request for limb amputation. Indeed, the doctor would be prohibited from performing these procedures because of his duty of nonmaleficence to prevent serious harm.

In sum, doctors should respect the beliefs of patients from non-Western cultures and be sensitive to alternative meanings of such terms as "benefit" and "health." But there are limits. If a patient requests a treatment that falls outside of the goals of medicine, broadly construed, then a physician has no obligation to provide it. If the treatment clearly harms the patient, then the physician is prohibited from providing it. Doctors are obligated to respect competent patients' refusal of treatment on religious or cultural grounds, even when this results in harm. But doctors are prohibited from providing a requested treatment that directly harms a patient, regardless of the reasons for the request.

What Sort of Doctors Do We Need?

When we become sick and need medical care, what qualities do we look for in doctors? Earlier, we noted the importance of empathy and compassion in disclosing information about diagnosis and prognosis to patients. In life-threatening conditions, though, compassion will not meet our acute needs. We want doctors who are competent and can treat these conditions effectively. The more acute the condition, the more competence matters. If I am brought to the emergency room with a life-threatening injury, competence means everything to me and compassion very little. But if I have a chronic and controllable condition, compassion may mean more to me than competence. Generally, doctors should be both competent and compassionate. These are the qualities we look for in a doctor who manages a chronic disease such as diabetes. Empathy and compassion are perhaps most important at the end of life, when a condition has become irreversible and aggressive life-sustaining treatment is replaced with palliative care to control pain and suffering. But even here it is important that doctors have expertise in pain management. They should be able to administer opioid analgesics in a way that will control pain while allowing patients to retain their mental capacities and dignity as much as possible.

Ideally, physicians should be competent in clinical care, compassionate, and knowledgeable about current research. A practitioner who is aware of clinical trials is more likely to know of promising new treatments for his or her patients' conditions. Yet, as we will discuss in the next chapter, there is a potential conflict for a physician who sees patients as research subjects and at the same time as individuals needing therapeutic treatments. Paying too much attention to clinical trials yielding scientific knowledge for future patients runs the risk of not meeting the physical and emotional needs of present patients. Medical research may perpetuate and accentuate the trend toward specialization and impersonalization within the medical profession.

The sort of doctors we want, and the qualities we look for in them, will depend upon the nature of our needs. Patients have different types and degrees of need at different stages of their lives. Meeting these needs requires different qualities in physicians. Depending on whether our medical needs are acute, chronic, or palliative, we may want and need different sorts of doctors. This is not a reflection of specialization in medicine, but of the fact that no doctor realistically can meet all of a patient's needs at all the stages of the patient's life.

Near the end of a patient's life, his or her needs may be more psychological or spiritual than physiological. A doctor's general duty to patients is to restore them to normal physical and mental functioning. If this is not possible, then the doctor has a duty to relieve pain and suffering. Suffering is a subjective response to pain. It involves the feeling of losing control over the body. Yet because suffering is a subjective response to pain or loss of control over the body, it is unclear whether, beyond relieving pain, doctors have an obligation to relieve suffering. Are there some things that patients want or need that are beyond the limits of what physicians are obligated to do for them? Should these acts be optional, beyond the call of the duty of beneficence, and thus more appropriately characterized as altruistic?

As a rule, physicians should not be considered altruistic when acting in their patients' best interests. This is because they do not have the choices in acting that we ordinarily associate with altruism, which is not motivated by any sense of duty or obligation. Doctors have professional duties to patients that they cannot discharge as a matter of choice. To be sure, becoming a doctor and thereby entering into a professional relationship with patients is an optional act. Once a doctor enters into this relationship, however, he or she cannot choose obligations. A doctor can choose not to treat a particular patient in a particular situation if doing so would compromise personal and professional integrity. But the doctor must ensure that the patient's care is transferred to another physician. Once one becomes a physician, one promises to promote the best medical interests of one's patients. This is not optional, but obligatory.

Physicians who join groups like *Médecins Sans Frontières* ("Doctors without Borders") do act altruistically in the sense that they are not obligated to put themselves in danger in order to treat patients with whom they have no special ties in unstable parts of the world. Also, a physician who makes a house call to a poor patient who has difficulty finding transportation acts altruistically because he or she goes beyond the boundaries of professional obligation. But these examples are the exception rather than the rule.

At the end of a patient's life, the line between beneficence and altruism for a physician is not so clearly defined. A patient who is religious may ask a doctor to pray with him because he believes that it will relieve his suffering. Is the doctor obligated to do this? Or is it optional? Being compassionate and empathetic can benefit patients and is part of a doctor's duty to them. But this duty does not imply an obligation to do anything that a patient asks. Forming too strong an emotional bond with a patient may impede the physician's ability to benefit other patients and may conflict with professional integrity. This is illustrated by the example of Dr. Rieux in Albert Camus's allegorical novel *The Plague*. Unable to cure his patients of the plague or treat their symptoms, Rieux empathizes with but restrains his feelings toward them. He realizes that becoming too close to his patients may adversely affect his ability to be effective in treating all of his patients in the long term. Dr. Rieux maintains an even keel between his feelings and his professional obligation in the face of a deadly epidemic. We want our doctors to have empathy, not just detached concern. But there are limits to what doctors are obligated to do in this regard.

Some might insist that doctors should respond to the requests of sick or dying patients in a less restrained way. Spending extra time with a patient or his or her family is a generous act that can help allay fear and relieve suffering. Still, this is optional, something that a physician is permitted but not obligated to do. And if the extra time with one patient means spending less time discharging more basic duties to other patients, then it may even be prohibited. Provided that they act respectfully and compassionately toward patients and their families, and are willing to talk with them about their disease, hopes, and fears, doctors are not obligated to do anything more.

Conclusion

The patient-doctor relationship over the years has moved from a model of physician paternalism to one of patient autonomy. The patient's right to informed consent, to disclosure of medical information, confidentiality, and the right to refuse treatment all fall under the principle of autonomy. Doctors have an obligation to respect patient autonomy. Nevertheless, some aspects of autonomy can be overridden when a patient's condition poses a significant risk of harm to other people.

In cross-cultural relationships between patients and doctors, respect for autonomy means that doctors should be sensitive to the beliefs and values of patients. They should also try to accommodate different meanings patients might attach to the concepts of "health" and "disease." In addition, doctors have an obligation to recognize that acting in the best interests of these patients may include factors that are not limited to medical conditions alone. These complicating issues go beyond the question of whether the patient is competent. In some cases, these differences can be resolved and Western doctors and non-Western patients can come to a mutual agreement about treatment goals. In other cases, conflicts may not be resolved. When the goals of Western medicine are incompatible with the beliefs and wishes of a patient, and the patient refuses a given treatment, the physician is obligated to respect the patient's wishes and not override the refusal. Yet there is an important asymmetry in a cross-cultural patient-doctor relationship, which is not fundamentally different from the same relationship in an intra-cultural context. Doctors have an obligation to respect a competent patient's refusal of even life-saving treatment. But they do not have an obligation to respect a competent patient's request to receive any treatment. If such a treatment falls outside the goals of medicine and will harm the patient, then a physician is not obligated and may be prohibited from providing it.

The model of patient and doctor in a cooperative relationship of shared decision making is being threatened in the United States. Managed care has introduced a third party mediating between doctor and patient and has altered the concepts of autonomy and informed consent. Physicians are fiduciary agents for their patients. At the same time, they are often employees of managed care organizations (MCOs). Physicians have a duty to their employer to control costs by limiting tests and referrals to specialists. This leads to two potential conflicts in the patient-doctor relationship. First, if physicians limit expensive diagnostic tests and referrals to specialists because of financial incentives, then they may not be acting in the best interests of their patients and may be failing to fulfill their responsibility to them. Second, if physicians do not fully disclose to patients which services the MCO does and does not cover, then physicians may be undermining patients' informed consent to various treatments. In both instances, the physician may be acting as a "double agent" who has conflicting obligations to the MCO, on the one hand, and to patients, on the other. Whether these conflicts can be resolved, and whether honest, shared decision making between doctors and patients can be preserved, will depend on the policies that we as a society adopt regarding the delivery of health care.

Selected Readings

Angel, M. "The Doctor As Double Agent." *Kennedy Institute of Ethics Journal* 3(1993): 279–286.

Buchanan, A., and Brock, D. *Deciding for Others: The Ethics of Surrogate Decision Making.* New York: Cambridge University Press, 1989.

Emanuel, E., and Emanuel, L. "Four Models of the Physician-Patient Relationship." *Journal of the American Medical Association* 267(1992): 2221–26.

Faden, R., and Beauchamp, T. *A History and Theory of Informed Consent.* New York: Oxford University Press, 1986.

Halpern, J. *From Detached Concern to Empathy.* New York: Oxford University Press, 2001.

Jecker, N., Carrese, J., and Pearlman, R. "Caring for Patients in Cross-Cultural Settings." *Hastings Center Report* 25(1995): 6–14.

Katz, J. *The Silent World of Doctor and Patient.* Baltimore: Johns Hopkins University Press, 2002.

Macklin, R. *Against Relativism: Cultural Diversity and the Search for Universals in Medicine.* New York: Oxford University Press, 1999.

Pellegrino, E., and Thomasma, D. *For the Patient's Good: The Restoration of Beneficence in Health Care.* New York: Oxford University Press, 1988.

Veatch, R. *The Patient-Physician Relation: The Patient As Partner.* Parts 1 and 2. Bloomington: Indiana University Press, 1991.

CHAPTER 3

Medical Research on Humans

Introduction

The Nuremberg Code was drawn up in 1946 as part of the judgment against physicians who conducted medical experiments on inmates in Nazi concentration camps. The Code consisted of ten ethical principles. Foremost among these was the requirement that human subjects give voluntary informed consent before participating in research. Another important principle was that there should be an appropriate ratio of benefits to risks in the research. These two principles form the core of ethical policies governing medical research on humans.

In 1964, the World Medical Association (WMA) adopted the Declaration of Helsinki, which added three important points to the Nuremberg Code. The first point was the distinction between therapeutic research, whose aim is to benefit patients, and nontherapeutic research, whose aim is not to benefit patients but to generate scientific knowledge. The second point was that an institutional mechanism should be in place to ensure that the main ethical principles were followed. The third point was the provision for proxy consent by family members when subjects such as children could not consent on their own. Shortly after the Helsinki Declaration, Harvard anesthesiologist Henry Beecher published an article in the *New England Journal of Medicine* exposing twenty-two unethical clinical investigations involving human subjects. Furthermore, in the early 1970s it was revealed that for forty years the U.S. Public Health Service had sponsored a study in which poor African-American men in Tuskegee, Alabama, were deprived of treatment for syphilis so that the course of the untreated disease could be studied.

In the wake of these and other revelations, Congress created the National Commission for the Protection of Human Subjects of Biomedical and Behavioral Research. The Commission issued the Belmont Report in 1979. It identified respect for persons as autonomous agents, beneficence, and justice as necessary principles for any research to be justified. The principle of respect for persons led to the requirement of informed consent. The principle of beneficence led to the requirement of a favorable risk-benefit ratio. And the principle of justice led to the requirements of an equitable selection of research subjects and a fair distribution of risk among them. To be ethical, all medical research on humans must conform to these requirements.

Physicians are obligated to promote the best interests of their patients. Those who are researchers are also obligated to generate scientifically valid knowledge about the causes of or treatments for diseases. In this capacity, they have an obligation to recruit patients who will serve as subjects in clinical trials. Yet if a doctor has a duty to protect patients from harm, and medical research exposes them to the risk of harm, then it seems that the doctor has an obligation to discourage them from participating in research. But this conflicts with his or her duty as a researcher to promote science and the health of future patients. Research in childhood leukemia, for example, has yielded more effective treatments and a significant reduction in mortality over the last twenty years. The physician-researcher must strike a delicate balance between these two obligations to patients-subjects. The problem is especially acute given the general nontherapeutic purpose of research. It promises no direct benefit to present patients, but uses them to test such things as drug toxicity so that more effective treatments can be developed for the benefit of future patients. Jay Katz (1993), one of the pioneers in the ethics of medical research on humans, captures the gist of the problem in raising the following question: "When may a society, actively or by acquiescence, expose some of its members to harm in order to seek benefits for them, for others, or for society as a whole?" (p. 34).

In this chapter, we will discuss different aspects of this general ethical problem. These aspects include equipoise, randomization, and the use of placebo controls in clinical trials. They also include problems with informed consent, whether special protections are required for vulnerable groups, and whether greater protections should be in place for healthy subjects over sick ones in research. In discussing these issues, we will be guided primarily by the second formulation of Kant's categorical imperative. In research involving human subjects, researchers have a duty to treat these subjects not only as means, but also as ends-in-themselves. But can we ensure that they will always be treated in this way?

Design of Clinical Trials

Generally, five conditions must be met for clinical trials to be ethically acceptable. First, voluntary informed consent must be obtained from subjects. Second, the research must involve a favorable benefit-risk ratio. The subjects must not be exposed to undue risk, and the potential benefit of learning whether a drug or surgical procedure works must be worth any potential risk to the subjects. Third, there must be an equitable selection of subjects that rules out any exploitation and adequately represents both sexes and all social groups. Fourth, the privacy of the subjects must be protected. Fifth, the confidentiality of the data yielded by the research must be protected. Independent review groups such as institutional review boards (IRBs) have the authority and responsibility to monitor research protocols to ensure that these five conditions are met.

Most clinical trials are designed to test the safety and efficacy of a drug or surgical procedure before it is used on patients in a clinical setting. These trials will follow tests using animal models. All clinical trials involving human subjects consist in the same four-phase approval process.

In a Phase I drug trial, researchers aim to test the toxicity of a drug, the highest dose human subjects can tolerate. Subjects in Phase I noncancer trials are usually healthy volunteers. In contrast, volunteers in Phase I cancer trials are sick and must have exhausted all therapeutic options and have a life expectancy of at least three to four months. Some volunteers may enter these trials for altruistic reasons, knowing that their participation will not benefit them but may benefit future patients. In many cases, though, patients enter these trials out of a desperate hope or mistaken belief that the drug will benefit them. In Phase II trials, researchers try to estimate an optimal dosing regimen and to find the experimental conditions that will allow the third phase of the trial to yield a definitive result. It is also here that the end points of the trial are specified, such as the five-year survival rate using a drug to treat a certain form of cancer. Phase III trials involve the largest number of subjects. The aim here is to learn whether the treatment is effective and what its side effects are. Phase IV trials take place once the drug has been approved by the Food and Drug Administration (FDA) and has been marketed. These trials are used to monitor a drug's side effects and to collect more information for possible additional uses. Phase III and Phase IV trials may be therapeutic because they can benefit subjects in addition to generating scientific knowledge.

Because Phase I and Phase II trials are nontherapeutic, the researcher's main moral obligation is to protect subjects from harm, which could be in the form of severe side effects or even death. Because Phase III and Phase IV trials may be therapeutic, the researcher's main moral obligation is to ensure that there is an appropriate risk-benefit ratio for subjects in the trials. Any potential risks of the experimental treatment to the subjects must be commensurate with the potential benefits to them.

The design of the trial becomes especially important in the second phase. At this stage, the control group is introduced as a point of comparison with the intervention group receiving the experimental treatment. In a placebo-controlled drug trial, the control group receives a placebo, a biologically inert pill or substance. *Placebo controls* should not be confused with the *placebo response*, the physiological changes in our bodies that occur because we expect them to occur. In an active-controlled trial, the control group receives the standard proven treatment. Many trials are randomized in the sense that subjects are assigned by chance to either the treatment group or the control group. Randomized controlled clinical trials are considered the "gold standard" in medical research in determining whether a proposed treatment is safe and effective. Many trials are blinded, in the sense that neither the researcher nor the subject knows to which group the subject has been assigned. A computer assigns the subjects to one group or the other. Blinding is necessary to factor out bias in the researcher and the subjects. These are called double-blind (placebo-controlled or active-controlled) clinical trials. Most clinical trials are prospective.

Subjects consent to participate in and are assigned to the control or treatment group in advance of the trial. But in some trials consent can be given only retrospectively, as in testing new treatments in emergency. For safety or other reasons, not all trials can be blinded. And a trial may be stopped before its originally intended date of completion. This can occur if the experimental treatment causes significant adverse events in subjects or if the benefits of the treatment conclusively demonstrate its efficacy.

Equipoise, Randomization, and Placebos

The main ethical issues in clinical trials concern equipoise, randomization, and the use of placebo controls. Equipoise refers to the attitude of a researcher, or group of researchers, involved in a randomized controlled clinical trial. A researcher is in equipoise when he or she does not know whether one treatment is more effective than another. A research community is in equipoise when there is genuine disagreement within the community about the comparative merits of the experimental and control arms of the trial. The available evidence offers no reason for saying that one arm is superior to the other. This disagreement justifies starting and continuing a clinical trial. A researcher may prefer one type of treatment to another. But, provided that there is uncertainty about the data underlying this preference, the researcher is still in equipoise. Preferences or hunches can be tested objectively when the researcher is part of a research community, as well as by the design of the trial.

The therapeutic relationship between doctor and patient is most beneficial when the doctor believes in the efficacy of the treatment he or she is giving to the patient. This in turn promotes the patient's trust in the doctor. But if the patient is a subject in a trial and receives a treatment for which the doctor does not have a preference, then arguably the doctor is not acting in the patient's best interests by encouraging participation in the trial.

One could respond to this claim by pointing out that the trial may show that the doctor's preference for a particular treatment was unfounded and that, in fact, it was not the better treatment for the patient. Furthermore, once a doctor informs the patient about the potential risks and benefits of entering the trial, the patient has the freedom and responsibility to decide whether or not to become a research subject. Entering a patient in a trial by itself does not mean that the doctor is acting contrary to the patient's best interests. If the doctor is truly uncertain about the two treatments and has no preference for one over the other, then recruiting the patient for the trial is the best way for the doctor to act in the patient's best interests. The trial will determine the better or best treatment for the patient's condition. If the experimental treatment is shown to be more effective than the standard treatment or a placebo, then even patients in the control arm will benefit from receiving effective therapy once the trial has been stopped. Alternatively, if the experimental treatment causes adverse events, then stopping the trial can prevent additional harm to subjects in the active arm. This can also prevent harm to subjects in the control arm who would have received the treatment if it had been approved.

The point here is that medical practice must not get ahead of medical science. A good example of this was a major trial sponsored by the National Institutes of Health (NIH) and the Women's Health Initiative testing the risks and benefits of hormone replacement therapy. For years, therapy combining estrogen and progestin had been prescribed to millions of women to treat symptoms of menopause. Yet in results published in July 2002, the trial showed that the risks of hormone treatment outweighed the benefits. Indeed, the evidence was so conclusive that the trial was stopped three years before its intended date of completion. On the other hand, a trial in which an experimental treatment has been effective in early stages should not be stopped too soon. Some treatments lose their efficacy over time and may result in unforeseen long-term adverse events. Researchers can determine whether the benefits of an experimental treatment outweigh the risks only by completing all phases of a trial.

Randomization initially raises some of the same ethical worries as equipoise. But, again, if there is uncertainty about the efficacy of any given treatment, a randomized trial is the best way to yield objectively valid results. It will tell the doctor which treatment is better for the patient. So, recruiting a patient to be a subject in a randomized clinical trial does not by itself compromise the researcher's duty as a doctor to care for the patient. The better treatment will be determined by the results of the trial. In fact, patients can benefit more from a research setting than from standard clinical care because they receive more attention with the resources available to the research team. By entering a patient in a random-ized controlled clinical trial, a doctor is treating the patient as a means for the sake of generating scientific knowledge. But the doc-tor is also treating the patient as an end by obtaining consent to participate in the trial and by ensuring that the potential risks are commensurate with the potential benefits. The physician is at once fulfilling the primary duty of a doctor to the patient and the sec-ondary duty of a researcher to the research subject.

An example will illustrate that entering a subject in a clinical trial is consistent with the doctor's duty of care to patients. There has been some debate about whether lumpectomy or mastectomy is the better treatment for early breast cancer. In lumpectomy, only a tumor and some surrounding tissue are surgically removed. The breast itself is left intact. In mastectomy, the entire breast is re-moved. Suppose that a surgeon is unsure about this question and recommends that her patients enter a clinical trial designed to yield a definitive answer. The surgeon is not treating her patients only as means for the sake of deriving scientifically valid data. She is also treating them as ends, offering each patient a 50 percent chance of receiving the better treatment, which is not yet known. Because the surgeon is uncertain, the best way to act in her patients' best interests is to follow randomization. If she prefers lumpectomy and recommends it to her patients without waiting for more objectively valid data on the comparative merits of mastectomy, then she might be exposing her patients to unknown risks and denying them ben-efits. Entering her patients in such a trial means that each of her patients will be better off than if they had been offered only one of the two treatments.

The use of placebos in clinical trials raises more troubling ethi-cal questions. Placebo-controlled trials are scientifically superior to active-controlled trials. Without a placebo, researchers cannot know whether a new treatment causes an improvement in a con-dition or whether the improvement would have occurred without an active intervention. This is especially the case if the active drug has never been proved against a placebo. So the results derived from placebo-controlled trials are more scientifically robust and promote greater potential benefits to future patients. Moreover, placebo-controlled trials require a smaller group of research sub-jects, making it more likely that the trial will be completed within a shorter period of time. In these two respects, placebo-controlled trials are superior to active-controlled trials.

But sick patients receiving placebos may be exposed to greater risks, because for a period of time they are not receiving any active treatment for their condition. Proponents of placebo controls respond to this objection by insisting that such trials should be for only a limited period of time. In addition, escape mechanisms involving active treatment should be in place to ensure that the patients' condition does not deteriorate. In 2000, the World Health Organization (WHO) revised the Declaration of Helsinki to say that any new treatments under study should be tested against "the best available treatments." Placebos could be used ethically only when "no proven treatment exists." Some might claim that this requirement presents an obstacle to determining the best treatment because only a placebo, not standard treatment, can accurately determine the efficacy of a new intervention. Even if it has been proven effective, available treatment might not be the "best" treatment. In general, deontological and consequentialist reasons support the WHO recommendations on placebos. The risk of harm to sick patients in the placebo arm of a trial may be significant enough to outweigh any potential benefits to them and violate a doctor's duty to protect her patients from harm. A placebo would not pose a significant risk if the medical condition in question were relatively mild, however. Although the placebo would delay treatment for such a condition, it would not undermine the effectiveness of the new treatment once the trial ended.

There are some conditions for which placebos are permissible, if not required, because only placebos can determine which treatment is best for patients. This is especially the case in psychiatry and neurology. Studies show that double-blind placebo-controlled trials provide the most reliable evaluation of antipsychotic agents for schizophrenia. Furthermore, in depression the difference in improvement rates between drug-treated and placebo-treated patients is not significant enough to make a placebo control unethical. And in trials involving drugs for Alzheimer's disease, placebo controls are clearly preferred to active controls. Specifically, cholinesterase inhibitors such as tacrine or donepezil cannot be called "standard" or "effective" therapy because only a small percentage of Alzheimer's patients have benefited from this type of drug. Placebo controls in clinical trials can be ethical with four provisos: (1) no effective therapy for the condition exists; (2) the trial cannot last too long; (3) the placebo cannot expose patients to unacceptable risk; and (4) patients must be adequately informed about the nature and risks of a placebo-controlled trial and give full voluntary consent to participate.

Because surgical interventions generally expose patients to greater risks than drug interventions, it is more difficult to justify placebo controls in surgical procedures. Even if randomized placebo-controlled trials are clinically superior, the risks of using placebos in surgical trials raise the question of whether they are ethical. These trials involve incisions into patients' bodies; patients are not aware of what the surgeon is doing, and they may have to undergo general anesthesia. Let's consider the use of a placebo control in a clinical trial testing the efficacy of fetal-cell transplantation to treat Parkinson's disease. The rationale for this trial was the belief that transplantation of fetal cells into the brains of Parkinson's patients might be more effective than drugs such as levodopa, which have significant side effects. Parkinson's patients suffer from a deficit of the neurotransmitter dopamine, which regulates the brain's motor control system. A deficit of dopamine causes involuntary bodily movements and general neurological deterioration. Fetal cells transplanted into the brain in theory could generate dopamine and thus control or alleviate the symptoms of the disease. The efficacy of the transplants could be tested more accurately if the control group did not receive drug therapy.

The NIH sponsored such a trial in 1999. Patients in the intervention group received general anesthesia. Burr holes were drilled in their skulls, penetrating the inner cortex of the brain, where the fetal tissue was implanted. Patients in the control group also received general anesthesia. But the burr holes did not penetrate the cortex. Both groups received a low dose of the immunosuppressive drug cyclosporine for six months and continued to receive medical therapy. To ensure that the trial was blinded, the surgical and evaluation sites were in separate locations. The surgeon was the only member of the research team aware of an individual subject's group assignment.

Even if drug therapy for Parkinson's is ineffective, can the benefits from learning whether the surgical procedure works justify exposing research subjects to its risks? If fetal-cell transplantation proves to be effective, then many patients suffering from Parkinson's might benefit from the research. If the procedure proves to be ineffective, then many patients will be spared the risks and financial burdens of an unproven operation. But the risks to subjects in the trial are significant. General anesthesia can lead to respiratory failure. Also, subjects might become infected from the burr holes and have their immune systems weakened by the cyclosporine. The patients who received the implants were exposed to greater risk because of the needle penetration to the brain. The risks to both groups seem significant enough to morally outweigh any potential benefits to them or to future patients. A doctor has a primary duty to protect patients from harm. Because entering them into such a trial entails enough risk of harm to violate that duty, it would seem that the doctor should not ask Parkinson's patients to participate in such a trial. In addition, some might claim that the "sham" surgery for patients in the placebo group is unethical because the surgeon is deliberately deceiving these patients. Nevertheless, only such a surgical trial can determine whether fetal-cell surgery is more effective in treating Parkinson's than drug therapy. The trial could yield results that eventually might lead to better treatments for the disease and thus benefit future patients.

The result of the trial in question was that fetal-cell transplants were not more effective than drug therapy for Parkinson's disease. A more recent trial in 2002 showed that arthroscopic surgery for arthritis of the knee did not improve knee function. These two examples illustrate the clinical significance of placebo-controlled surgical trials. But the Parkinson's trial also illustrates an equally significant ethical point. It shows the conflict between the researcher's duty to use research subjects to generate valid scientific knowledge and the doctor's duty to protect patients from potential harm. When the risk of harm in a trial is significant, obtaining consent from patients alone does not justify entering them in the trial. Even if a patient exercises autonomy and consents to participate in research, doctors have a duty to protect patients from significant harm that may befall them as research subjects. Exposing them to risk solely for the sake of scientific knowledge is using them as means but not also as ends-in-themselves. If no patients enter these and other trials, however, then better treatments for Parkinson's patients will not be developed and they will continue to suffer from the disease. Is there any way to resolve this dilemma?

The most defensible position for the doctor-researcher to take in these and other trials is to fulfill the duty to protect present patients from undue risk, but remain open to the needs of future patients. Although the duty to care for one's present patients is primary, it does not prohibit one from using patients in research to generate scientific knowledge that might benefit future patients. Indeed, a researcher has an obligation to recruit patients for this purpose, provided that the research exposes patients only to a minor risk of harm. While discharging their primary duty to prevent harm to their patients, doctors need to explain to them that existing treatments developed as a result of past research on patients who were willing to serve as research subjects. These patients were motivated not only by the desire to benefit from new treatments, but perhaps also to benefit other patients who would have similar diseases later on. Many patients refuse to participate in research because of their perception of risk. Yet one could argue that they could take some responsibility for improving medical treatment and be willing to make some sacrifice in accepting minimal risk as research subjects. Researchers could not use this idea in recruiting subjects, though, because it could be a form of coercion. Participation in research must always be voluntary rather than obligatory, consistent with the principle of autonomy emphasized in the Belmont Report.

Whether a doctor asks patients to participate in a clinical trial should depend on his or her assessment of the risks the trial entails. Assessment of the risks will depend on whether the doctor is more duty based or goal based in his or her beliefs about medical research on humans. In the first case, the doctor will be motivated more by deontological considerations and will give more weight to respecting patients' right not to be harmed. In the second case, the doctor will be motivated more by consequentialist considerations and will give more weight to the scientific knowledge generated by having patients take part in the research. Those who argued that the clinical trial for Parkinson's using the placebo control was unethical did so along deontological lines. Those who argued that it was ethical did so along consequentialist lines. The position a doctor takes on the ethics of clinical trials will depend on how he or she weighs the duty of a doctor to present patients against the duty of a researcher to science and future patients.

Problems with Consent

In therapeutic research, subjects may not always understand the information presented to them about a clinical trial. They may misunderstand the meaning and implications of randomization and placebo controls. Moreover, patients may agree to participate in a trial because they trust their doctor, who has a research interest in the trial. Participating in a trial may not entirely be a patient's own decision, as he or she may be subtly coerced or unduly influenced by the doctor. This raises the question of whether the consent is truly voluntary. Questions about how voluntary consent really is also arise when patients who have not responded to existing therapies pin their only hope of controlling their disease on an experimental treatment. Patients with severe symptoms of Parkinson's disease may ignore the risks in surgical trials and agree to participate for this reason.

This does not mean that no patients with severe disease ever truly consent to participate in clinical trials. It may be reasonable for a patient to try an experimental medicine, even if its chances of working are not very good. Some patients with severe disease may give valid consent to an experimental medicine, believing that, for *them*, the potential benefits outweigh the potential risks. Nevertheless, full voluntary consent to participate in research may not be as common as is generally thought.

Obtaining consent from healthy volunteers in Phase I noncancer trials may not seem ethically problematic. Because they are healthy, volunteers are not motivated to participate out of a desperate hope for life-saving treatment. They are more likely to be competent, to rationally assess the information in the consent form, and to give full voluntary consent on the basis of the information. While some of these volunteers may be motivated by the monetary compensation they will receive from participating in a trial, others may be motivated by altruism. They knowingly and willingly expose themselves to risk in order to benefit others. Any benefit they receive is only psychological, not physiological. But the number of altruistic participants in clinical trials is likely very small. Many more will volunteer because they are financially desperate or simply naive. They may believe that being paid for participating in research is equivalent to being paid for doing their job. Still, nontherapeutic trials must address not only consent, but also the degree of risk to which subjects can be exposed. The fact that they are healthy might lead us to think that there should be a higher standard of protection for them than for volunteers who are sick. We will discuss this issue later in this chapter.

Problems with consent are especially acute in Phase I cancer trials. Although consent forms explicitly state that these trials aim to measure dose toxicity of cancer drugs, and that no therapeutic benefit is expected, many patients fail to understand the purpose of these trials. Many of these patients are desperate and cite hope of remission or cure as their main reason for entering the trial, even though it contradicts what is written in the consent form. Some cancer patients might seize upon the mention of "benefit" in the form or by their physician, ignoring the fact that what they have read or have been told is "you are not likely to receive any benefit from participating in this trial." Response rates in these trials are extremely low, remissions are rare, and some deaths result from drug toxicity. The fact that so many patients enrolling in nontherapeutic cancer trials confuse hope with medical fact suggests that they are not giving full voluntary informed consent when they enter these trials. If these patients cannot benefit from but can only be harmed by the research, and if they participate in it without giving true informed consent, then it seems that the research is unethical and should not be conducted. The trials violate the two main requirements for research to be ethical. By recruiting patients for these trials, doctors fail to protect patients from harm and fail to obtain informed consent from them. So it seems that doctors should be prohibited from recruiting patients for these trials.

Yet, if Phase I cancer trials were prohibited, then crucial information about drug dose toxicity would be lacking. This would preclude subsequent Phase II and Phase III trials from testing the efficacy of new drugs. With medical research suspended or limited, there would be no improvement in treatments for cancer and other diseases. Future patients would be deprived of effective treatments that would enable them to control or cure their diseases and to improve the quality of their lives. Again, doctors who are researchers have to strike a delicate balance between their obligation to protect their patients from harm and their obligation to generate scientific knowledge for the benefit of future patients. A favorable risk-benefit ratio is necessary for a clinical trial to be ethical. If it offers no potential benefits and has significant risks, then it is unethical and should not be conducted. Yet consent from research subjects is also necessary for a trial to be ethical. This condition holds independently of considerations of risk.

Even if prospective subjects for Phase I cancer trials misunderstand the nature of these trials, can we deny them one last chance of responding to an untested drug? Isn't a small chance better than no chance? Shouldn't doctors construe "informed consent" more loosely and give patients one last chance? On the other hand, if doctors believe that their patients will not benefit in any way from a trial, would encouraging them to enter the trial only create false hope? Would they be treating patients as mere instruments for the sake of science?

A study conducted at the University of Chicago in 1995 shows the depth of the problem. Thirty cancer patients enrolled in a Phase I trial were surveyed. Although 93 percent said that they understood the information given to them, only 33 percent were able to state that the purpose of the trial was to determine toxicity, tolerability, or the safest dose of the drug that was administered. Less than one-third of participants said that the research team discussed the option of no treatment with them. Significantly, 85 percent said that they had decided to participate for the reason of possible therapeutic benefit.

Misunderstanding in these cases is due not only to desperation, fear, or hope, but also to confusion surrounding the link between the doctor-patient relationship and the researcher-subject relationship. While these two types of relationship can overlap in therapeutic research, they are distinct in nontherapeutic research. In the latter, the researcher must clearly explain the distinction between therapy and research to the prospective subject. The doctor has an obligation to point out that the aim of the trial is not to benefit subjects like the patient. At the same time, the researcher must not exploit the patient's trust as a way of encouraging participation in the trial. Not participating in the trial must be presented as one of two options in honest and open dialogue between the doctor-researcher and the patient-subject.

To prevent a subject from having unreasonable expectations in volunteering for a Phase I cancer trial, he or she must be made aware that such a trial is nontherapeutic. Knowing this ahead of time, the patient is less likely to be psychologically harmed later upon learning that hope for remission or cure cannot be realized through the trial. Also, if the oncologist explains the nontherapeutic aim of the trial to the patient before participation, then he or she is more likely to retain the patient's trust when the patient does not respond to the drug. This is another respect in which psychological harm to the subject can be prevented.

More generally, these steps can help to ensure that subjects really do consent to participate in a Phase I cancer trial. Oncologists must not trade on patients' hopes in interventions that will not cure or control their particular type of cancer. Instead, they must respect patients' capacity for autonomous reasoning and decision making. They can do this by emphasizing the distinction between therapy and research, and explaining that by participating subjects can benefit only science and future patients, not themselves. But researchers should also emphasize the social importance of this benefit. Honesty in explaining the aim of a clinical trial to a potential subject is as obligatory for a doctor as is full disclosure about a patient's diagnosis and prognosis. Oncologist Matthew Miller goes to the core of the problem:

> We cannot continue to claim that, since the novel agents under investigation have never before been used in humans, any dose is potentially therapeutic. The opposite is true. Unless and until we know whether a given drug is effective, under what conditions, for which malignancies, and at what dose, these trials remain non-therapeutic and ought to be spoken of as such. (2000, p. 40)

Some might argue that there never can be true voluntary informed consent in nontherapeutic research because patients' beliefs and emotions cannot be factored out of their reasoning and decision making. In some cases, researchers may unwittingly contribute to this by seeing and projecting themselves as compassionate physicians at the same time that they are acting in the service of dispassionate science. To be sure, the process of obtaining or giving informed consent will never be perfect. Nevertheless, better communication between researchers and subjects, and between physicians and patients, can help to reduce the degree of misunderstanding that is an obstacle to informed consent. Improvements in the way consent forms are written can help in this regard too. In particular, because "understanding" is inherently vague and often a matter of degree, it may be preferable to use "the design, aims, benefits, and risks of the trial have been explained to me," instead of "I understand the design, aims, benefits, and risks of the trial." This shift can facilitate a context of shared responsibility between researcher and research subject. One is responsible for ensuring that all the important features of the trial are explained clearly. The other is responsible for making a rational decision on the basis of the information presented. Provided that the research is explained as nontherapeutic, and that the risks are clearly spelled out to the subject, the informed consent the subject gives in such a case is sufficient to meet this ethical requirement.

Vulnerable Populations

Patients in Phase I cancer trials represent a special class of vulnerable research subjects. They are vulnerable because they are very sick and often desperate for any intervention that might have some therapeutic benefit. They are also distinct from other subjects because the research in which they participate is nontherapeutic. In therapeutic and some nontherapeutic research, *children* and the *mentally ill* are vulnerable because they cannot consent to participate on their own. The *poor* who are uninsured and lack medical care have the decisional capacity to consent. But this capacity may be compromised by their need for costly diagnostic and therapeutic interventions, and clinical trials may offer the only opportunity to receive them. Finally, clinical trials for better antiretroviral drugs (ARVs) to treat AIDS and other diseases are conducted on *people in developing countries*. Yet these trials may not offer the best available treatment for subjects in the control arm. In fact, many of these trials do not offer treatment in the control arm but are forced to use placebos because AIDS drugs are prohibitively expensive. Lack of access to these drugs may make more people more susceptible to the disease. Each of these four groups presents a unique set of ethical issues, and we will consider them in turn.

Earlier, we mentioned the success of medical research in understanding the cause of and developing treatment for childhood leukemia. This would not have occurred if children had not entered clinical trials as research subjects. At the earliest stage of these trials, children were participating in nontherapeutic research testing new chemotherapeutic drugs for toxicity. They were exposed to risk and did not receive any physiological benefit. In spite of this, the children did not consent to being research subjects in these trials. Parents consented on their children's behalf. The Belmont Report concluded that children should be the last social group on which medical research should be permitted, because they are the most vulnerable. It further recommended that, when the research involves no more than a minor increase over minimal risk, and it does not offer the prospect of direct therapeutic benefit, then the IRB overseeing the protocol can allow it only when the following conditions hold: (1) the research must be commensurate with procedures that others with the same disorder ordinarily undergo; (2) it must offer the prospect of a significant benefit to future children who will be at risk of or suffer from the disorder; and (3) if the research involves more than a minor increase over minimal risk, then it can be permitted only when it presents an opportunity to better understand or prevent a condition affecting the health and welfare of children in general.

There are deontological, communitarian, and consequentialist arguments for and against permitting children to be research subjects. Because the child cannot give informed consent, his or her parents must act as surrogates who consent for the child. Parents have a duty to promote the best interests of and not harm their children. By exposing their children to risk, they are acting in violation of their duty. Moreover, insofar as children cannot benefit from research, allowing them to enter a nontherapeutic protocol is not in their best interests. The child is being treated only as a means and not also as an end-in-itself. Thus the participation of children in research should be prohibited. This is one deontological argument against using children as research subjects. A second deontological argument supports the use of children in research. Parents have an obligation to instill an attitude of unselfish service to others. This can promote their child's moral development. Participating in research that can benefit others enables children to think beyond narrow self-interest and to take into account the interests and needs of other children who are or will be sick. A child who participates in nontherapeutic research is treated as a means to promote scientific knowledge. But the child is also treated as an end when his or her parents promote moral development. Of course, this will not be the case when the child's condition is imminently fatal.

The communitarian argument says that children should be considered as social beings who are members of a greater good that transcends self-interest. When a child's participation in research serves this greater social good, it is permissible. But if this were extended to adults, then it could violate individual autonomy and the ethical requirement of voluntary consent. It would be difficult to justify anything more than an imperfect obligation to put oneself at risk in order to benefit future patients. The obligation is imperfect because it depends on the degree of risk to oneself. When the risk to oneself is greater, the obligation to others will be weaker. Consistent with the concepts of autonomy and imperfect obligation, one should always have the choice to agree or refuse to enter a clinical trial, regardless of the promise it holds for benefiting other people.

The consequentialist argument is similar to the communitarian one, in the sense that it is framed in terms of promoting the general social good. Unlike communitarianism, though, consequentialism is not motivated by shared social values. Instead, the reason for participating in research and sacrificing some of one's own interests is to maximize benefits and minimize harms for patients in general. This end will be achieved by entering clinical trials that will help to better understand the causes of diseases and lead to the development of more effective treatments for them. Without the participation of some children in medical research, other children would continue to suffer from diseases. Also, without appropriately conducted nontherapeutic trials, harmful side effects of drugs would appear later and adversely affect more people.

Any one of the three arguments in favor of permitting children to participate in research can be defended, provided that the children are not exposed to more than a minor increase above minimal risk. Some have defined "minimal risk" as commensurate with risks children ordinarily encounter in everyday life. But this definition is open to conflicting interpretations. There must be regulations in place that clearly spell out what is meant by both minimal risk and a minor increase over minimal risk. This is the only way to avoid variation in interpretation among parents and researchers and to specify what the responsibilities of parents and researchers are so that children will be adequately protected.

The mentally ill constitute another vulnerable group in research. Like children, they cannot make voluntary decisions about whether to participate in research testing new drugs or surgical treatments. The National Bioethics Advisory Commission has recommended that surrogate decision makers could permit incapacitated persons to participate in research that involves a minor increase over minimal risk. There is at least one important difference between children and the mentally ill, however. Whereas children will become autonomous decision makers, in many cases the mentally ill have lost, or never will have, the capacity to make rational, informed decisions about research and other important matters. So the deontological argument for moral development through participation in clinical trials is not plausible for the mentally ill. On the contrary, the deontological argument for the duty to protect the vulnerable from risk of harm seems persuasive enough to prohibit these subjects from participating in research. But knowledge about the causes of mental disorders and better ways of treating them cannot be obtained in any other way than through clinical trials. In this respect, the consequentialist argument for conducting research as a way of benefiting patients with mental disorders is much more persuasive. Still, there would have to be some chance of at least indirect benefit to those who participate.

It would be difficult to justify the participation of the mentally ill in nontherapeutic research if they lack the capacity to be aware of the needs and interests of others. Ordinarily, participation in this type of research is justified because autonomous subjects believe that they are benefiting future patients, despite the risks to which they are exposed. Surrogates making decisions for the mentally incapacitated may very well have this capacity. But the capacity does not transfer from one party to the other. This raises the question of whether surrogates are entitled to make such decisions. If nontherapeutic research on the mentally ill is to be justified, then nothing more than minimal risk should be allowed. The reason for this is that these subjects cannot experience or understand the risks of ordinary life in the same way as competent individuals. These are the risks with which the notion of minimal risk in research is compared. The inability of the mentally ill to adequately assess these risks, combined with their inability to consent on their own, is what makes them vulnerable. For these reasons, IRBs must be especially vigilant in monitoring research protocols involving the mentally ill.

Poor volunteers in research are vulnerable in different respects. Because many of them lack medical insurance and access to basic health care, they do not have a therapeutic relationship with a doctor. They only have a relationship with a researcher, who does not have the same duty of care to them as he or she would have with subjects who are also his or her patients. The indigent subject may confuse the roles of researcher and physician and perceive the researcher as engaging in a therapeutic relationship. This perception can generate expectations in the subject that cannot be met. Moreover, the poor are often motivated to become research subjects by the desire for remuneration, which could be coercive. Some might counter this point by saying that the poor receive better care in a trial than they would receive in a typical doctor-patient relationship. Also, because poor volunteers do not have a relationship with a primary-care physician, they cannot be unduly influenced to enter a trial. Yet the poor may be exposing themselves to risk out of a critical need for medical care, and this too could be considered coercive. But if this is the only way for the poor to receive medical care, can we object to it on ethical grounds? We will respond to this question in the next section when we discuss the just allocation of risk in research.

The last vulnerable population to consider is subjects in therapeutic trials conducted in developing countries. In particular, these are people enrolled in trials testing the efficacy of drugs for HIV-AIDS. Trials in the United States and Europe have demonstrated that such ARVs as zidovudine (AZT) can significantly reduce the incidence of AIDS in newborn infants when taken by infected pregnant women. In Asia and especially sub-Saharan Africa, these drugs have not been widely available because of their high cost. Some have argued that placebo-controlled trials offer the best way of determining which drugs will be most effective in preventing the transmission of AIDS. They also have argued that, because AZT is prohibitively expensive, other less expensive drugs could be used in the intervention arm of these trials. This seems doubly unethical. If AZT is a more effective drug than any alternative, then subjects are not receiving the best available treatment. Furthermore, given the fact that AIDS is transmissible to newborn infants, many will be exposed to high risk if their mothers are in a placebo arm with no treatment at all. Because so many pregnant women are infected, the probability and magnitude of harm to children will be very high. On the other hand, it might be paternalistic to prevent trials in developing countries unless controls are governed by an international standard of care. This might deny people the only opportunity they have of receiving even an experimental drug.

In any case, it is unfair for subjects in these trials not to have access to the same ARVs as subjects in developed countries. It is equally unfair for infected women to receive placebos in the control arm of these trials, given the risk of viral transmission to their children. There is an unfair distribution of risks between these subjects and their counterparts in developed countries. Can the balance be redressed?

Protections and Justice

In June 2001, twenty-four-year-old Ellen Roche died after inhaling a chemical designed to induce asthmatic symptoms. This occurred in a nontherapeutic trial at the Johns Hopkins University. Roche entered the trial for altruistic reasons, wanting to benefit science in general and asthmatic patients in particular. Because she was healthy, some have claimed that subjects like her deserve greater protection in research than sick subjects. Presumably, healthy subjects deserve greater protection because they have more to lose. Becoming sick or dying from an experimental drug or surgical procedure is worse for a healthy person than for one who suffers the same fate but is sick to begin with. The loss for healthy subjects between the starting and end points of the trial is greater than the loss for sick subjects. Yet, because they are worse off than the healthy when they enter a nontherapeutic trial, the sick are more vulnerable to begin with than the healthy and thus require special protection. Can we compare these two distinct senses of being worse off and determine which protections should be in place so that risks can be allocated fairly between the two groups?

In nontherapeutic research, the issue is not whether benefits to one group morally outweigh risks to another, since there is no direct benefit to volunteers. Rather, the issue is whether it is obligatory for researchers to provide greater protections for healthy volunteers over sick ones, or vice versa. What should matter morally is not the difference between the starting and end points of the trial, but the outcome. On an absolute scale of health, a trial that results in morbidity or mortality is just as bad for a healthy subject as it is for a sick one. Instead of providing greater protections for healthy or sick volunteers, equal weight should be given to their distinct claims not to be harmed. IRBs have the responsibility to provide these protections by ensuring that the trial minimizes risks for both healthy and sick subjects. Because exposure to risk can harm these two groups in distinct ways, fairness in the distribution of risks does not involve comparing the claims of one group against the other. It involves respecting the rights of all research subjects not to be harmed and thus not to be exposed to undue risk.

A just solution to the problem of poor volunteers in therapeutic research is to ensure universal access to a basic package of medical benefits to all citizens. Roughly forty-three million Americans have no health coverage. If everyone had basic medical coverage, then the incidence of chronic disease might be lower, and it might be less likely that people entered clinical trials as the only way to receive medical treatment. Furthermore, if medical coverage to the poor were adequately subsidized and they did not have to spend a large portion of their income for medication, then they might be less inclined to volunteer for nontherapeutic research solely for remuneration. A fairer or more just distribution of risks in research between the economically better off and worse off would be more likely to come through universal health care. Such a medical system would not entirely solve the problem of fairness, however. For example, there is disparity between blacks and whites in access to medical services in the U.K. and the U.S. military, both of which claim to offer universal health care.

Fairness in the allocation of risks from AIDS will come by ensuring that people with the disease in developing countries have the same access to the most effective ARVs as infected people in developed countries. Indeed, access to these drugs should be easier than in developed countries, given the higher incidence of the disease in developing countries. People in sub-Saharan Africa have a greater need and thus a stronger claim to the drugs. In this case, fairness is a function of degree of need. A fair distribution of the drugs is one that will give more weight to stronger claims of need. Similarly, we can argue that only active-controlled, not placebo-controlled, trials should be conducted in these countries. Because more women are infected in these countries than in developed countries, the risk of mother-to-child transmission is greater, and only active-controlled trials can minimize or reduce the risk. The high cost of the drugs could be alleviated if the WHO and United Nations spent more money on programs to prevent mother-to-child transmission of AIDS. They could make less expensive drugs like nevirapine more widely available and persuade pharmaceutical companies to freeze or lower prices on more expensive and potentially more effective AIDS medications like combivir.

Conclusion

In this chapter, we focused on three ethical requirements to protect human research subjects. First, voluntary informed consent must be obtained from subjects. Second, there must be an appropriate risk-benefit ratio in clinical trials. Third, there must be a fair distribution of risks between different groups participating in research. It is the responsibility of IRBs and, at a higher level, government regulatory agencies to ensure that these ethical requirements are met in every clinical trial. We also discussed the potential conflict for one who is both a physician and a researcher. The physician's obligation to benefit and not harm patients in a therapeutic relationship is distinct from the obligation to recruit research subjects in order to generate valid scientific knowledge. Whether or to what extent the physician emphasizes one obligation over the other will be a reflection of whether he or she is more duty based or more goal based in thinking. Either way, the physician-researcher must treat volunteers in clinical trials as both subjects and as patients— not only as means, but also as ends-in-themselves.

There has been an increasing blurring of boundaries between the pharmaceutical industry and academic medicine. As a result, there are now more potential conflicts of interest as academic researchers serve as both investigators and as sponsors or patent holders of products of research. Collaboration with a pharmaceutical company or self-interest in obtaining a patent may unduly influence researchers as they recruit subjects for clinical trials. Patients might be used as mere means to a financial end, and there could be an erosion of public trust in medical research. The long-term scientific benefits of research could be compromised.

To prevent this, as well as to prevent the deaths of volunteers like Ellen Roche, all phases of clinical trials must be monitored to ensure that researchers comply with all ethical requirements in conducting these trials. As former U.S. Health and Human Services Secretary Donna Shalala has argued:

> We must work together to reform the current system . . . so that it can guarantee the greatest possible protection for every human subject. We have been the beneficiaries of an extraordinary golden age of biomedical research. We want that research to continue to flourish and make this century one of scientific discovery and progress. (2000, p. 810)

Selected Readings

Angel, M. "Investigators' Responsibilities for Human Subjects in Developing Countries." *New England Journal of Medicine* 342(2000): 967–69.

Beecher, H. "Ethics and Clinical Research." *New England Journal of Medicine* 274(1966): 1354–60.

Brody, B. *The Ethics of Biomedical Research: An International Perspective.* New York: Oxford University Press, 1998.

Foster, C. *The Ethics of Medical Research on Humans*. Cambridge, Eng.: Cambridge University Press, 2001.

Freedman, B. "Equipoise and the Ethics of Clinical Research." *New England Journal of Medicine* 317(1987): 141–45.

Katz, J. " 'Ethics and Clinical Research' Revisited: A Tribute to Henry K. Beecher." *Hastings Center Report* 23(1993): 31–39.

Katz, J., Capron, A., and Glass, E., eds. *Experimentation with Human Beings*. New York: Russell Sage Foundation, 1972.

Miller, M. "Phase I Cancer Trials: A Collusion of Misunderstanding." *Hastings Center Report* 30(2000): 34–42.

Ross, L. F. *Children, Families, and Health Care Decision-Making*. Oxford: Clarendon Press, 1998.

Shalala, D. "Protecting Research Subjects: What Must Be Done." *New England Journal of Medicine* 343(2000): 808–10.

CHAPTER 4

Reproductive Rights and Technologies

Introduction

In the 1973 case of *Roe v. Wade,* the U.S. Supreme Court recognized a constitutional right of women and their doctors to end pregnancies substantially free from state restrictions. But states could prohibit abortions beyond the point of fetal viability. Since 1973, the right to an abortion before fetal viability has consistently been upheld. The Court has maintained that a pre-viable fetus is not a person as interpreted under the Fourteenth Amendment and therefore does not have the same right to life as persons generally guaranteed by the Constitution. In contrast, Common Law doctrine (as practiced in the United Kingdom and Canada) treats only those individuals who are born alive as legal persons. On this view, even second- and third-trimester fetuses do not have the same right to life as infants. This gives women broader reproductive rights over their bodies.

The development of assisted reproductive technologies introduced a new set of biomedical, legal, and ethical issues. In 1978, Lesley Brown in the United Kingdom gave birth to a daughter named Louise. Louise became the first person whose life was traced to an embryo that had existed for a time outside the mother's body. Lesley was infertile because her fallopian tubes were blocked. An egg was retrieved from her ovary and was fertilized with her husband's sperm in a laboratory glass dish (*in vitro*). The resulting embryo was then transferred to and implanted in Lesley's uterus, and

it developed into Louise. In vitro fertilization (IVF) has enabled
many couples to have children when they were unable to do so
through natural biological means.

In 1985, the high-profile case of "Baby M" raised ethical issues
regarding surrogate pregnancy. A woman was artificially inseminated using the sperm of a man who, with his wife, contracted the
woman to have a child for them. The surrogate's egg was fertilized and she carried the fetus in her womb until the baby was born.
This instance of gestational surrogacy showed that there could be
a separation of genetic, gestational, and social mothers. The mother
who contributes the egg can be different from the mother who carries the fetus during pregnancy, who can also be different from the
mother who raises the child. At the same time, the biological father who contributes sperm may be distinct from the social father
who raises the child. Techniques such as amniocentesis, sperm sorting, and preimplantation genetic diagnosis (PIGD) can determine
the sex of the embryo or fetus. These techniques give prospective
parents the ability to choose children on the basis of gender preference. Presently, the most fiercely debated form of reproductive
technology is therapeutic cloning. This involves cloning embryos
to derive embryonic stem (ES) cells that might rejuvenate tissues
and organs damaged from degenerative diseases.

In this chapter, we will discuss whether aborting a fetus is
morally permissible or impermissible. In addition, we will discuss
whether embryos have moral status, and what this implies about
what we are allowed to do with IVF embryos existing outside the
womb. We will also consider moral arguments for and against surrogate pregnancy and the grounds on which sex selection can or
cannot be morally justified. In surrogacy, which mother (genetic,
gestational, or social) has a stronger claim to and responsibility for
the welfare of the child? Does surrogacy exploit women or lead to
the commodification of children? Does sex selection further insti-
tutionalize discrimination against women? Are there cases in which
sex selection might be permitted as a way of preventing harm to
children? Finally, we will examine both therapeutic and reproductive cloning. If cloned embryos have moral status, then does this
mean that they should never be created for medical research and
treatment, no matter how beneficial the result might be? Or are the
potential benefits of therapeutic cloning so great that they outweigh
any value embryos have in virtue of being nascent human life? If
reproductive cloning did not physically harm human beings,

would it still be morally objectionable on the ground that it violated something essential to our humanity?

Abortion

Conservative opponents of abortion maintain that a human being exists from the time of conception and has the same right to life as any other human. A more moderate position is that a fetus does not have an equal right to life until it has reached viability, the capacity to survive outside the womb. A similar position holds that a right to life depends on sentience, the capacity to experience pleasure and pain. The most liberal view on abortion says that an individual has a right to life only at birth and thereafter. On this view, abortion is morally permissible even in the later stages of pregnancy. Despite their differences, each of these positions makes its claims and arguments about abortion on the basis of the moral status of the fetus. Moral status is a property that gives individuals a claim on others, who in turn have an obligation to treat these individuals in a certain way. For conservatives on abortion, a fetus has moral status because it is a human life. Moderates define moral status in terms of viability or sentience. And liberals define moral status in terms of the capacity for self-conscious awareness.

The most influential positions on abortion aim to show that the conclusions in arguments presented for or against the practice do not follow from the premises. Judith Jarvis Thomson argues that, even if the fetus is a person with a right to life, it does not follow that abortion is impermissible. In contrast, Don Marquis argues that, even if fetuses lack the capacity for self-conscious awareness, it does not follow that abortion is permissible. Thomson's argument is a challenge to the conservative position on abortion, while Marquis's argument is a challenge to the liberal position.

Thomson calls the view that abortion is impermissible, even in order to save the mother's life, the "extreme view" and builds her case against it. This view assumes that a fetus is a person with a right to life, which presumably entails the right of the fetus to use the pregnant woman's body to be brought to term. But Thomson holds that one right does not entail the other. This is because no one is morally required to make large sacrifices to keep another person alive. Allowing a fetus to use the woman's body to develop to term would involve such a sacrifice. So no woman is morally required to allow a fetus to develop to term. Hence, aborting a fetus and detaching one's body from it is morally permissible.

To test your moral intuitions about abortion, Thomson asks you to imagine that you wake up one morning and find yourself back-to-back with an unconscious violinist. He has a fatal kidney ailment, and you have a compatible blood type. The Society of Music Lovers has kidnapped you and plugged the violinist's circulatory system into yours so that your kidneys can function as a dialysis machine for him. The hospital director tells you that the staff could not have prevented this from occurring. Because it has occurred, there is nothing they can do for nine months. If they unplugged the violinist from you, he would die. The director goes on to say that all persons have a right to life, and the violinist is a person. You have a right to decide what happens to your body. But the violinist's right to life morally outweighs what happens to you and your body. Therefore, it would be wrong for you to be unplugged from him.

Thomson says that most of us would find this argument outrageous. She extends it by analogy to the right to life of a fetus and claims about the impermissibility of abortion to show that these claims are untenable. The violinist has no right against you that would entail an obligation for you to give him continued use of your body. He could only have such a right if you gave it to him as an act of kindness or generosity. He would benefit from your being a Good Samaritan. Similarly, the fetus has no right against you that would entail an obligation for you to give it the use of your body. You may allow it this use. But you would not "owe" it to the fetus, since there is no moral obligation to be a Good Samaritan. If the pregnant woman is not obligated to keep the fetus attached to her body, and if the fetus threatens the woman's life, then she is permitted to separate herself from it through abortion.

The violinist example is analogous to a case of pregnancy due to rape. One might present a different argument and raise a different question about pregnancy and the permissibility of abortion. If a woman voluntarily engages in sexual intercourse, knowing that it can result in pregnancy, and she becomes pregnant, then she is responsible for the fetus inside her. Unlike rape or incest, wouldn't this responsibility imply an obligation to ensure that the fetus' right to life is respected? Thomson's response is that the distinction between rape and responsible pregnancy shifts the focus from the fetus' right to life to the pregnant woman's responsibility for the fetus. But a fetus' right to life does not depend on the nature of the event that resulted in pregnancy. If this right depends on whether pregnancy resulted from a voluntary or involuntary sexual act, then unborn persons whose existence is due to rape have no right to use their mothers' bodies. Those resulting from responsible pregnancy do have this right. Yet no property intrinsic to the fetus justifies this distinction. Insofar as an individual's right to life does not depend on how that individual came into existence, the argument from responsibility is not a successful argument against Thomson's defense of abortion.

Thomson makes two important qualifications to her position. First, she argues that abortion is generally permissible, not that it is always permissible. She distinguishes between a frightened fourteen-year-old who aborts a pregnancy due to rape and a woman who aborts in the seventh month of pregnancy to avoid postponing a trip abroad. While the reason for abortion in the former case supports its permissibility, the reason in the latter case does not. Second, Thomson argues that, although it is permissible to detach one's body from the fetus through abortion, it is not permissible to guarantee the death of a baby once it is born. The right to an abortion does not entail a right to commit infanticide.

Thomson's argument relies on the distinction between negative and positive rights. A negative right of one individual implies an obligation for other individuals not to interfere with the expression of that right. A positive right implies an obligation for others to support or facilitate its expression. Negative rights outweigh positive rights because the right not to be burdened or harmed has more moral weight than the right to be benefited. The pregnant woman has a negative right not to be burdened or to take on risk. She therefore has a right to not allow the fetus the use of her body. The fetus' presumed right to life and right to use the woman's body are positive rights. Because the fetus' positive rights threaten or violate the woman's negative right to bodily noninterference, and negative rights outweigh positive rights, the woman has a right to abort the fetus.

A variant of the earlier argument from responsibility against Thomson can sidestep questions about fetal and maternal rights. If pregnancy results from voluntarily engaging in sexual intercourse, then the woman and her partner could be responsible for the welfare of the fetus and obligated to bring it to term. This is not due to a fetus' putative right to life, but to the responsibility for accepting the consequences of one's voluntary actions. On the other hand, if a fetus resulting from a voluntary sexual act has a known abnormality that would lead to severe disease in a future child, then the parents might be obligated to abort the fetus in order to prevent harm to the child. In either case, whether one is responsible for bringing a fetus to term or for aborting it does not depend on whether the fetus has a right to life.

Marquis begins his argument by assuming that whether or not abortion is morally permissible stands or falls on whether a fetus is the sort of being whose life it is seriously wrong to end. What explains the wrongness of killing an adult human being is that it deprives one of all the experiences, activities, projects, and enjoyments that would have constituted one's future. A fetus' future includes these same features. Because the reason for the wrongness of killing adults also applies to fetuses, abortion is prima facie morally wrong. For Marquis, abortion is prima facie morally wrong, not absolutely wrong. In some instances, the harm resulting from failing to abort may be just as great as the alternative. An example would be carrying to term a severely deformed fetus with a future life of severe disability, pain, and suffering as a person.

The crucial part of Marquis's argument is the claim that the wrongness of killing adults extends to the wrongness of killing fetuses. But there are significant differences between adults and fetuses, which casts doubt on whether the argument goes through in the second case. Killing is wrong because it deprives the victim of a valuable future. But the future is not valuable in itself. It is valuable only for individuals with the capacity for experiences, activities, and projects if they live or continue to live. The capacity to value experiences presupposes the capacity for self-conscious awareness. This capacity emerges at the earliest in infancy. Fetuses lack the mental capacity to have interests in and to value the future. Aborting a fetus does not deprive it of any value; it does not suffer any loss of a future like ours (adults). Therefore, abortion is not morally wrong. Marquis asserts that the idea of having a valuable future like ours is independent of the category of personhood. Yet the capacity to have an interest in and to value future experiences presupposes the capacity for self-conscious awareness, and this is what defines personhood. For Marquis, the moral permissibility of abortion hinges on the moral status of the fetus. A fetus has this status when it possesses the property of having a valuable future. But because fetuses lack the mental capacity to have an interest in the future, one can question whether this is a property that a fetus can possess and thus whether a fetus has any moral status.

Marquis's antiabortion argument can be characterized as an argument from potential. A fetus has moral status because of its potential to become a person. But we need to distinguish between two senses of "potential." Jeff McMahan distinguishes between identity-preserving potential and non-identity-preserving potential. The first type of potential is identity preserving in the sense that the fetus and the neonate are two phases of one individual who persists through the changes from the earlier to the later phase. The second type of potential is non-identity-preserving in the sense that the fetus and neonate are distinct individuals. In the first case, the potential is intrinsic to the fetus because it is realized from within. In the second case, the potential is extrinsic to the fetus because it requires factors external to the fetus to be realized. Only intrinsic, identity-preserving potential can give a fetus an interest in living and a moral status that make it wrong to kill it.

Late-stage fetuses have developed the structures and functions of the brain necessary for the potential for consciousness. Because this potential can be realized by the fetus becoming a neonate without a substantial change in its properties, the realization of this potential is identity preserving. And because this potential is identity preserving and gives the fetus an interest in living, it is wrong to kill a late-stage fetus. In contrast, early-stage fetuses lack the structures and functions of the brain necessary for the potential for consciousness. Any potential an early-stage fetus has is non-identity-preserving, since such a fetus cannot become a neonate without a substantial change in its properties. Because it has only non-identity-preserving potential in becoming a neonate and lacks the capacity for consciousness, it cannot have an interest in living. And because it cannot have an interest in living, it is not wrong to kill an early-stage fetus. If one accepts the distinction between these two senses of potential, then Marquis's antiabortion argument is persuasive for late-term fetuses, but not for early-term fetuses.

On balance, Thomson's case for the permissibility of abortion is more persuasive than Marquis's case for the impermissibility of abortion. Still, it would be unwarranted to draw a more general conclusion about the morality of abortion from their arguments because there are positions on abortion other than the two Thomson and Marquis defend. In particular, the moderate position that defines moral status in terms of viability or sentience may offer the most reasonable and broadly supported argument for when abortion is or is not permissible. On this view, killing early-stage fetuses would be permissible, but killing late-stage fetuses would not be permissible. This moderate position would also block any move from the permissibility of abortion to the permissibility of infanticide.

Against this position, Mary Anne Warren argues that abortion and infanticide are both prima facie permissible because neither fetuses nor neonates are persons. Fetuses and neonates lack the capacity for self-conscious awareness that makes one a person and gives one moral status. Apart from the revulsion many people feel at the thought of infanticide, there are at least two principled reasons for prohibiting it. First, the potential of a neonate to develop self-conscious awareness appears to be identity-preserving potential. If it is, and if this potential is sufficient for an interest in living and moral status, then killing infants is wrong. Second, it is unclear at what point after birth an infant develops self-conscious awareness. So it is unclear when an infant develops an interest in living and moral status and at what point an infant can be harmed or wronged by being killed. On these grounds, the moral distinction between the permissibility of abortion and the impermissibility of infanticide can be upheld.

There is one more perspective on abortion that we should consider. Ronald Dworkin claims that moral objections to abortion rest on people's belief in the sanctity of human life. He focuses on a secular interpretation of this idea, though it is not fundamentally different from religious interpretations. The sanctity of life principle says that every human life has intrinsic value, independent of whether it is valued by or is good for anyone. A fetus is a human life with intrinsic value. Killing even an early-stage fetus violates the sanctity and value it embodies and therefore is wrong. Yet if something does not have the capacity for interests or rights, then it is difficult to understand how it could be harmed or wronged. Life has value for individuals, not independently of them. Sanctity of life may support an argument against abortion of late-stage fetuses, because they may have the capacity for interests and rights. But it does not support an argument against abortion of early-stage fetuses, because they lack this capacity.

The Moral Status of Embryos

Many opponents of abortion apply the same reasoning to embryos that they apply to fetuses. They argue that embryos have the potential to become persons and that this potential gives a moral status to embryos that protects them from being destroyed or created for the purpose of stem-cell research. The claim that an embryo has the potential to develop into a human being or person seems to assume that the embryo can realize this potential on its own. Its potential is an intrinsic property that can be actualized independently of such extrinsic properties as the embryo's location within the uterus. Yet the embryo needs the uterus and other biological structures such as the placenta in order to develop. So the development of an embryo depends on extrinsic properties, not on its intrinsic properties alone. The issue of potential is more problematic in the case of IVF embryos. Even with much assistance in the laboratory, the chances are roughly 20 percent that such an embryo will develop into a live birth. Because embryos lack identity-preserving potential and moral status, it would not be wrong to prevent their development into fetuses and persons.

Let's assume that an embryo's potential includes both intrinsic and extrinsic properties, and that these together confer moral status on it. This status gives it a right to develop into a human being. There still would be a problem for those who rely on the idea of potential to explain the wrongness of destroying embryos. An unfertilized egg also has the potential to develop into a human being, given the right biological circumstances. The inclusion of genetic material from sperm in the egg is one of many events and processes necessary for the egg's further development. There is no reason to suppose that, while the fertilized egg has the potential for further development, the unfertilized egg does not. As a matter of consistency, if both embryos and male and female gametes have the potential to develop into human beings, and if preventing embryos from further development is morally wrong, then contraception is also morally wrong. The argument from potential provides no good reason for not tracing the reproductive process all the way back to the gametes.

Yet some might argue that we *can* stop at the embryo rather than at the gametes. The reason they might give is that the potential of embryos to become persons is much stronger than the potential of gametes to become persons. But it would be difficult to defend the claim that this potential is identity preserving. For the identity of one and the same embryo through time cannot predate the first cell division of the fertilized ovum and, arguably, cannot begin until monozygotic twinning is no longer possible. This is when a zygote splits into two numerically distinct zygotes at around fourteen days after fertilization. The original zygote ceases to exist beyond this point. Clearly, in these cases the potential of the original zygote cannot be identity preserving. The potential of the post-fourteen-day embryo to become a person is not identity preserving either, given the substantial difference in properties between embryos and persons. So the argument from potential does not support the case for the moral status of an embryo at any stage of its development.

IVF embryos present a different sense of "potential" and a unique set of ethical problems. In the process of fertilizing ova with sperm in a laboratory dish, genetic mutations or other biological abnormalities might result from the transfer of genetic material. Or abnormalities might develop during cryopreservation, where embryos are frozen and stored indefinitely in liquid nitrogen. In both cases, the abnormalities might cause disease and disability in the people who develop from them. Also, several or more embryos might implant and result in multiple births. These tend to be delivered prematurely and have a higher risk of developing various disorders than full-term births. In these respects, IVF embryos have the potential to result in harm to people.

The point here is not that IVF embryos themselves have an interest in not undergoing genetic mutations. Rather, the point is that, once they exist, the people who develop from these embryos have an interest in not experiencing disease and disability as consequences of mutations. In this sense, the moral status of an embryo depends on its extrinsic properties. Events or processes in the laboratory dish or liquid nitrogen container can damage embryos and adversely affect future people. An embryo has moral status, not in the intrinsic sense of a right to life, but in the extrinsic sense of a person's right not to be harmed by the consequences of events occurring at the embryonic stage.

As a form of assisted reproduction, IVF enables infertile couples or women to have children when they cannot do so through natural biological means. Transferring IVF embryos from the petri dish to the uterus involves some risk to the woman. The procedure is also expensive. Indeed, the cost of the procedure can make it inaccessible to many women and couples. Yet this may seem unfair to those who cannot afford a procedure that offers them the only way to have natural biological children. For example, they might argue that the cost of the procedure should be covered by extended Medicaid benefits.

Crucially, the argument from fairness regarding access to IVF technology presupposes that reproductive rights include the right to bring people into existence. Negative reproductive rights consist in the right to bodily noninterference in general and not to be forced to carry a fetus to term in particular. But one can question whether there is a corresponding positive reproductive right, the right to be aided in bringing people into existence. Two points motivate this question. Bringing more people into existence would only add to the problem of global overpopulation. If people wanted to have a child, they could choose adoption as an alternative to reproduction. A right to reproduce seems weak when there are already too many people in the world. One might object that this places an unfair burden on infertile couples to adopt because, unlike fertile couples, they do not have the choice between unassisted reproduction and adoption in having children. We can respond to this objection with a second, more controversial, point: There is no right to cause people to exist. As a positive right, a right to reproduce involves a claim on others and an obligation that they facilitate the expression of that right. Medical professionals may have an obligation to ensure that people's positive reproductive rights are realized. But the exercise of this right results in an individual who could not consent to being brought into existence. Children are affected directly by the exercise of a positive reproductive right. Yet they have no voice when the right is exercised. The claim that a woman's reproductive right entails responsibility for the consequences of its expression means that there is an obligation to promote the welfare of the child, once it exists. But this does not alter the fact that the child cannot consent to being born and exposed to the risk of harm in the events of human life. So the right to reproduce is at most a prima facie right.

Some might go further and take these points to imply that reproduction is not a right, but a privilege. If having children is not something to which people are entitled, then the argument from unfairness for access to IVF collapses. Unequal access to a reproductive technology between different groups of people is unfair only if everyone is entitled to what the technology allows. If couples are not entitled to IVF, then they would not be wronged by being denied the procedure because of an inability to pay for it. This argument could be supported further by the claim that the right to have access to medical procedures pertains only to the treatment of diseases, and the inability to reproduce is not a disease. It is important to emphasize, though, that these points are plausible only if the negative right to an abortion and bodily non-interference can be separated from the positive right to reproduce. Many would reject this distinction, holding that these two reproductive rights are inseparable. But we should consider the full implications of causing people to exist before rejecting this distinction out of hand.

It has been argued that the potential of an embryo to develop into a human being does not give it a moral status that would entail a right to life. If it does not have such a right, then there is no moral obligation to ensure that it develops to that end. But does it follow from this that embryos have no moral status at all and that we can do whatever we want with them? Do embryos possess any properties that constrain us in the way we treat them? The fact that "spare" embryos not implanted in the uterus for pregnancy are eventually destroyed suggests that there are no moral constraints. Yet even if they lack moral status, embryos seem to have moral value, a symbolic value for what they represent. This value may prescribe limits on what we are permitted to do with them. Specifically, it could mean permitting research on existing IVF embryos for therapeutic uses, but prohibiting the creation of new embryos for research. Nevertheless, the moral value of an embryo is not an intrinsic property of the embryo, but an extrinsic property falling under the procreative autonomy of its genetic parents. As an expression of this autonomy, parents may consent to allow their embryos to be used for therapeutic research. When there is a conflict between the genetic parents of embryos, the right not to use embryos for reproduction outweighs the right to use them for this purpose.

This was the conclusion of a ruling by the Supreme Court of Tennessee in a legal case involving disputed IVF embryos in 1992 (*Davis v. Davis*). Mary Sue and Junior Lewis Davis divorced after producing seven embryos through IVF. The embryos were then cryogenically preserved. Mary Sue originally asked for control of the frozen embryos, with the intention of having them transferred to her uterus in a post-divorce effort to become pregnant. Junior Davis objected, saying that he preferred to leave the embryos in the frozen state until he decided whether he wanted to become a parent outside the bounds of marriage. The trial court awarded "custody" to Mary Sue and directed that she be permitted to have the opportunity to bring the embryos to term through implantation. But the Court of Appeals reversed the decision, finding that Junior Davis had a constitutionally protected right not to beget a child when no pregnancy had taken place. Procreative autonomy consists in two equally significant rights: the right to procreate and the right to avoid procreation. When these two rights conflict, the second overrides the first. This rests on the view that negative moral and legal rights outweigh positive moral and legal rights. Accordingly, Junior Davis's right to prevent implantation of the embryos outweighed his ex-wife's right to have them implanted and develop into births.

Because each genetic parent is causally responsible for the existence of the embryo, each has a right to determine how an embryo is used. If embryos are to be used for research, for example, then both genetic parents must consent to allow them to be used for this purpose. If the length of time frozen increases the likelihood of genetic or other biological damage to embryos, then they should be destroyed beyond a certain period of time. Despite any reproductive property rights of parents, this practice can be justified on the ground that it prevents harm to the future people who would develop from these embryos.

Surrogate Pregnancy

Another form of assisted reproduction to which a woman or couple may turn is surrogate pregnancy. Typically, a woman is artificially inseminated with the sperm of a man to whom she is not married and is asked to carry the resulting fetus to term. When the baby is born, she relinquishes her claim to the baby and gives it to the person or persons who contracted for it. Alternatively, one woman contributes the egg that is artificially inseminated and is the genetic mother. A different woman is the surrogate and the gestational mother. When the surrogate contributes the egg from which the fetus and baby develops, she is both the child's genetic mother and its gestational mother.

The two most common reasons for a woman or a couple to seek a surrogate are female infertility and a potentially high-risk pregnancy. In the latter case, a woman is able to have a child through natural biological means. But she has an existing medical condition that poses a significant risk to her health. Such a condition could rule out IVF. Once the embryo has been fertilized in the petri dish, it is transferred to and implants in the uterus of the same woman who contributes the egg. This process could adversely affect the woman's medical condition. In the "Baby M" case, Elizabeth Stern, one of the contracting parents, had multiple sclerosis and feared that pregnancy might exacerbate her disease.

There are three main ethical questions regarding surrogate pregnancy. We mentioned these in the chapter introduction; but they are worth repeating. Is the surrogate the rightful mother of the child, and does she deserve custody? Does surrogacy lead to the commodification of children? Does surrogacy exploit women? As we have noted, surrogacy requires distinguishing among genetic, gestational, and social mothers. It also requires distinguishing between genetic and social fathers. The distinction between the genetic and the gestational mother is crucial to the question of who is the rightful mother of the child. This question arises when the surrogate changes her mind and decides that she does not want to give up the baby. Mary Beth Whitehead was both the genetic mother who contributed the egg and the gestational mother who carried "Baby M" to term. Thus, it would seem that she would have a stronger claim to the child than either William Stern, who was only genetically related, or Elizabeth Stern, who was neither genetically nor gestationally related to the child. Nevertheless, the social mother (or father) is arguably more important than genetic or gestational mothers, because the social mother is responsible for the welfare of the child from birth onward. Although it cannot be determined at the time when a surrogacy contract is formalized, at some point during pregnancy the surrogate may express an intention to be the social mother as well. If this occurs, then it may give more weight to the claim of the surrogate over the claim of the genetic father and his partner to have custody of and raise the child.

In the "Baby M" case, William and Elizabeth Stern agreed to pay Mary Beth Whitehead $10,000 to be a surrogate and bear a baby conceived through artificial insemination. Whitehead refused to surrender the child at birth, claiming that she was the child's natural mother. Some have argued that she reneged on her part of the contract and was obligated to turn the baby over to the Sterns. The legality of the surrogacy contract notwithstanding, Whitehead's genetic, gestational, and intended social relationship to the child were enough to make her the rightful mother. Although the New Jersey Supreme Court granted custody to Mr. Stern, it overturned the decision by the State Superior Court. The lower court had concluded that the terms of the surrogacy contract precluded White-head from being the rightful mother. Significantly, Whitehead re-fused the money offered in the contract. If she had accepted the money and effectively remained a surrogate, then she would not have had any claim to be the child's mother. Although the State Supreme Court argued that commercial surrogacy was baby-selling and unethical, this was not a convincing moral reason for upholding Whitehead's claim. Rather, her claim to be the child's rightful mother was supported by the biological and social factors that we have mentioned.

Some might insist that surrogacy is equivalent to selling babies. To be sure, there were no social connections between the Sterns and Whitehead. If the fetus were abnormal, then arguably the Sterns would have reneged on the surrogacy contract or would have demanded an abortion. Still, this does not mean that a sur-rogate like Whitehead is simply selling a baby. Instead, one could say that she is making available her biological services so that oth-ers can have a child. By entering a surrogacy contract, the surro-gate does not buy the right to treat the child as a commodity or property to be used as she pleases. When the surrogate accepts the money specified in the contract and delivers the child to the con-tracting parent or parents, she is giving up her parental right to have a relationship with that child. And if the contracting social parents act in the child's best interests, the child will not be treated merely as their property. Child abuse and neglect laws help to en-sure this. Understood in this way, there is nothing unethical about paid contractual surrogacy.

Ultimately, the main ethical concern is the welfare of the child, and nothing about the practice of surrogacy or a surrogacy con-tract obviously harms a child. The welfare of the child will depend not only on legal events and biological processes that precede birth, but also on what happens after birth. This reinforces the earlier point that it is the social mother, more so than the genetic or ges-tational mothers, who is most important. The social environment in which the child is raised affects his or her welfare at least as much as the uterine environment in which the fetus develops be-fore birth. This is not determined by the surrogacy contract or the practice of surrogacy itself. So the argument that surrogacy would lead to the commodification of children is not convincing.

Does surrogacy exploit women? Some feminists find this question offensive. They support the practice of contractual pregnancy as con-

sistent with reproductive autonomy. As an extension of the right to
have an abortion, surrogate pregnancy is one more instance of a
woman's control over her body. Other feminists contend that women
may be exploited because, in certain social situations, they will turn
to surrogacy out of economic necessity rather than real choice. Furthermore, they may claim that surrogacy turns women into reproductive vessels. For these reasons, surrogacy should be banned. But
the reasons for saying that surrogacy exploits woman are not convincing. The vast majority of woman who have been surrogates have
not done so out of financial necessity. For example, Mary Beth Whitehead wanted to pay for her children's private education, which is
valuable but not a necessity. Against this, one could argue that surrogacy would amount to exploitation for those who are not well-off
financially. Their financial status would give them fewer choices to
decline financial offers, which could be coercive. But most surrogates
emphasize that their decision was an informed, autonomous choice,
and that it would be insulting and demeaning to claim that they
were unduly influenced by factors beyond their control.

Restricting or prohibiting surrogacy on grounds of potential exploitation could limit other forms of reproductive choice, such as
egg donation, and turn back many of the gains in women's reproductive autonomy made over the past thirty years. Unless it can
be shown that a woman's decision to be a surrogate is not informed
or not voluntary, there is no good reason to think that surrogate
pregnancy is clearly exploitative of women. On the contrary, it may
be taken as one expression of a woman's freedom to do what she
wants with her own body.

Sex Selection

Sperm sorting, PIGD, amniocentesis, and ultrasound can all reveal
the sex of the developing embryo or fetus. It is one thing to know
that a future child will be male or female. It is quite another to
abort a fetus or terminate an embryo on the basis of this knowledge. Some point out that this practice usually involves selecting
males over females and reinforces discrimination against women.
Sex selection may also lead to unequal sex ratios and significant
demographic problems in developing countries.

Perhaps the most disturbing example of sex selection occurs in
China. Too many Chinese families allow male fetuses to develop

to term, but abort female fetuses. Family planning rules now permit couples in rural areas to have a second child if the first is a girl. But they forbid more than two children. Recent studies show that in 92 percent of cases where couples already had a girl, pregnancies were aborted when prenatal ultrasound revealed that the next child would also be a girl. Sex selection is morally repugnant when it means the elimination of unwanted females. There is no conceivable justification for such a practice when it is based on the idea that women are valued less than men.

There are some cases in which sex selection may be morally permissible on medical grounds. Duchenne muscular dystrophy and hemophilia are genetic diseases that affect male children almost exclusively. These diseases are traceable to distinct mutations on the X chromosome. A woman who carries one of these mutations will pass on the mutation and the disease it causes to half of her male offspring. Half of her daughters will carry the mutation but will be unaffected. There is no cure for these diseases, and each involves varying restrictions on the quality of life of the people who have them. If PIGD or amniocentesis revealed that a male embryo or male fetus had the genetic mutation that caused either of these diseases, then parents would be permitted to terminate the embryo or fetus. The reason would be to prevent harm to a child who would have the disease if he were born. Parents would be permitted to select only female embryos or male embryos without the mutations. Indeed, because of the severity of Duchenne's, parents might even be obligated to select against male embryos with the mutation causing this particular disease.

Using sex selection for family balancing may seem more difficult to justify. Parents who already have a boy might select against male embryos or fetuses in order to have a girl. Conversely, if they already have a girl they might want to select against female embryos or fetuses in order to have a boy. A parent's experience in raising a girl can be very different from the experience in raising a boy, and having both may make parenting a more rewarding experience. Because parents have children for a variety of reasons, it seems arbitrary to focus on the desire for family balancing as morally objectionable. There is no justification for saying that this practice is immoral. On the contrary, it is supported by the idea that families are autonomous units, where parents have the right to determine the composition of the family. More importantly, what matters morally is the welfare of the child once it exists, and this depends on how the child is raised rather than on whether it is male or female.

Some parents may opt for sex selection because they believe that being of one sex rather than the other will offer better lifetime opportunities. If families are autonomous units, and if parents believe that having a child of a particular sex will promote the child's welfare, then selecting a male over a female child is morally permissible. In Western industrialized nations, women and couples may use sex selection in order to have a child of each sex. Some will prefer to have sons. Given the general desire for family balancing, though, the number of sons selected in the West will probably not produce a large disparity in the ratio between males and females. Warren (1999) suggests that sex selection may have biological and moral benefits: "it is possible that in some instances sex selection will prevent severely *declining* sex ratios in the future, e.g., if natural sex ratios at birth decline due to environmental contaminants that are differentially lethal to male fetuses, or androgenic spermatozoa" (p. 141).

The strongest objection to sex selection of males over females is that it reinforces discrimination against and oppression of women. But it is not obvious that sex selection causes the oppression of women, even if there is a correlation between the two. Correlation is not equivalent to causation. There may be other factors that account for oppression; sex selection alone does not explain it. This counterargument is similar to the one saying that, just because there is a correlation between men who read violent pornography and men who commit crimes against women, it does not prove that the two are causally connected. Data showing that most couples in developed countries prefer family balancing seem to confirm that any disparity between the sexes will not become too large. But a correlation between a disproportionate selection of males and the adverse impact it has on women provides a moral argument for regulations on sex selection in developing countries.

Cloning

Among the new medical technologies, cloning is the most ethically controversial. This is largely because some conservative thinkers and policy makers conflate cloning and the ethics and politics of abortion. While there has been considerable public debate on the ethics of *reproductive cloning*, most of the recent debate has focused on *therapeutic cloning*. First we will consider arguments for and against therapeutic cloning, and then go on to examine arguments for a ban on reproductive cloning. Although there is disagreement on whether the first type of cloning should be permitted, most people argue that the second type should be prohibited.

Cloning involves inserting the nucleus of an adult human somatic cell into a human egg whose nucleus has been removed. This is also called somatic-cell nuclear transfer. Somatic cells of the body are distinguished from germ cells of the sperm and egg. In nuclear transfer, an egg genetically reprograms an adult somatic-cell nucleus into a totipotent state. This means that the created cell can develop into many different cell types and can become an embryo as well. It may develop into the type of cell that constitutes tissue of the heart, kidneys, or skin. Once the egg has become a five-day-old embryo and has reached what is called the blastocyst stage, ES cells can be mined from the embryo. These cells can then be grown in culture and develop into embryonic stem-cell lines. Korean researchers announced in February 2004 that they had successfully cloned a human embryo and extracted a stem-cell line from it. In addition to totipotence, what makes ES cells distinctive is their ability to regenerate tissue. This type of cloning is called "therapeutic" because of its potential to rejuvenate tissues or even replace organs damaged from such degenerative diseases as Parkinson's, diabetes, and heart disease. ES cells might cure or at least alleviate the symptoms of these and other diseases that adversely affect the quality of many people's lives.

Those who object to therapeutic cloning argue that it is morally wrong to create embryos solely for the sake of research leading to therapy. What they specifically object to is the fact that, once ES cells have been mined from the cloned embryos, the embryos will be destroyed. This would amount to destroying potential human life. Insofar as the potential of an embryo to become a human being gives it a right to life, therapeutic cloning would violate this right and therefore should be prohibited. Another objection is that creating embryos for research violates the sanctity of human life from the time of conception. Some have tried to sidestep these moral issues by promoting research on adult stem cells, which are not derived from embryos. Yet, although some types of adult stem cells are plastic, or capable of generating many different cell types, they are not as capable of generating as many cell types as ES cells are. Moreover, ES cells are less likely to provoke an adverse immune response when injected into the body. So, adult stem cells would not be as versatile or as safe as ES cells in treating degenerative diseases. In any case, many scientists claim that research on both adult and embryonic stem cells is necessary to determine whether they are equally plastic and equally regenerative, or whether ES cells are superior in these respects.

Suppose that the potential of embryos to become persons gives them a right to life. Would this be a reason for banning therapeutic cloning? Some argue that therapeutic cloning should be banned because it blocks the embryo's potential to become an actual person. It is wrong to create embryos for this purpose, even if therapeutic cloning could improve the lives of existing people suffering from degenerative diseases. But others could argue that because embryos are nothing more than a nonintegrated clump of cells, they cannot have interests or rights. If embryos cannot have interests or rights, then they cannot be harmed or wronged by not becoming persons. The argument to ban therapeutic cloning rests on an absolute claim that embryos' right to life outweighs any potential benefit to existing people. But while embryos cannot suffer from and be harmed by not realizing their potential, existing people can suffer from and be harmed by disease. These people could benefit from treatments resulting from therapeutic cloning research. Embryos cannot be harmed or wronged by being created for this research.

Earlier, we raised the question of whether the idea of the sanctity of life could give moral status to fetuses. Suppose, for the sake of argument, that embryos embody the sanctity of human life. Creating and using embryos for research and therapy is morally wrong because it violates this sanctity. Would this be a reason for banning therapeutic cloning? Like embryos, existing people also embody the sanctity of life. In this regard, embryos and people have equal moral status. Yet, what makes them unequal is that embryos cannot suffer, while existing people can suffer. The combination of sanctity and suffering seems to have more moral weight than sanctity alone. If the suffering of existing people is morally worse than creating and destroying embryos, then we should be more concerned about alleviating the suffering of existing people. If embryos cannot be harmed, and if therapeutic cloning can alleviate suffering, then therapeutic cloning should be permitted. This argument is based on the idea that we should do more to meet the actual

needs of existing people than the putative needs of merely potential people (embryos).

Reproductive cloning involves the same procedure of somatic-
cell nuclear transfer as in therapeutic cloning. But it does not merely
aim to mine ES cells from embryos created in this way. Instead, it
aims to create full-fledged human beings from these embryos.
There is less general disagreement about the ethics of reproductive
cloning than there is about the ethics of therapeutic cloning. Most
people argue that the first type should be banned because it is
morally objectionable for many reasons. Some of these reasons are
less persuasive than others, however.

The strongest reason for banning reproductive cloning is that it
would result in physical harm to a cloned child. This concern has
been borne out in part by the case of the sheep cloned in 1996.
"Dolly" aged at an accelerated rate. She developed severe arthritis and progressive lung disease, which led to her being euthanized
in February 2003. The reprogramming of genetic material transferred from the donor-cell nucleus to the enucleated egg may cause
mutations leading to premature aging and disease. Although the
biological reasons for these mutations are not fully understood,
sexual forms of reproduction seem more able than asexual forms
to limit the incidence of genetic mutations in the cells of a developing embryo and fetus. Furthermore, the donor-cell nucleus may
already have mutations in its DNA before it is transferred to the
egg. This could also accelerate aging and disease. There may be so
many mutations in the cells of a cloned embryo or fetus that it
would spontaneously abort or be born as a severely deformed
child. These biological reasons against reproductive cloning support moral reasons for banning the practice. The potential for physical harm to a cloned child is too great to justify its use. But if we
could reduce the incidence of genetic complications and thus minimize the risk of harm, then we could morally justify reproductive
cloning.

Weaker reasons for banning reproductive cloning are that it
amounts to genetic reductionism and determinism and that it
would violate our dignity and humanity. The genes that a cloned
child inherits from a parent or sibling may very well influence the
psychological properties that constitute the child's identity. But
genes alone cannot determine the nature or content of one's desires, beliefs, and emotions. These mental states depend at least
partly on how one responds to the social and physical environ-

ment. Moreover, there are different probabilities of genetic penetrance in different people. Even within families, a genetic trait in a
parent may not be passed on to a child; it may skip one or more
generations before expressing itself again. Similarly, genes that are
expressed as identifiable traits in the donor might not be expressed
in the clone. Having the same genes as the person from whose cell
one is cloned does not mean that the clone will be identical to the
donor in physical or other relevant respects. Nor does cloning itself restrict one's autonomy. Rather, what restricts one's autonomy
is a parent's refusal or inability to allow a child to develop his or
her own life plan and values and instead impose the parent's plan
and values to control the child's life. This is all too common among
families. But surely it is not limited to those that would have cloned
children. All of these points show that genetic determinism and genetic reductionism are false. This should allay any fears that cloning
would mean producing an exact replica of a person who already
exists.

A deeper objection is that cloning would undermine something
essential to our humanity. As an asexual form of reproduction,
cloning would be unnatural and thus violate what it means to be
human. But it is difficult to see how the difference between sexual
and asexual reproduction would imply this. If cloning is morally
objectionable because it is contrary to natural means of reproduction, then IVF and artificial insemination would be unnatural and
thus morally objectionable as well. By extension, would artificial
insulin injections to control diabetes be considered unnatural and
also objectionable? It is unclear where a line could be drawn between unnatural procedures that threaten our humanity and those
that do not.

Concerns about cloning violating human dignity are misguided
because they focus too much on the biological means through
which we come into existence. We possess dignity because we are
persons with autonomous desires, beliefs, and intentions that are
not entirely functions of our biology. To be sure, biology has a necessary role in our mental life insofar as our bodies and brains generate and sustain our capacity for mental life. But biology cannot
account for all the qualitative features of our psychology that make
us persons. Whether one is conceived and comes into existence
through an asexual form of reproduction like cloning, or through
sexual reproduction, has little to do with what makes one a person worthy of self-respect and respect from others. So the claim

that cloning violates our humanity and dignity can be refuted as well. The only compelling reason for banning reproductive cloning is that it could result in physical harm to individuals who might be cloned.

Conclusion

We have examined arguments for and against the permissibility of abortion, surrogate pregnancy, sex selection, and cloning. Some of these arguments hinge on the question of the moral status of human embryos, both those produced inside the womb and those produced outside the womb through IVF. Advances in reproductive technology over the past thirty years have broadened the landscape of reproductive ethics beyond the abortion debate generated by *Roe v. Wade*. The debate now involves not only issues about a woman's right to control her own body and whether embryos and fetuses have a right to life. It also involves the interests of future people who will be born as a result of using these technologies and who may benefit from or be harmed by them.

Decisions about whether to abort or bring a fetus to term, as well as decisions to use assisted forms of reproduction, can have a significant impact on the welfare of a child. Accordingly, any positive reproductive right to cause people to exist must be weighed against the right of these individuals to not be harmed once they are born. If there is a positive reproductive right, then it is at most a prima facie rather than an absolute right. If a future child would be harmed by the exercise of such a right, then the child's right not to be harmed would outweigh a woman's positive reproductive right. With respect to therapeutic cloning, creating embryos for stem-cell research has both medically and ethically significant implications because it can have a positive impact on the lives of people suffering from degenerative diseases.

Some of the topics discussed in this chapter overlap with genetics and share some of the same ethical concerns. Many reproductive decisions depend on genetic factors. A case for permitting (and perhaps obligating) sex selection against males would be one in which a male embryo had a genetic mutation that would result in disease or disability to the child born from it. PIGD was one of the techniques mentioned that could determine this. We also noted the possibility of genetic mutations resulting from the transfer of genetic material between the somatic-cell nucleus and the enucleated egg in reproductive cloning. Other issues in genetics raise additional ethical questions. These issues need to be considered separately and in greater detail, which we will do in the next chapter.

Selected Readings

Boonin, D. *A Defense of Abortion*. New York: Cambridge University Press, 2002.

Dworkin, R. *Life's Dominion*. New York: Alfred A. Knopf, 1993.

Harris, J. " 'Goodbye Dolly'?: The Ethics of Human Cloning." *Journal of Medical Ethics* 23(1997): 353–60.

Kass, L. "The Wisdom of Repugnance: Why We Should Ban the Cloning of Humans." *The New Republic*, 2 June 1997, 17–26.

Mahowald, M. B. *Women and Children in Health Care: An Unequal Majority*. New York: Oxford University Press, 1993.

Marquis, D. "Why Abortion Is Immoral." *Journal of Philosophy* 86(1989): 183–202.

McMahan, J. *The Ethics of Killing: Problems at the Margins of Life*. Oxford: Oxford University Press, 2002.

Steinbock, B. *Life Before Birth: The Moral and Legal Status of Embryos and Fetuses*. New York: Oxford University Press, 1992.

Thomson, J. J. "A Defense of Abortion." *Philosophy and Public Affairs* 1(1971): 47–66.

Warnock, M. *Making Babies: Is There a Right to Have Children?* Oxford: Oxford University Press, 2003.

Warren, M. A. *Moral Status: Obligations to Persons and Other Living Things*. Oxford: Clarendon Press, 1997.

Warren, M. A. "Sex Selection: Individual Choice or Cultural Coercion?" In *Bioethics*, edited by P. Singer and H. Kuhse, 137–42. Oxford: Blackwell, 1999.

Weissman, I. "Stem Cells—Scientific, Medical, and Political Issues." *New England Journal of Medicine* 346(2002): 1576–79.

CHAPTER 5

Genetics

Introduction

Ever since James Watson and Francis Crick discovered the molecular structure of DNA in 1953, people have been fascinated by genes and their implications for health and disease. The Human Genome Project was created in 1989 with the goal of mapping and sequencing the entire human genome. To oversee this project, the National Institutes of Health established the National Center for Human Genome Research. One of its mandates was to use a small percentage of the Human Genome Project's funds for assessment of and education about the ethical, legal, and social implications (ELSI) of human genetic research. ELSI has funded the study of ethical issues in such procedures as presymptomatic genetic testing and screening of adults and children, preimplantation genetic diagnosis (PIGD) of embryos, and different forms of gene therapy.

Genes are stretches of nucleotide base pairs along strands of the DNA molecule, the major component of each chromosome. They specify the amino acid sequences of the proteins that largely control the physiological processes of our bodies. In June 2000, researchers announced that they had mapped and sequenced a first draft of the entire human genome. One of these researchers, Francis Collins (1999), claimed that this achievement would make possible "a new understanding of genetic contributions to human disease and the developments of rational strategies for minimizing or preventing disease phenotypes altogether" (p. 28). This claim is driven by the belief that there is a direct causal connection between genotypes and disease phenotypes, between genes and the observable physical and mental traits associated with disease.

Diseases with a genetic cause can be divided into three types: *monogenic, polygenic,* and *multifactorial.* The first type of disease is caused by a mutation in a single gene. Examples include cystic fibrosis, Tay-Sachs, and Huntington's. The second type of disease is caused by mutations in several or more genes. Some forms of cancer appear to be polygenic. The third type of disease is caused by the interaction of several or more genes and the environment. Most diseases are multifactorial.

There are three main types of monogenic disorders. *Autosomal dominant* disorders, such as Huntington's disease, are caused by a mutation in one copy of a gene and may be inherited from either parent. They affect one in two children of a parent with the mutation. *Autosomal recessive* disorders, such as cystic fibrosis, are caused by a mutation in two copies of a gene. An affected child inherits one mutated copy from each parent. These disorders affect one in four children of the two carrier parents. *Sex-linked* disorders are traceable, not to any of the twenty-two autosomes, but instead to the sex chromosomes X and Y. Most of these disorders are X-linked, meaning that one in two male children of mothers who carry the mutation will be affected. Half of the daughters of these mothers will be unaffected carriers. Duchenne muscular dystrophy and hemophilia are examples of X-linked disorders.

Only a small percentage of diseases are caused by a mutation in a single gene. The majority of diseases with a genetic component are not monogenic. Thus, claims that genetics will revolutionize medicine by focusing on specific genes are exaggerated. Monogenic diseases like cystic fibrosis and Huntington's have virtual complete penetrance. This means that having a mutation in a particular gene entails close to a 100 percent chance of getting the disease. For most diseases, though, genes have varying degrees of penetrance. There is rarely a direct causal link between a mutation and a disease. Having a mutation does not necessarily mean that one will develop the disease associated with it. This underscores the ambiguity in the genetic component in most diseases.

These considerations raise the following ethical questions about different forms of genetic intervention in humans. Can testing individuals for high-penetrance genetic mutations that cause diseases later in life be justified if there are no treatments for these diseases? Should we select against embryos with mutations that might cause disease and disability in the people who would develop from them? Would we be obligated to terminate these embryos if the disease and disability were severe? Do the potential benefits of somatic-cell gene therapy and germ-line intervention outweigh the risks? If we could enhance people's cognitive capacity by manipulating genes in the brain, would it make all of us better off by providing us with more opportunities in life? Or would it only exacerbate existing social and economic inequalities? Are presymptomatic genetic testing of children and adults, PIGD of embryos, gene therapy, and genetic enhancement all various forms of eugenics? Do they discriminate against people with disabilities and devalue their lives? We will discuss these and other ethical questions about human genetics in this chapter.

Genetic Testing and Screening

Genetic *testing* is designed for individuals who are known to be at increased risk of having a genetic disorder with a familial mode of inheritance. Genetic *screening* is designed to test members of a particular population for a disorder for which there may be no family history or other evidence of its presence. Testing and screening are often presymptomatic, in the sense that they are done on people before they show any symptoms of disease. Some testing is for clinical diagnosis of a condition after the onset of symptoms. The reason for testing and screening is to prevent harm to people who would develop genetic diseases during their lives. Causing people to exist with these diseases can harm them by defeating their interest, once they exist, in living without pain, suffering, and limited opportunities.

One of the dangers of testing individuals for a genetic predisposition is that insurers or employers might discriminate against them on the basis of the genetic information. Because insurance operates on the idea of pooling risks, and the genetically better off may not want to pool their risk of disease with the genetically worse off, the latter might be rejected in applying for health insurance. Moreover, if genetic information were required when applying for work or to keep a job, employers who pay the health care premiums of their employees might refuse to consider or might dismiss people who have tested positive for a mutation that predisposes them to a given disease. But a predisposition to a disease is no guarantee that one will develop it. Just because a genetic mutation entails some risk of disease does not mean that it will cause the disease. Given the uncertainty about what it means to have a genetic mutation or to be genetically predisposed to a disease, there is little justification for discrimination in these cases. Legislation, such as the Genetic Information Nondiscrimination Act of 2003, rightly prohibits insurers and employers from discriminating against individuals on the basis of ambiguous genetic information about nonmonogenic diseases. Yet employers and insurers *would* have a legitimate interest in knowing whether a person had a high-penetrance mutation for a severe disease. In that case, the genetic information would not be ambiguous. It could have a significant impact on one's ability to work and could make one more likely to file insurance claims.

The main reason for testing and screening for monogenic diseases is that the procedures can prevent physical and psychological harm to people. Suppose that a man with a family history of Huntington's disease suspects that he may have the disease after developing jerky bodily movements. A mutation in a single gene is enough to cause this ultimately fatal disease. It is characterized by irreversible motor and mental degeneration and considerable pain and suffering for those affected by it. A person with Huntington's will transmit the mutation and the disease to half of his or her offspring. For those who have the mutation, there is virtual 100 percent penetrance, meaning that they will develop the disease. Unfortunately, by the time symptoms appear an affected person may already have had children and unwittingly transmitted the mutation and the disease to some of them. There is a test that can determine whether an individual has the mutation, even before symptoms appear. Given the predictive power of genetic testing, would the man in our example have an obligation to be tested, despite the fact that there is no treatment for the disease?

Let's assume that the man's symptoms and family history strongly indicate a diagnosis of Huntington's. Given that he understands how the mutation is inherited, its degree of penetrance, and the severity of the disease, he would be obligated to be tested and inform his children of the result. Testing would confirm the diagnosis and clarify to each of his children their 50 percent risk of having the mutation. From the children's perspective, the differ-

ence between a 0 percent and 50 percent risk is significant and could
influence important life choices. The father would be obligated to
be tested and share the information with his children because it
would prevent harm in two respects. First, by having precise information about the risk, his children may decide not to have children of their own and thus not transmit the gene and the disease
to additional people. Second, the information would serve his children's prudential interests, enabling them to plan other aspects of
their lives accordingly. The point is to offer those at risk of having
a severe disease the opportunity to make informed choices. This
will depend on how they assess the risk of having the mutation,
as well as the likelihood of developing the disease if they do have
it. People with the Huntington's mutation are not merely predisposed to a disease. They are at a very high risk of developing a disease that can result in significant physical and psychological harm.

Considerations of harm also apply to testing for mutations in the
BRCA1 and BRCA2 genes. These mutations involve a significantly
high risk of breast (up to 85 percent) and ovarian (up to 60 percent) cancer over a lifetime. Children of people with these mutations (which include men as well as women) have a 50 percent
chance of also having them. Suppose that a woman in her forties
whose mother and grandmother both died from breast cancer at a
relatively early age suspects that she has one of the mutations. If
she has no sisters or children, then she would have no obligation
to be tested and to confirm whether she has the mutation. The only
concern would be a prudential one. It would depend on the
woman's own interests and whether knowing that she was affected
served these interests. For example, she might decide to undergo
frequent mammography testing starting at an earlier age. But if the
woman has been diagnosed with breast cancer and has siblings or
children, then she would be obligated to be tested and confirm that
the cancer was caused by the BRCA mutation. This information
would clarify the risk for her family. The obligation would be
grounded in the high risk of breast cancer entailed by the mutation, as well as in the high risk of morbidity and mortality associated with the disease. Still, the woman's obligation would not be
as strong as that of the man with Huntington's. This is due to the
difference between the 50–85 percent and 100 percent probabilities
of having the diseases, given the mutations in question.

A different example supports the justification for preconception
genetic screening within certain populations. This involves screen-

ing of couples intending to have children. There is a much higher incidence of Tay-Sachs disease within the Ashkenazi Jewish population. Babies affected by this disease appear normal at birth, but in the first year of life their nervous systems begin to degenerate, and they usually die by the time they reach age three or four. Tay-Sachs is a recessive disorder, where the affected child inherits one mutant allele, or copy of the gene, from each parent. The parents are only carriers of the trait and do not have the disease. Because of screening programs in a number of countries since the 1970s, there has been a significant reduction in the incidence of Tay-Sachs among the Ashkenazi Jewish population. This decrease is due to carriers within the Orthodox Jewish community avoiding marriage, carrier couples undergoing prenatal testing and terminating affected embryos or fetuses, the use of donor gametes, and adoption. Adolescents constitute a large percentage of those who have undergone screening. This has prudential and moral implications. Being screened at an early age allows people ample time to plan their future marriages and families in accord with their values. It also enables them to prevent harm to children who would be born with Tay-Sachs disease.

The most compelling case for genetic screening is for disorders that can be treated through nongenetic means. For example, phenylketonuria (PKU) is a recessive disorder in which the body fails to metabolize the amino acid phenylalanine. This can lead to severe mental retardation in affected children. But the condition can be avoided by a diet that limits the intake of phenylalanine. Neonatal genetic screening provides parents of children with PKU with the knowledge they need to administer the appropriate diet. It is a relatively straightforward way for parents to prevent harm to children who have the disorder.

Preimplantation Genetic Diagnosis

Mutations that cause severe early-onset genetic disorders, such as Tay-Sachs, and moderately severe disorders, such as cystic fibrosis, can be detected by testing the cells of embryos. On the basis of these tests, a prognosis can be given of the likely nature and severity of a genetic disease in the people who would develop from IVF embryos. These embryos are tested before they implant in the uterine wall for pregnancy. PIGD allows prospective parents to select among different embryos for implantation and subsequent birth on the basis of their genetic status. Given that gene therapy and other medical interventions have not been effective in treating most genetic disorders, parents may be morally obligated to select against embryos with the genetic mutations that cause the most severe of these disorders. This is a means of preventing diseases by preventing the lives of the people who would have them. Such a practice can be morally justified on grounds of nonmaleficence and justice. Nonmaleficence requires that we not harm people by causing them to experience significant pain and suffering over the balance of their lives. Justice requires that we not deny people the same opportunities for achievement and well-being that are open to others who are healthy or have only moderate diseases. Together, these principles imply that it can be morally wrong to cause a person to exist with a severe disease when it is possible to cause a different person to exist without the disease.

We should emphasize, though, that parents do not have an obligation to provide their children with the best possible life. They have an obligation only to ensure that their children have a minimally decent life with adequate opportunities for achievement. The obligation is not grounded in the principle of perfectionism, but in the principles of nonmaleficence and justice.

Would parents be obligated to select against embryos with genetic abnormalities that result in a late-onset disease such as Huntington's, Alzheimer's, and amyotrophic lateral sclerosis (ALS)? These conditions make the question of whether we are obligated to prevent lives on the basis of genetics more ethically controversial. This is because, unlike early-onset disorders that affect people for most or all of their lives, in late-onset disorders people are healthy for many years before the onset of symptoms.

The onset of symptoms in people with Huntington's can range anywhere from age thirty to sixty. Symptoms include progressive loss of muscle control and dementia. Generally, people die within fifteen years after the first symptoms appear. Prior to this time, they usually have high levels of cognitive and physical functioning for a considerable number of years. In trying to determine whether people's lives are worth living on the whole, we need to evaluate the quality of their lives in terms of all of the stages in them. Quality of life is a function of the presence or absence of pain and suffering, and of the cognitive, physical, and emotional ability to have opportunities for achieving a decent minimum level of well-being. Obviously, this determination will be subjective to a certain degree. Nevertheless, by setting a low threshold of what counts as a decent minimum, there can be reasonable objective agreement about lives that are not worth living because they fall below the threshold. With late-onset diseases such as Huntington's, however, the difference between cognitive and physical functioning before and after the onset of symptoms makes it difficult to assess overall quality of life for the people who have them.

One way of measuring lifetime quality in severe late-onset genetic diseases is to compare the level of normal functioning per year lived with the level of pain, suffering, and disability per year lived. The more severe the pain, suffering, and disability caused by a disease, the earlier the onset of symptoms, and the longer the period between onset and death, the stronger will be the reason for saying that the life is not worth living on the whole. If there is a high risk that a mutation will cause a severe disease, then there may be a decisive reason for preventing such a life by not selecting an embryo with that mutation. For a person who first experiences the degenerative physical and cognitive symptoms of Huntington's at thirty-five and who dies at fifty-five, the severity of these symptoms in the last twenty years of life may be enough to outweigh the good functioning in the first thirty-five years. The level of lifetime well-being may fall below the decent minimum.

This assessment is influenced by the idea that we have a bias toward the future. We care more about what we will experience in the future and less about what we experienced in the past. Most people prefer a life that matures to one that degenerates, a life that starts poorly and gets better to one that starts well and then goes progressively downhill. If this is correct, then the subjective value of our last stage of life may be disproportionate to the value of other stages in terms of its overall quality. The suggestion is that a long and painful final stage of life may have enough disvalue to make the life not worth living on the whole. Thus, if parents could foresee this progression of a diseased life through PIGD of an embryo, then arguably they would be obligated to not select that embryo for implantation. They would be obligated to prevent the life of the person who would have the disease.

Consider Alzheimer's disease. A mutation in the amyloid precursor protein (APP) gene on chromosome 21 has been implicated as a cause of this disease, which is by far the most common form of dementia. Those who have an autosomal dominant mutation of the gene have a very high likelihood of developing Alzheimer's at an early age. Suppose that a person with this mutation begins to have symptoms at age forty or earlier. If her condition deteriorated gradually over a period of twenty years, then one could argue that the balance between burdens and benefits in that person's life as a whole would make it not worth living. There would be a decisive reason for preventing a similar life in the future.

This was the rationale of a thirty-year-old California woman who wanted a child and used PIGD to select against IVF embryos with the APP mutation. As reported in February 2002 in the *Journal of the American Medical Association*, the woman did not yet have any symptoms of the disease when she was tested. But she knew that she had the mutation and that she would develop the disease on the basis of predictive testing, which she underwent because of a family history of early-onset Alzheimer's. She also knew that she would pass the disease on to any child developing from an embryo with the mutation. Once normal and affected embryos were identified, the woman selected a normal embryo for implantation, pregnancy, and birth. By selecting against the embryos with the mutation, she avoided bringing a person into the world who would suffer the same fate with the disease as she. With Alzheimer's, it is not so much the final stage of the disease that is harmful to those affected by it, since they may no longer be aware that they have it. Rather, the harm consists more in the suffering associated with experiencing the gradual deterioration of one's mental and physical functioning over a prolonged period.

Some might be disturbed by the idea of making decisions about selecting embryos on the basis of the probability of developing a disease, given a genetic mutation. Even with a family history of a disease with a genetic component, the gene in question may not express itself in every member of the family. Moreover, one can inherit a genetic mutation and have a risk of developing a disease, yet prevent it through diet and lifestyle. These two points are supported by the incomplete penetrance of genotypes, the fact that there is rarely a direct causal connection between a mutation and a disease that is not monogenic.

Three criteria have been cited in assessing whether a life is worth living on the whole. The probability of penetrance is a further criterion that must be included in judging whether a life should be prevented. So, assuming that a defective gene can be detected in an embryo, four criteria will determine whether a life should be prevented by not selecting that embryo for implantation and subsequent birth: (1) the probability of genotypic penetrance, or how likely it is that a genetic mutation will cause a disease; (2) the severity of the symptoms of the disease; (3) the time of onset of symptoms; and (4) the time between onset and death.

As we have noted, people with the autosomal dominant form of the APP mutation have a very high chance of developing Alzheimer's at a relatively early age. This provides a decisive reason and thus an obligation not to allow embryos with these mutations to implant in the uterus and to develop into a birth. It also justifies the decision of the California woman and explains why she had an obligation not to allow a particular embryo to become a person. Similar reasoning could be applied to embryos with mutations causing the neurodegenerative disease ALS. Between 5 and 10 percent of ALS cases involve a genetic mutation, with a penetrance that is close to 100 percent. If PIGD could accurately detect the mutation, then prospective parents might be obligated not to select an embryo with the mutation.

But consider the case of the physicist Stephen Hawking. He illustrates that a person can suffer from severe physical disability with ALS and still maintain a high level of cognitive functioning and quality of life. It would be difficult to find reasons for preventing his life, which is very much worth living for him. On the other hand, for people who value physical functioning very highly (e.g., athletes, dancers), severe physical disability might lead them to judge that their lives on balance are not worth living. These considerations suggest that how a late-onset genetic disorder with variable symptoms affects a person's quality of life will depend on the type of life plan that person already has chosen and cultivated before the onset of symptoms. It also depends on one's willingness and ability to adjust to change. The quality of a person's life in progress is shaped by his or her values and preferences. These cannot be predicted on the basis of genetic testing of embryos. So decisions about preventing lives with late-onset diseases should not be made lightly.

There is a deeper objection to the practice of embryo selection on the basis of genetics. If parents have an obligation to select a genetically normal embryo over a genetically abnormal one, then this seems to imply that parents would be obligated to always select the embryo with the best genetic profile. On this view, they would be obligated to select against embryos that would develop into people with only moderate disease or disability. The suggestion is that we should always select only embryos with the best predictable health status, not simply those with adequate predictable health status.

But there would be no obligation to make this selection. If one embryo had no genetic abnormality, and a different embryo had an abnormality involving susceptibility to a treatable condition like mild hypertension, then there would be no decisive moral reason for choosing one over the other. The people developing from each of these embryos would be at or above a decent minimum of health for the balance of their lives. Still, parents would be permitted to choose the better of the two. There would be no decisive moral reason against this choice. Yet, if the embryo with the abnormality would develop into a person with a severe, untreatable disease, then the parents would be obligated to select the better embryo. This particular obligation would be grounded in the more general obligation to prevent harm to the people we cause to exist.

Even if there were no strict obligation to select against a genetically abnormal embryo, there would not be an obligation to select a genetically normal embryo for implantation and subsequent birth. Presumably, such an obligation would be grounded in the principle of beneficence. But we cannot benefit a person by causing him or her to exist. We benefit a person by making him or her better off than before, which requires a comparison between two states of affairs in which the same person exists. Yet we cannot coherently compare a person's existence with his or her nonexistence. If we cannot benefit persons by causing them to exist, then there cannot be an obligation to do so.

The claim that prospective parents have an obligation to prevent lives has been restricted to lives that would have severe pain, suffering, and disability. By this line of reasoning, it is permissible to bring about lives with moderate to moderately severe disease or disability. But would it be permissible to *deliberately* select an embryo with a genetic mutation that would cause a moderate to moderately severe disability in a person? Suppose deaf parents want to have a deaf child. They produce several embryos through IVF and select one with a mutation that would cause deafness in a future child. Their decision is motivated by their belief that the family is an integrated unit, and that the child's interests cannot be separated from the interests of the parents. One could cite the defense of sex selection from Chapter 4 to support family autonomy and the right of the parents to have a deaf child. Also, the case at hand is different from that of the Jehovah's Witness parents in Chapter 2, whose refusal to allow a blood transfusion for their child could be overridden because of the risk of death to the child in not having it. Deafness is not a matter of life or death.

Nevertheless, deafness restricts a person's opportunities in life. Although parents have an obligation only to ensure that their children have adequate life opportunities, the deliberate restriction of these opportunities is morally objectionable. Parents have considerable autonomy in determining the values of their family; but it is not absolute. They do not have the autonomy to make deliberate decisions that automatically restrict their child's opportunities for the child's entire life. Parents cannot assume that their child's best interests always will be defined in terms of their own. To do so is to violate the child's right to an open future. The character Lara in the 1997 German film *Beyond Silence*, whose parents are deaf but who is not deaf herself, illustrates that one can have greater opportunities in life by being allowed to be part of these two worlds of experience.

Gene Therapy

Somatic-cell gene therapy involves correcting a mutated copy of a gene or inserting an additional normal copy of a gene into the cells of a person's body. The aim is to treat genetically caused diseases in existing people. In contrast, germ-line genetic alteration involves modifying the cells of gametes (sperm and egg). The aim of this second type of genetic intervention is to delete or correct mutations that would be passed on to offspring. In this regard, germ-line genetic intervention is a form of disease prevention rather than therapy.

Gene therapy is not yet feasible for treating most diseases with a genetic component. There are different reasons for this. Gene therapy is primarily relevant to single-gene disorders, and multifactorial diseases such as cancer involve interactions between several or more genes and environmental factors. Furthermore, chromosomal disorders causing mental retardation, such as Down's and Fragile X syndromes, involve large segments of DNA that are too difficult to alter. The single-gene disorders that in principle might be amenable to gene therapy are recessive rather than dominant. Recessive disorders might be treatable because inserting one normal copy of the gene into the affected cells would be enough to ensure proper cell function. Dominant disorders would be treatable only by replacing the mutated copy of the gene with a normal copy. Replacing a defective gene would be superior to adding a normal copy of a gene because its potential to correct mutations could prevent both dominant and recessive disorders. Unfortunately, it is not presently possible to correct mutations but only to insert normal copies of genes into affected cells. Even so, to date only a few genetic diseases have been treated with this type of gene therapy.

In theory, a recessive disorder such as cystic fibrosis could be treated by inserting a normal copy of the critical gene into the affected cells. This would ensure that the pancreas produced the necessary enzymes for food absorption and that the glands in the lining of the bronchial tubes functioned properly. In an X-linked disorder like hemophilia, a normal copy of the gene coding for the proteins that control blood clotting (Factors VIII and IX) could be delivered through injections. In practice, researchers have not found a suitable vector that can deliver therapeutic genes into cells and ensure their proper functioning. Viral vectors have been the most common form used. These may consist of inactivated adenoviruses that carry pieces of DNA into cell nuclei. Yet this method has been largely unsuccessful because these stripped-down viruses do not provide a stable platform for the genes to operate efficiently. Some of these viruses are not large enough to carry a complete gene with all of its functions.

Vectors consisting of retroviruses are more effective in inserting genes into cells. Like adenoviral vectors, though, retroviral vectors can provoke an adverse immune response. This has occurred with genetically engineered proteins in some new drugs. For example, some hemophiliacs react to the anemia drug Eprex as if the protein were a germ, and their immune systems try to destroy it. As a result, their anemia is worse than it would have been without the drug. In these cases, the immune system makes antibodies that attack the protein, making it less effective as a drug. This is likely because the body can tell the difference between a natural and a genetically engineered protein.

The risk of harm to individuals undergoing gene therapy has become evident in the wake of recent deaths resulting from adverse immune responses to retroviruses. Jesse Gelsinger had a mild form of ornithine transcarbamylase (OTC) deficiency. In this disorder, the liver cannot process ammonia, a toxic by-product of food. He died in 1999 while participating in a clinical trial that used a retroviral vector at the University of Pennsylvania. Around the same time, an individual died after receiving gene therapy involving vascular endothelial growth factor (VEGF) for heart disease in Boston. Citing these deaths, some physicians, researchers, and ethicists called for a moratorium on most forms of gene therapy until the risks of the procedure could be reduced.

Gene therapy using retroviruses has shown some success in treating children with severe combined immune deficiency (SCID). But even this treatment has risks. Two French children treated in 2000 with gene therapy for SCID have developed a condition resembling leukemia. This led the FDA to suspend twenty-seven gene-therapy trials in January 2003. In spite of the risk that gene therapy can cause some cancers, an American advisory panel has recommended that gene-therapy experiments proceed with close monitoring and some restrictions. The rationale for proceeding with these experiments is that they offer hope to children with fatal immune and other genetic conditions. More generally, others argue that the promise gene therapy holds, not only for monogenic disorders, but also for autoimmune diseases, heart disease, and many cancers, is too great to stop or severely restrict research. Instead of dooming gene therapy, the diseases and deaths that have resulted from it thus far could provide clues to designing safer viruses as vectors. With adequate scientific and ethical oversight of research and clinical trials, the potential benefits of gene therapy outweigh the risks.

The principle of beneficence specifies an obligation to move forward with gene therapy research, provided that it is balanced by the principle of nonmaleficence specifying an obligation to minimize risks. If research subjects are exposed to no more than minimal risk, this recommendation is consistent with what we said about permissible risk in Chapter 3. Many people suffering from various diseases could benefit from gene therapy. In cancers, for example, most tumors involve a mutated tumor suppressor gene. Replacing this gene with a normal copy might suppress the growth of tumor cells. If it were safely designed, gene therapy might control the rate of cell division and thereby prevent the growth of tumors responsible for many cancers. Gene therapy research might also lead to the development of vaccines to prevent viral infections such as HIV-AIDS.

Germ-line genetic intervention might seem more attractive than somatic-cell genetic intervention. Deleting or correcting a mutation in germ cells would ensure that the mutation would not be passed on to future generations. It could eliminate the mutation within certain populations. Such a practice would be more desirable than gene therapy to treat disease because, by intervening at the germ line, we would be preventing genetic diseases from occurring in the first place. Still, germ-line genetic intervention might not be desirable from an evolutionary perspective. Some genetic mutations are necessary for species to adapt to changing environmental conditions. And some genetic disorders involve alleles that confer a survival advantage on certain populations sensitive to these conditions. Perhaps the best example of this phenomenon is the allele associated with sickle-cell anemia, which at the same time provides greater resistance to malaria in populations native to equatorial Africa. Altering a gene or genes at the germ line to correct one disorder might lead to other disorders that could harm many people in successive generations. Any unwanted effects would not remain within the bodies of individuals, but would be passed on to their offspring. This might involve knocking out tumor suppressor genes that control the proliferation of cancer cells or damaging genes controlling other mechanisms of disease.

We still do not know what effects germ-line intervention would have on genes. If anything were to go awry as a consequence of this intervention, then it could result in more disease and harm in future people. In the light of this possibility, the scientifically and ethically reasonable course of action is to postpone such intervention until we know more about these genetic mechanisms. Genes interact in complex ways. Because of this complexity, it would be difficult to weigh the potential health benefits of germ-line intervention to people in the present against any health burdens of this intervention to people in the future. Their interests in not being harmed by disease, once they exist, have as much moral weight as the same interests of people who already exist. This concern is not enough to justify a prohibition on germ-line research. But it does justify a precautionary approach that recommends proceeding slowly until the safety and efficacy of this type of genetic intervention can be assessed more accurately.

Genetic Enhancement

Gene therapy must be distinguished from genetic enhancement. The first is an intervention aimed at restoring physical and mental functioning to an adequate level. The second is an intervention aimed at improving already adequate functioning. Genetic enhancement augments functions and capacities that otherwise would be considered normal. Insofar as the goals of medicine are to treat and prevent disease and thereby restore and ensure adequate functioning, gene therapy falls within these goals. Genetic enhancement falls outside of them.

Some claim that it is mistaken to think that a clear line can be drawn between treatment and enhancement because many forms of enhancement are employed to prevent disease. The most frequently cited example in this regard is "boosting" the immune system through immunization against infectious disease. Yet, because the goal of immunization is to prevent disease, strictly speaking it would not be enhancement. Genetically intervening in the immune system would be a way of maintaining it in proper working order. It would be better able to protect the body from life-threatening pathogens. Thus the idea of "boosting" the immune system offers no reason to give up the distinction between treatment and enhancement.

Admittedly, there is a gray area near the baseline of adequate functioning where it may be difficult to distinguish clearly between treatment and enhancement. Accordingly, we should interpret the baseline loosely enough to allow for some deviation above or below what would be considered normal functioning. An intervention aimed at raising one's functioning *to* the baseline would be a treatment. An intervention aimed at raising one's functioning *above* the baseline would be an enhancement. For an athlete with a normal blood count, taking the hormone erythropoietin (EPO) to produce more oxygen-carrying red blood cells and make himself more competitive in his sport would be an enhancement. For a child with severe anemia and the risk of bone abnormalities and heart failure, giving EPO to correct the condition would be a treatment.

The main ethical concern about genetic enhancement of physical or cognitive traits is that it would give some people an unfair advantage over others with respect to competitive goods like beauty and intelligence. Enhancement would be unfair because only those who could afford the technology would have access to it. Many people are financially worse off than others through no fault of their own. Not having access to technology that could improve people's physical and cognitive traits would put some at a competitive disadvantage compared to others. Some might argue that the same concern applies to gene therapy, which also would be expensive and not affordable by all the people who need it. If gene therapy became an effective intervention, then there would be a compelling reason for federal subsidies so that all people who could be treated could afford it. As a form of disease prevention or treatment, gene therapy would fall within the goals of medicine. But there would be no compelling medical or ethical reason to subsidize genetic enhancement, because it neither prevents nor treats disease. Unlike gene therapy, genetic enhancement pertains to people's preferences rather than to their needs. More importantly, genetic enhancement could exacerbate inequality between rich and poor, because only those who could afford the technology would have access to it. The problem is that the goods that would be enhanced would not be basic, noncompetitive goods like adequate health. They would be competitive goods like beauty and intelligence.

Suppose that genetic enhancement became universally accessible. Presumably, many competitive traits that some people had over others would be cancelled out. Any competitive advantages would gradually erode, and there would be more equality among people in their possession of the relevant traits. But this would not ensure complete equality. Different parental attitudes toward social goods such as education would mean differences in the extent to which cognitive enhancement was utilized. Some parents would be more selective than others in sending their children to better schools or in arranging for private tutors. These factors would mean unequal outcomes of genetic enhancement, despite equal access to it. Some might take the inability to control these outcomes as grounds for the permissibility of genetic enhancement. They might say that it is inconsistent to prohibit parents from seeking the best for their children genetically, if we permit them to seek the best for their children in other ways.

Even if we could neutralize competitive goods through universal access to genetic enhancement, the process could end up being self-defeating on a collective level. One probable side effect of boosting every child's cognitive capacity would be brain damage and mental impairment in some of the children who underwent the procedure. The net social cost of using the technology could outweigh the social advantage of everyone having access to it. No child would be cognitively better off than others, and some children would be cognitively worse off than they were before the procedure. The net social disadvantage could provide a reason for prohibiting universal genetic enhancement.

It could be argued that inequalities above the baseline of adequate physical and cognitive functioning are of no great ethical significance and may be neutral on the question of fairness. Although equality and fairness are closely related, one does not necessarily imply the other. Equality pertains to how some people fare relative to others. Fairness pertains to meeting people's needs in terms of an absolute measure of health. A fair distribution of a good is one that gives greater weight to those with greater needs. But when people's basic needs have been met, inequalities between people above the decent minimum might not be unfair. On this view, there would be nothing unfair or morally objectionable about enhancements that made some people better off than others. After all, enhancements improve what are already normal functions or traits. Thus, if those without access to enhancements fall at the baseline of normal cognitive and physical functioning, then any claims to having enhancements would pertain to their preferences rather than their needs. There would be little or no moral force to these claims.

Nevertheless, all of this could undermine our belief in the importance of equality, regardless of how well off people are in terms of an absolute measure of health. Equality is one of the social bases of self-respect, which is essential for social harmony and stability. Allowing inequalities in access to enhancement technology might erode this basis and the harmony and stability that rest on it. Although it would be difficult to measure quantitatively, this type of social cost might constitute another reason for prohibiting genetic enhancement.

Imagine that we could manipulate certain genes to enhance our noncompetitive virtuous traits, such as altruism, generosity, and compassion. Surely, these would contribute to a stable, well-ordered society. Nothing in this program would be incompatible with the prevention and treatment of disease. Yet it would threaten the individual autonomy essential to us as moral agents who can be candidates for praise and blame, punishment and reward. Autonomy consists in the process of critical reflection on and identification with the motivations that issue in our actions. This capacity for self-control enables us to take responsibility for our actions and to be held responsible for them. Given the importance of autonomy, it would be preferable to have fewer virtuous dispositions that we can identify with as our own than to have more virtuous dispositions implanted in us through genetic enhancement. These would undermine our autonomy and moral agency because they would derive from an external, alien source.

Even if our genes could be manipulated to make our behavior conform to a morally perfect course of action in every situation, it is unlikely that we would want it. Most of us would rather make autonomous choices that turned out not to lead to the best course of action. This is because of the importance of moral growth and maturity that come with making choices under uncertainty. The dispositions that we cultivate on our own, imperfect as they are, make our lives valuable to us. All of these considerations may not be enough to constitute reasons for prohibiting genetic enhancement. But they raise troubling questions about permitting it.

Eugenics

Some may characterize the types of genetic intervention that we have been discussing as eugenics. Literally meaning "good creation" in Greek, eugenics can be defined as the use of science to improve the human genome. "Eugenics" is almost universally regarded pejoratively. This is due mainly to its association with the human experimentation in Nazi Germany and the sterilization programs in the United States and Canada earlier in the twentieth century. Yet there is a broader conception of eugenics that does not have the repugnant connotation of improving the human species. This requires drawing a distinction between negative and positive eugenics. To the extent that the aim of genetic testing and screening, PIGD, and gene therapy is to prevent or control disease, they are forms of negative eugenics. To the extent that the aim of genetic enhancement is to improve people's normal traits and capacities, it is a form of positive eugenics. If there is a decisive reason and thus an obligation to prevent or control diseases, then we are obligated to practice negative eugenics. If there is no decisive reason and thus no obligation to improve normal capacities, then there is no obligation to practice positive eugenics. Indeed, some would argue that positive eugenics should be prohibited, though we have reserved judgment on this question with respect to genetic enhancement. More importantly, it must be emphasized that positive and negative eugenics are distinct practices motivated by distinct aims.

Forms of eugenics not involving direct genetic intervention have been practiced since antiquity. For example, in Plato's *Republic* and *Laws*, an ideal society would encourage "judicious matings." Mating between people in the ruling and mercantile classes was discouraged. Only those people most likely to produce the "best" offspring would be encouraged to mate, and these would be limited to the ruling class. This example of positive eugenics seems morally objectionable because it involves discrimination on the basis of social class. Yet many people today select mates with whom they believe they will have children with favorable physical and cognitive traits, giving them a competitive advantage over others for social goods. This is also a version of positive eugenics, even though it does not involve genetic intervention. Nor would most people acknowledge it as such.

Selecting a mate in order to have children with certain physical or cognitive traits by itself is not morally objectionable. If it is not part of a state-sponsored program, does not involve any coercion, and does not give some an unfair advantage over others in having children, then there would be no reason to prohibit it. We can defend this position on grounds of parental autonomy and because it does not result in any harm to any person. Besides, owing to the uncertainty surrounding the transmission of genetic traits from one generation to the next, it cannot be predicted precisely which traits a child will inherit from his or her parents.

Suppose that a couple wants to have children. Each partner is aware of being a carrier of the mutation associated with cystic fibrosis. The partners also know that, if they have children, then there will be a 25 percent risk of each child inheriting both copies of the mutation and having the disease. The decision not to have natural biological children would be a defensible form of negative eugenics. Similarly, a rabbi may advise a couple who are Orthodox Ashkenazi Jews and carriers of the Tay-Sachs mutation not to marry or not to have children. Provided that the rabbi's advice was not coercive and the couple made a voluntary, informed decision, this too would be a defensible form of negative eugenics. In both cases, the aim would be to prevent harm by eliminating the risk of having a child with a serious genetic disease.

PIGD and gene therapy are both forms of negative eugenics. The purpose of the first is to prevent genetic disease by preventing the existence of people who would have it. The purpose of the second is to treat genetic disease in people once they exist. PIGD is motivated by the principle of nonmaleficence, while gene therapy is motivated by the principle of beneficence. Genetic enhancement is a form of positive eugenics. Given that its purpose is to improve normal genetic traits, it is motivated by the principle of perfectionism. Because disease treatment and prevention, on the one hand, and enhancement, on the other, are distinct aims resting on distinct principles, there is no reason to be concerned about the first collapsing into the second.

Disabilities rights advocates might reject the distinction that we have just drawn and discussed. They might argue that, no matter how one slices it, PIGD, gene therapy, and genetic enhancement are all forms of eugenics that devalue the lives of people with disabilities. In PIGD, selecting against embryos with genetic mutations causing disabilities would reduce the number of people with disabilities. Consequently, public support for people living with disabilities would erode, and there would be further social discrimination against them. One could respond by saying that it is not the *people* with disabilities we devalue, but rather the *disabilities*. Yet many people with disabilities identify with their disabilities and would maintain that the two cannot be separated so neatly.

This point does not have much force if we are considering whether to select against an embryo that would develop into a diseased and disabled person. The properties of an embryo and the properties of a person are so distinct that it would be implausible to suppose that they are simply earlier and later stages of the same individual. In particular, embryos lack the biological structures to support the capacity for mentality that is necessary for personhood. Nor do embryos have the potential to develop these structures on their own. Thus, any moral decisions about embryos cannot be logically extended to persons. Embryos do not have disabilities; only persons do. Since embryos are not identical to persons, and since only persons can be harmed, selecting against or terminating an embryo does not harm anyone. On the contrary, if an embryo has a genetic abnormality that would result in a severe disability, then selecting against it would prevent harm by preventing the existence of a person who would experience the pain, suffering, and limitations associated with it. This is supported by the principles of nonmaleficence and justice. In Allen Buchanan's words: "We devalue disabilities because we value the opportunities and welfare of the people who have them—and it is because we value people, all people, that we care about limitations on their welfare and opportunities" (1996, p. 33).

Disabilities rights groups have been successful in securing necessary legal protection through political means, as the 1990 Americans with Disabilities Act attests. Some insist that preventing the existence of people who would have disabilities will increase discrimination against people who already have disabilities. But there is something disturbing about this idea. It suggests that those brought into existence with disabilities might be treated as mere means for the ends of others. This would be difficult to justify on moral grounds, even if it brought about political and legal gains for those living with disabilities. Moreover, one could argue that, if the number of people coming into existence with disabilities were smaller, society would be better able to meet their needs. In particular, it might help to ameliorate the problem that many school systems have in paying for nurses, physical therapists, psychologists, and special buses for severely disabled children. This could be done without sacrificing the less urgent, but still significant, needs of many other students. In an era of limited budgets for education and social services, this issue cannot be ignored. More generally, even if there is no obligation to select against embryos that would develop into people with disabilities, this does not mean that there is an obligation to allow these embryos to develop into people. Indeed, there is no obligation to allow even genetically normal embryos to develop into people. The reason is that we cannot benefit embryos in this or any other way.

Conclusion

In this chapter, we considered the ethical implications of different forms of genetic intervention. We discussed presymptomatic genetic testing and screening and how the information derived from these procedures should and should not be used. In addition, we presented arguments for selecting against embryos with mutations that could cause severe early- and late-onset diseases on the basis of PIGD. We then addressed somatic-cell gene therapy and germ-line genetic alteration. Despite some significant risks, the potential of gene therapy to treat many diseases and improve the lives of many people provides a strong reason for research to continue in this area. On the other hand, because any adverse effects of germ-line alteration would be passed on to future generations, it is best to adopt a precautionary approach with this technology. We also noted that because genetic enhancement does not aim to prevent and treat disease, there are only weak reasons for defending it. Finally, we distinguished between positive and negative eugenics and argued that, as forms of disease prevention and treatment, most of the negative eugenic interventions we examined are morally permissible. Some may even be obligatory.

Genes play an important role in shaping our physical and cognitive traits and determining whether we have healthy or diseased lives. But we are more than our genes. Our bodies and our minds are not completely determined by our genotype. The incomplete penetrance of genotypes makes the link between genes and most diseases a probabilistic rather than a deterministic one. Apart from the relatively rare monogenic diseases, the presence of a genetic mutation does not necessarily mean that one will have a disease associated with it. Moreover, there may be varying degrees of severity with the same genetic disease. These phenomena are reflections of the complex interaction between genes and the environment. The goals of better disease prevention and treatment will be realized by studying genes within a broader causal framework that includes behavioral, environmental, and other biological factors. While acknowledging the significance of genetics, these considerations should temper any expectations about what genetic research can achieve in affecting the nature and improving the quality of our lives.

Selected Readings

Baird, P. "Altering Human Genes: Social, Ethical, and Legal Implications." *Perspectives in Biology and Medicine* 37(1994): 566–75.

Buchanan, A. "Choosing Who Will Be Disabled: Genetic Intervention and the Morality of Inclusion." *Social Philosophy and Policy* 13(1996): 18–46.

Buchanan, A., Brock, D., Daniels, N., and Wikler, D. *From Chance to Choice: Genetics and Justice.* New York: Cambridge University Press, 2000.

Collins, Francis. "Medical and Societal Consequences of the Human Genome Project." *New England Journal of Medicine* 341(1999): 28–37.

Draper, H., and Chadwick, R. "Beware! Preimplantation Genetic Diagnosis May Solve Some Old Problems But It Also Raises New Ones." *Journal of Medical Ethics* 25(1999): 114–20.

Holtzman, N., and Marteau, T. "Will Genetics Revolutionalize Medicine?" *New England Journal of Medicine* 343(2000): 141–44.

Kitcher, P. *The Lives to Come: The Genetic Revolution and Human Possibilities.* New York: Simon & Schuster, 1996.

Marteau, T., and Richards, M., eds. *The Troubled Helix: Social and Psychological Implications of the New Human Genetics.* Cambridge, Eng.: Cambridge University Press, 1996.

Parens, E., ed. *Enhancing Human Traits: Ethical and Social Implications.* Washington, D.C.: Georgetown University Press, 1998.

Rothstein, M., ed. *Genetic Secrets: Protecting Privacy and Confidentiality in the Genetic Era.* New Haven, Conn.: Yale University Press, 1997.

CHAPTER 6

Medical Decisions at the End of Life

Introduction

Ending a human life may be the most momentous decision one could ever make. This decision will depend largely on what death means to us. Until the second half of the twentieth century, death was defined in relatively simple terms. A person who ceased to breathe and whose heart stopped beating was declared dead. But the use of the mechanical ventilator in the late 1960s and early 1970s forced a change in the cardiopulmonary definition and diagnosis of death. This new technology made it possible to sustain breathing and heartbeat, even when the brain stem controlling these processes had ceased to function. Mechanical ventilation, cardiopulmonary resuscitation (CPR), artificial hydration and nutrition, and drugs that could sustain blood pressure enabled medical professionals to extend lives that would have ended without these interventions. Early on, however, it became evident that these interventions could have undesirable and indeed tragic consequences.

One of these consequences was the case of Karen Ann Quinlan. In April 1975, this twenty-one-year-old woman arrived comatose at a New Jersey hospital after ingesting drugs and alcohol. She was put on a respirator to assist her breathing, but gradually fell into a persistent vegetative state (PVS). Individuals in such a state are wakeful but not consciously aware of their surroundings. Karen's parents wanted the breathing tube removed; but her doctors refused. The New Jersey Supreme Court ruled in March 1976 that, given her irreversible condition, mechanical life-support could be disconnected, even if it resulted in her death. The Court ruled that this action was permitted on grounds of a privacy right guaranteed by the Constitution, and that Karen's parents were the appropriate surrogates to exercise that right for her. Once the breathing tube was removed, Karen unexpectedly began to breathe spontaneously. She lived in a PVS until June 1985, when all of her bodily functions permanently ceased and she was declared dead.

Doctors and other medical professionals often must decide whether to withhold, withdraw, or continue life-sustaining interventions. These decisions are difficult to make because it is difficult to know in advance what the long-term burdens and benefits will be for patients. Determining *when* a patient dies can also be controversial in some cases. These and related issues at the end of patients' lives raise the following questions: How can we formulate a definition of death that will be acceptable, not only to clinicians and academics, but to the general public as well? What are the implications of the definition of death for justifying such practices as procuring organs for transplantation? Is there a morally relevant distinction between withholding and withdrawing treatment, between intending and foreseeing a patient's death, and between killing a patient or letting her die? Can these distinctions help us to determine the permissibility or impermissibility of euthanasia and physician-assisted suicide (PAS)? Can a physician justifiably discontinue life-support on grounds of medical futility? Or is futility a value-laden concept that is interpreted differently by doctors and patients' families? How can conflicts about treatment between these parties be resolved? By addressing these questions in this chapter, we will explore different ethical dimensions of medical decisions at the end of life.

Defining Death

Prior to 1968, the only criterion used to determine death was the irreversible cessation of cardiopulmonary function. The loss of heart and lung function entailed the loss of brain function, and vice versa. But the ventilator enabled patients to continue breathing and have a heartbeat even though they lacked brain function. This raised the question of whether brain death should be equated with the death of the patient.

To sort out these matters, in 1968 an ad hoc committee at Harvard Medical School formulated a new brain-based set of criteria for determining death. They stated that a patient could be declared dead when all brain functions, including those of the cerebral cortex and brain stem, had permanently ceased. Shortly thereafter, the President's Commission for the Study of Ethical Problems in Medicine and Biomedical and Behavioral Research drafted a similar definition. It stated that the permanent loss of all brain functions should be the main criterion for determining death, because these functions are necessary for the integrated functioning of the organism as a whole. Since then, the "whole-brain" criterion of death has been widely accepted by the general public and adopted in legal and clinical practice. But this criterion has been challenged on at least two fronts.

Some have argued that the whole-brain criterion is physiologically inaccurate. The standard account suggests that the brain controls and integrates all bodily processes. Yet many of these processes are neither mediated nor controlled by the brain. In fact, some of the body's integrated functions can continue for some time after the brain has ceased to function. For example, although the brain mediates breathing and nutrition, these bodily functions are not reducible to or completely controlled by the activity of the brain. So brain death should not be equated with the death of the organism as a whole. Others have argued that death should not be defined in terms of the whole brain, but instead when the higher brain necessary for consciousness permanently ceases to function. Proponents of this "higher-brain" definition of death distinguish persons from human organisms. They hold that, although persons are constituted by their bodies and brains, they are not identical to them. Persons are defined in terms of the capacity for consciousness, which depends on the activity of the cerebral cortex. The permanent cessation of cortical function is sufficient for the death of a person. But if the brain stem and structures other than the cortex continue to be active, then a human organism can continue to live after a person has died. For many, this idea has the counterintuitive implication that a human being is dead when he or she is still breathing and his or her heart is still beating.

Commonsense intuitions notwithstanding, there are sound philosophical reasons for distinguishing between persons and their bodies regarding death. If death is a biological phenomenon, and persons are not essentially biological but psychological beings, then death pertains only to the body. On this view, death occurs when all integrated functions of the body and the brain permanently cease. But if persons are defined essentially in terms of the capacity for consciousness, then a person dies when the region of the brain that generates and sustains this capacity permanently ceases to function. Perhaps we should say that there are two definitions of death: one for persons and one for human organisms. More importantly, what matters morally is not so much how we define death, but the fact that only persons and not their bodies can have interests. The capacity for consciousness is necessary to have interests. Persons but not their bodies have this capacity. Because only persons can have interests, and because benefit and harm are defined in terms of satisfying or defeating interests, only persons can be benefited or harmed by what happens to their bodies. A body without the capacity for consciousness cannot have any interest in what happens to it and therefore cannot be harmed.

If one accepts this position, then one can argue that a patient who has lost all cortical function and the capacity for consciousness is beyond harm. Admittedly, some patients can emerge from prolonged comas. In some cases, it can be difficult to determine whether the loss of the capacity for consciousness is permanent. In most cases, though, beyond a certain point it can be determined conclusively that the loss of this capacity is permanent. When this occurs, it seems permissible to take organs from a patient's body for transplantation, even if respiration and heartbeat are still present in the body. The only scenario in which the patient could be harmed in such a case would be if, at an earlier time, he expressed a wish that his organs not be harvested once he permanently lost the capacity for consciousness. This may have been expressed verbally to an intimate or more formally in an advance directive such as a living will. Ignoring this directive would be a violation of consent and a form of posthumous harm. It harms the patient in the sense that it ignores his interest in what happens to his body after he dies. The interest survives his death, and the subject of harm is the person whose interest it was.

Yet thinking of death in the way we have just described it remains at odds with the commonsense intuitions that ground the legal and clinical understanding of death. In particular, the idea that a patient cannot be harmed if organs are taken from his or her body when some bodily functions are still intact is difficult for most people to accept. For this and other reasons, it is unlikely that the philosophical account of death, and the higher-brain criterion it recommends, will influence public debate and lead to changes in the law and policy on organ transplantation. It is more likely that these will continue to be based on the whole-brain criterion and the associated "dead donor rule." This rule says that organs can only be taken from the bodies of patients who have been declared dead. It has been upheld in order to avoid killing people by taking their organs. Significantly, this view assumes that being alive or dead is defined in strictly biological terms. But it is unclear how the concept of harm can be described and defended in biological terms alone, without some reference to the psychological properties of persons. This problem is merely one example of the difficulty in defining and diagnosing death, which remains a matter of considerable controversy.

Of the three criteria of death that we have considered, both the cardiopulmonary and whole-brain definitions ground clinical and legal practice and are more socially acceptable than the higher-brain definition. The whole-brain criterion is useful for procuring organs for transplantation. It supplements, rather than supplants, the cardiopulmonary criterion. Still, the whole-brain criterion has broader legal and social importance. As Stuart Youngner and Robert Arnold (2001) point out, it allows doctors to turn off respirators without fear of legal consequences. It also allows organ procurement without violating the dead donor rule. They further note that "no one has seriously considered repealing the laws recognizing brain death; nor has any national professional organization or religious group called for their abandonment or even modification" (pp. 532–533).

But the whole-brain definition leaves the main moral problem concerning death unresolved. By focusing on human organisms rather than persons, it cannot explain how patients can be harmed by what is done to them at the end of their lives. Although the definition proposed by the Harvard Committee in 1968 has been challenged, it has not been refuted by either of the alternatives we have considered. The higher-brain criterion of death is more philosophically satisfying. But the whole-brain criterion is more clinically, legally, and socially acceptable. For this reason, it is not likely to be replaced in the foreseeable future.

Withdrawing and Withholding Treatment

Many believe that there is a morally significant difference between withdrawing and withholding life-sustaining treatment. The decision to stop treatment seems weightier than the decision not to initiate treatment. When a doctor removes a respirator from a patient who cannot breathe on her own, he causes the patient's death. In contrast, if a doctor does not put the same patient on the respirator and she dies, then presumably the cause of death is an underlying disease process running its normal course. In the first case, the doctor causes an event to occur. In the second case, he allows an event to occur. If withdrawing treatment is the cause of a patient's death, then the person who performs that action is responsible for the death. But if withholding treatment does not cause the patient's death, then the doctor is not responsible for it.

Closer analysis shows that the presumed moral significance of this distinction is unfounded. Actions and omissions both can play a causal role in a sequence of events and the outcome of such a sequence. One can have and exercise causal control over and thus ensure that a certain outcome occurs by acting or omitting to act. If a patient goes into cardiac arrest and a physician fails to give CPR, then by not acting the physician plays a causal role in how the respiratory and cardiac failure result in the patient's death. When the doctor could have prevented the death by intervening, he ensured the outcome by not acting. In this regard, the doctor plays a causally and morally significant role in the patient's death and can be held responsible for it. His omission affected the sequence of events resulting in the patient's death. One can exercise causal control over and thus ensure an outcome either by intentionally acting or by intentionally omitting to act, when one can foresee that either the action or the omission can lead to that outcome. So, an appeal to intention alone cannot motivate a moral distinction between actions and omissions. To be sure, one's intention in acting or failing to act can be benevolent in one case and malevolent in another. This intention can influence the degree to which one is praiseworthy or blameworthy for what one does or fails to do. But causal and moral responsibility for outcomes does not depend on the distinction between actions and omissions. Thus, there is no causally or morally relevant distinction between withdrawing and withholding treatment when both can lead to a patient's death.

Some have described the distinction between actions and omissions in end-of-life decision making in terms of killing the patient versus letting the patient die. But we can raise the same question here that we raised with the first distinction. If a doctor has causal control over a sequence of events resulting in a patient's death, and can exercise this control and ensure the patient's death either by killing him or letting him die, then it is unclear how the distinction between killing and letting die is morally significant.

What is morally relevant is not withdrawing and withholding treatment as such, but rather how an action or omission benefits or harms the patient. Obviously, this is much more difficult to estimate before a decision about whether to treat is made than it is once treatment has been initiated. Even in the latter case, there is always some degree of uncertainty about whether the patient's condition is reversible. Some patients brought to emergency are put on a ventilator with the belief that mechanical ventilation is necessary to get them through a critical period of trauma and restore them to normal functioning. Yet, if a patient's condition deteriorates and shows no sign of being reversible, then at some point a decision must be made about the benefits and burdens of remaining on the ventilator. The moral issue pertains not to withdrawing ventilation itself, but rather to whether withdrawing it is in the patient's best interests. Withdrawing treatment because the burden of continuing it outweighs any benefit is morally equivalent to withholding treatment because the burden of giving it would outweigh any benefit. Just as a treatment can be permissibly withheld, it can be permissibly withdrawn. If a treatment is not likely to reverse a condition, then there is no duty to initiate it. Similarly, if an initiated treatment cannot reverse a condition, then there is no duty to continue that treatment. Indeed, a physician may be obligated to withdraw it if it is clear that it offers no benefit to and only harms the patient. The belief that withdrawing treatment is worse than withholding it can lead to greater harm because it may incline some to continue treatment long after it has ceased to be effective. By focusing on actions or omission themselves, rather than on how they affect patients, preventable harm can befall patients.

The distinction between withdrawing and withholding treatment, or between actions and omissions, is different in important

respects from the distinction between intending to act and foreseeing a consequence of an intentional action. The intending-
foreseeing distinction is at the core of the Doctrine of Double Effect (DDE), which is often invoked in discussions of euthanasia and
PAS. It will be helpful to examine DDE in some detail to see
whether it can help us in assessing the moral permissibility or impermissibility of these practices.

Double Effect

DDE specifies a moral distinction between intending a harmful effect by acting, and foreseeing a harmful effect as an unintended
outcome of a good action. It says that, although one cannot permissibly perform a harmful act to bring about a beneficial effect,
one can permissibly bring about a harmful effect as a result of a
beneficial act. In DDE, the distinction is not between actions and
omissions, or killing and letting die, but between direct and indirect agency. It concerns the difference between what we do and
what we bring about as a result of what we do. The idea of "double effect" refers to the fact that the same action can have good and
bad, beneficial and harmful, effects.

Four conditions must be satisfied for an action with a double effect to be justified: (1) the action must be good, independent of its
consequences; (2) although the bad effect can be foreseen, the agent
must intend only the good effect; (3) the bad effect must not be a
means to the good effect; and (4) the good effect must outweigh,
or compensate for, the bad effect. Saint Thomas Aquinas first formulated this doctrine in his analysis of justifiable homicide, where
he argued that it was justifiable for one to kill another when acting in self-defense. According to DDE, it is morally permissible to
give a high dose of morphine (or a similar narcotic) in order to relieve a patient's pain when a doctor foresees that it will hasten the
patient's death. But it is morally impermissible to give the drug in
order to bring about the patient's death. The physician cannot permissibly kill the patient as an intended means to the end of relieving pain.

But it is not obvious that the difference between intending a
harmful effect and merely foreseeing it is morally significant. This
is due mainly to two reasons. First, intentions are often complex.
One can intend two or more outcomes by performing one action.

In giving a high dose of morphine, a doctor may at once intend to relieve pain and intend to kill the patient, given the belief that no available medication can relieve the patient's pain and keep him or her alive. In a sequence of events that ends in a patient's death, a doctor may intend to bring about what is presumed to be a foreseen effect. Second, DDE focuses on the mental states and actions of the physician, ignoring the wishes and interests of the patient. What constitutes a benefit or harm to the patient is not something that can be determined by the physician. Nor can be it determined by whether the physician intends or merely foresees an outcome for the patient. If a patient's pain cannot be treated with any medication, then intentionally killing the patient may benefit him or her, provided that the patient wants and consents to it. The distinction between intending and foreseeing cannot tell us which treatments are beneficial or harmful to a patient. So DDE is not very helpful in determining when killing a patient is permissible or impermissible.

The main problems with DDE are that it assumes that it is always wrong to intentionally kill a patient and that death always harms the patient. But there are some cases in which killing a patient can be morally justified because it benefits the patient. In addition, DDE fails to acknowledge that killing a person is the same as causing his or her death, and that death can be caused by an action or an omission. Thus, whether a doctor intends a patient's death or merely foresees it when he or she acts will not tell us whether the doctor is morally justified in causing the death.

In the first version of the morphine example, death is a side effect of giving the medication. It is not the doctor's goal or reason for giving it, and in this sense it is not intended. Although the death is not intended, the doctor nonetheless kills the patient. She causes the patient's death by administering the morphine. One could defend the act by appealing to the idea of proportionality in DDE, maintaining that pain relief is a good that morally outweighs the badness of death. But is the difference between intending and foreseeing the death crucial to the permissibility of the act? As we noted earlier, the physician may both believe that the morphine will hasten the patient's death and intend to hasten it. The physician may believe that the patient's pain is resistant to all attempts to manage it and that any relief will be only temporary. In such a case, it seems that pain relief and killing are inseparable intended effects. If they are inseparable, then if we are to condemn intentionally bringing about death, we must condemn intentionally relieving pain when it results in death as well. The two issues seem to stand or fall together. On the other hand, if pain relief through high-dose morphine is permissible, and if intending pain relief is inseparable from intending the patient's death, then intentionally killing the patient is permissible as well.

The point here is not that killing a patient is permissible in all cases, only in *some* cases. Still, our analysis suggests that whether death is intended or foreseen is not the crucial issue, because one can cause the same outcome intentionally or unintentionally. Instead, what matters is whether the act or its outcome benefits or harms the patient. And there will be some cases in which killing a patient can benefit him or her. This line of reasoning suggests that there is no morally significant difference between giving a drug for pain relief that indirectly causes death, and giving a drug that directly causes death. Specifically, it suggests that it would not be wrong to give a neuromuscular blocker to some patients. This type of drug paralyzes a patient's muscles, preventing breathing and resulting in certain death. Giving such a drug would not be palliation but euthanasia. But if it is the *only* way to relieve the patient's pain, and if it benefits the patient by preventing the greater harm of continued pain, then it is not obvious that it should be prohibited.

Isn't it incoherent to say that death can benefit a person? If death eliminates the person, then how can it benefit him or her? Aren't we eliminating the potential beneficiary? We can respond to these questions in the following way. A person's life could contain only pain and suffering and no compensating goods beyond a certain point. Such a person would be better off having a shorter life containing less pain and suffering than a longer life containing more of these uncompensated bad experiences. By ending these bad experiences, the person's death benefits him. Death prevents him from having a longer and worse life. This is coherent because we are comparing shorter and longer lives of the same person and determining whether he would be better or worse off in one or the other. A notable exception to this view is the concept of redemptive suffering. This is when one finds meaning in one's pain and suffering by relating them to something larger, such as God, humanity, or the universe. Redemptive suffering can make life valuable for a person even if the last stage of that life contains considerable pain and suffering. In either case, the critical ethical issue is not whether a patient's death is an intended or unintended but foreseen outcome for a physician. Rather, the issue is whether this outcome is better or worse for the patient, given his or her values and interests.

But it is controversial to claim that in some cases it is morally permissible to intentionally kill a patient or to assist a patient in a suicide. Even if one understands benefit and harm along the lines we have described, deliberately ending a life seems to conflict with the physician's duty to heal patients. It violates what many take to be an absolute duty inscribed in the Hippocratic Oath: Doctors must not kill. Because they are controversial, the permissibility of euthanasia and PAS need further elaboration and defense.

Euthanasia and Physician-Assisted Suicide

Euthanasia (from the Greek: *eu* = good; *thanatos* = death) means death that benefits the person who dies. The act that results in death is performed by someone other than the patient, usually a physician or nurse. Euthanasia is illegal in the United States, though it is legal in Belgium, the Netherlands, and Switzerland. In PAS, the act that results in death is performed by the patient, who is assisted by a physician or someone else who provides the means through which the patient can take his or her own life. Oregon is the only state in the United States where PAS is legal (since October 1997).

There are three types of euthanasia. *Voluntary* euthanasia involves a patient making a voluntary and persistent request that someone actively cause his or her death. *Involuntary* euthanasia involves killing a patient against his or her expressed wishes to the contrary, or without consulting such wishes. *Nonvoluntary* euthanasia involves someone killing a patient who is incompetent and unable to express his or her wishes about wanting to live or die. As we will see shortly, the third type of euthanasia presents the greatest potential for abuse. In these cases, decisions about whether to bring about a patient's death often are made by surrogates. It is not always obvious that they fully understand or act in the best interests of the patient.

In our discussion of DDE, we sketched an argument for the permissibility of voluntary euthanasia. We can lay it out more precisely in four steps. (1) It is permissible to cause a patient's death as an unintended side effect of giving morphine for pain relief when pain relief is in the patient's best interests and thus benefits him or her. (2) There is no morally significant distinction between foreseeing death as a result of giving a lethal dose of morphine for pain relief and intending the patient's death by giving a lethal dose of the drug for pain relief. (3) In some cases, intentionally bringing about a patient's death by giving a lethal dose of morphine is the only way to relieve pain. (4) Therefore, when pain relief is in the patient's best interests and thus benefits him or her, and when a lethal dose of morphine is the only way to relieve pain, it is permissible to intentionally cause the death of the patient by giving the drug. In other words, sometimes it is morally permissible to intentionally kill a patient. Because this is an argument for voluntary euthanasia, the patient must consent to being killed for it to be sound. It should be emphasized that this is an argument for the moral rather than legal permissibility of euthanasia.

Some will reject this argument. They will point to research indicating that more efficient delivery of opioid analgesics can effectively relieve even the most severe pain. When death occurs, it is due more likely to the underlying disease than to the effects of pain medication. This would obviate the need to give lethal doses of opioids and would allay fears that doctors and nurses might have in administering this medication. Epidural or spinal delivery systems can control pain for longer periods without depressing respiration and without hastening death. Moreover, recent research suggests the possibility of using drugs in combination with opiates that can inhibit their tendency to depress breathing. So the instances in which euthanasia is justified are relatively rare.

But there will always be some cases where pain cannot be controlled by any means. Everyone reacts differently to narcotics like morphine, which may manage pain for some people but not others. Terminal sedation may be the only alternative. In this procedure, a patient is sedated until he or she becomes unconscious and no longer can feel pain. Often other treatments such as artificial hydration and nutrition will be withheld until the patient dies. This practice is legally and morally permitted because it involves giving medication considered necessary to relieve pain, and because it is done with the patient's consent. Nevertheless, terminal sedation is an intentional act that kills the patient. If terminal sedation is permissible, then it seems that intentionally killing a patient by the other means we have described should be permissible as well.

Many will insist that doctors have an absolute duty not to kill patients. Killing patients conflicts with their duty to relieve pain and suffering and to heal. From the claim that a doctor has a duty to relieve pain and suffering, it does not follow that a doctor has a duty to kill a patient, even if it is the only means of pain relief. Yet in the (admittedly rare) cases in which pain is intractable to all medication, it is not clear how a doctor can heal a patient because healing means to make the patient whole again, to restore the unity of mind and body that has been severed by pain. Untreatable pain makes this reintegration difficult, if not impossible, to achieve. Furthermore, the claim that doctors must not kill needs qualification. Those who endorse a prohibition on euthanasia presuppose that killing is an intentional act. But we have seen that, even when a doctor foresees that giving a certain dose of morphine will depress respiration and eventually cause death, this can be described as killing the patient, albeit unintentionally. Opponents of euthanasia likely mean that doctors must not intentionally kill, and this is consistent with the principles stated in the Hippocratic Oath. Yet when continued life is the greater evil and death is the lesser evil, strictly abiding by this prohibition may mean that in some cases doctors will not just fail to benefit patients. They will harm them by prolonging their pain and suffering.

The claim that euthanasia is permissible only when a patient consents to it must be qualified as well. In the four-step argument for euthanasia, it was asserted that intentionally killing a patient is permissible when death is the lesser evil, continued pain the greater evil, and pain relief is in the patient's best interests. This assumes that he or she rationally and voluntarily consents to being killed. When a patient does this, he or she effectively waives the right not to be killed. The waiver releases medical professionals who are treating the patient from their duty not to kill him or her. (This does not imply a duty to kill a patient, however, as we will explain shortly.) Yet a doctor's duty to a patient does not entirely depend on the patient's consent to have or forego treatment. In addition to the duty to respect patient autonomy and consent, doctors have a duty not to harm patients. The first duty does not necessarily entail the second. A competent patient may voluntarily consent to or request a procedure even when it is not in his or her best interests to have it. For example, if a patient who has had a heart attack consents to donating a kidney for a transplant, then allowing the patient to donate could harm him. Given his condition, undergoing surgery could entail a significant risk of morbidity or even mortality. Moreover, a volunteer in a clinical trial may consent to an experimental procedure that exposes him to risk. As we discussed in Chapter 3, even with a volunteer's consent the researcher is obligated to ensure that the volunteer is not exposed to undue risk. This brings us back to euthanasia and the doctor's duty to relieve pain and suffering. Euthanasia is justified only when the patient consents to it, when ending the patient's life is the lesser evil, and allowing continued pain and suffering is the greater evil.

Some might argue that it is not enough for a doctor to be morally *permitted* to kill a patient in these cases. The doctor would be morally *obligated* to kill the patient because he or she has a duty to relieve pain and suffering. If the only way to achieve this is by ending the patient's life, then the doctor is morally obligated to do this. But it is difficult to justify the move from the weaker claim about a moral permission to kill to the stronger claim about a moral obligation to kill.

To say that a doctor has an obligation to kill a patient, even one with untreatable pain, suggests a radical departure from the standard interpretation of nonmaleficence and beneficence that few would accept. It is difficult to defend the claim that there is a decisive reason to intentionally kill a patient. It is also difficult to assess a patient's experience of pain, or whether medication is being delivered in the right dose and manner to adequately treat it. Furthermore, if we are comparing lesser and greater evils in these cases, rather than lesser and greater goods, then some might take this to mean that a doctor has an obligation to bring about one of these evils. But surely a patient can benefit from not experiencing the harm that comes through continued pain and suffering. By ending the patient's life, the doctor is preventing further harm to the patient and is thereby giving the patient a net benefit. In this respect, ending the patient's life can be a good.

Significantly, if a doctor is not obligated to kill a patient, but is at most permitted to do so, then this casts doubt on the claim that a patient has a right to die. A patient's right to die would entail a doctor's duty to ensure that this right was realized by killing the patient. To say that a person has a right entails a duty of other persons to treat him or her in a certain way. But if a doctor does not have a duty to kill a patient, then a patient does not have a right to be killed by a doctor. Even the idea of a prima facie right to euthanasia is questionable because it means that a doctor has a prima facie duty to kill a patient. The idea that there is such a duty conflicts with the common understanding of the goals of medicine and the professional integrity of doctors. In the final analysis, the only claim that can be defended is that, in some cases, voluntary euthanasia is morally permissible. It is permissible when it is the only way to relieve pain and suffering.

More controversial is whether voluntary euthanasia is permissible in order to relieve suffering that is not caused by pain. Even with good pain management, a patient with a terminal illness may suffer because he or she feels a loss of control over life, or believes that his or her life no longer has any dignity. Would a doctor or nurse be permitted to terminally sedate such a patient in order to relieve suffering? A full complement of palliative care, including psychosocial support, may alleviate the patient's emotional state. But if these measures cannot achieve this, then it would be prima facie permissible to administer terminal sedation when it is the only way to relieve the patient's suffering.

Can the same argument for the permissibility of euthanasia be given for PAS? Recall that PAS involves a patient requesting assistance in dying from a doctor. The patient performs the final act that ends his or her life. The doctor only provides the means for the patient to kill him or herself. PAS has figured prominently in public debate about medical decisions at the end of life since the Supreme Court ruling on two right-to-die cases in 1997. The Court reversed decisions in the Ninth and Second Federal Circuit Courts of Appeals, holding that state laws prohibiting PAS in New York and Washington were unconstitutional. These decisions had left states free to prohibit or permit it. In its *Cruzan* decision of 1990, the Court held that there is a constitutionally protected liberty interest in foregoing life-sustaining treatment. In its 1997 ruling, the Court upheld a patient's legal right to forego life-support and to receive palliative care, even if it involved terminal sedation. But it distinguished these practices legally and morally from PAS. The Court's main objection to PAS was that it was wrong because it involved intending the patient's death. Presumably, this is unlike foregoing life-support and palliative care that hastens death because, in these practices, the patient's death is not intended. This objection, and the distinction between intending and foreseeing death on which it rests, have considerable intuitive appeal. There is also the concern that permitting PAS would lead to abuse, where patients would feel coerced by financial or family pressure to take their own lives. Let's consider each of these objections in turn.

It has been argued that there is no morally significant difference between intending and foreseeing death when one has causal control over the sequence of events that leads to death. A physician or nurse can cause a patient's death by not offering CPR or by not putting a patient in respiratory distress on a respirator. One can play a causal role in an outcome by intentionally performing an act or by intentionally not performing an act when one knows or believes that this will ensure the outcome. Similarly, it does not matter morally whether a physician intends a patient's death by prescribing a lethal dose of barbiturates or other medication for the patient, or whether he or she foresees the patient's death as a possible outcome of prescribing them. Instead, what makes the physician's action morally permissible is that the patient consents to it and it is in the patient's best interests.

A physician may have multiple intentions in prescribing a lethal dose of barbiturates. Although giving the patient the prescription may lead to an overdose and death, the doctor's intention may be only to relieve the patient's anxiety and allay his or her fears. Instead of intending the patient's death, the physician may intend that the patient have more choice and thus more control over the time and manner of death. Providing a patient with the necessary means to commit suicide does not imply that the physician intends the patient's death. Because a physician may not intend death by prescribing the means necessary for a patient's suicide in one instance, and because a physician may intend a patient's death by foregoing life-sustaining treatment in another instance, the difference between intention and foresight cannot justify a moral distinction between the two. If one is permitted, then the other should be permitted as well. So we can question the reasoning behind the Court's ruling in *Vacco v. Quill* and *Washington v. Glucksberg*.

Like euthanasia, PAS is morally permissible when a competent patient is terminally ill, makes a voluntary and persistent request for it, when it is in the patient's best interests, and when it is the only way to relieve pain and suffering. Put another way, PAS is permissible when death for the patient is the lesser evil and continued life is the greater evil. Provided that these conditions are in place, one can defend PAS against the claim that it violates a physician's duty to heal by relieving pain and suffering. Again, better pain management and palliative care may obviate the need for PAS in most cases. If optimal end-of-life care were available, then patients might not feel forced to turn to PAS.

Nevertheless, there will be some cases where this care is not available. Some patients will prefer not to endure a dying process they find worse than an earlier death. As we noted earlier, many people who seek either euthanasia or assisted suicide are motivated not by unbearable pain, but by factors such as indignity or loss of independence. Palliative care and PAS should be seen as complementary rather than conflicting. Having both options can enhance the sense of control patients have over the end of their lives and ensure that they have a humane and dignified death. As Dan Brock (1999) argues, rather than prohibit PAS, we should aim "*both* to galvanize efforts to improve the care of all dying patients *and* to make PAS available to those patients for whom PAS remains preferable to the best care available to them" (p. 543, emphasis added).

Opponents of PAS cite the potential for abuse as another reason for prohibiting the practice. Permitting doctors to assist patients in dying would put us on a slippery slope. At the bottom of the slope, patients would be coerced into ending their lives by anxiety over the cost of their care to others or otherwise feeling that they are a burden on others. The main area of potential abuse is when a patient is incompetent and a surrogate makes a life-ending decision for him. This is especially problematic if the patient has not expressed any preference for how he would want others to act if he became terminally ill or if the surrogate ignores the patient's expressed preference. But an advance directive formalizes such a preference. This directive can prevent abuse of PAS when it is based on open dialogue between the patient and the surrogate.

Additional safeguards can prevent abuse, too, and we have mentioned some of them already. Specifically, six conditions for PAS to be morally permissible. (1) There must be a diagnosis of terminal illness. (2) The patient must be suffering from an unbearable and irreversible condition. (3) The patient must be informed about the diagnosis and prognosis of his or her condition, as well as about alternatives to PAS, such as hospice care and other palliative services. (4) The patient who requests PAS must not be suffering from treatable depression. (5) The patient must make an enduring and voluntary request for assistance in dying. (6) When a patient dies as a result of PAS, the doctors who assist him or her must report it to the regulatory authorities. Oregon adopted these guidelines in 1997. The potential for abuse of PAS will never be eliminated, but the guidelines we have listed can significantly minimize this potential.

In the wake of the 1997 Supreme Court ruling on the two cases we have mentioned, a group of distinguished philosophers issued an *amicus curiae* ("friend of the court") brief. They urged the Court to uphold the decisions of the lower Second and Ninth Circuit Courts affirming that, in a limited class of cases, patients have a constitutionally protected right to secure the help of willing physicians in ending their lives. The main author of the brief, Ronald Dworkin (1997), stated that the brief defended the constitutional principle that "every competent person has the right to make momentous personal decisions which invoke fundamental religious or philosophical convictions about life's value for himself" (p. 41). Dworkin and his coauthors maintained that this principle supported a protected right to PAS because "death is, for each of us, among the most significant events of life" (p. 44). Dworkin and colleagues argued from the premise that it is permissible to forego or terminate treatment with the intention that the patient die, to the conclusion that it is permissible to assist a patient in dying with the intention that the patient die. If a doctor can permissibly turn off a respirator and thereby end a patient's life, then the doctor can permissibly prescribe pills that a patient may use to take his or her own life.

There may not be a morally significant difference between killing and letting a patient die when we consider the question in terms of the *doctor's intention*. But there does seem to be a morally significant difference between killing and letting die when we consider the question in terms of *patients' rights*. When competent patients refuse treatment, they are exercising a negative right to bodily noninterference. A patient may intend to die by refusing the treatment or might foresee that he or she may die by refusing it. More importantly, the physician would have a duty to respect the patient's exercise of this negative right and be prohibited from giving treatment. The alternative would be to force treatment on the patient, which would violate the negative right to noninterference. On the other hand, doctors do not have a duty to offer a treatment to a patient simply because he or she requests it. A patient has at most a positive right to receive treatment, and positive rights entail a weaker obligation for others to respect them than do negative rights. If lethal medication for suicide is considered a treatment that would satisfy a patient's positive right, then the physician is not obligated to prescribe it. If there is a duty here, then surely it is much weaker than the duty to respect the patient's right to forego treatment.

The alternative to letting die is forcing treatment, which is morally prohibited. The alternative to assisted suicide is doing nothing, leaving the patient alone. It would be difficult to argue that doing nothing in such a case should be morally prohibited. Forcing treatment on a patient is morally worse than failing to offer treatment that would not prevent death and might even hasten it. So there is an asymmetry in the moral evaluation of killing and letting die when we describe them in terms of a patient's negative and positive rights to refuse or have treatment. As F. M. Kamm (1997) puts it, leaving the patient alone often "does not violate any of his rights against us, and so we can, and sometimes we should be required to refuse to help because we disapprove of his goals" (p. 23). The patient's goal of taking his or her own life may conflict with the doctor's understanding of the goals of medicine, as well as his or her personal and professional integrity. Even if we cannot defend the stronger claim that a doctor is prohibited from helping a patient to die, we can defend the weaker claim that a doctor is not required to help a patient to die. If a doctor is not required and thus has no duty to help in this way, then we can question whether there is a right to PAS.

The duty to respect a patient's right to refuse treatment does not imply a duty to respect a patient's wish to be aided in suicide. Thus, we cannot move from the right to refuse treatment considered in *Cruzan* to the permissibility of assisted suicide considered in *Vacco v. Quill* and *Washington v. Glucksberg*. From the doctor's perspective, being obligated not to do something and being permitted to do something are morally distinct. The force of the reasons for or against foregoing or giving treatment is different in these cases. We can characterize PAS as a form of giving treatment. But it is one thing to claim that a doctor is permitted to assist a patient in dying. It is quite another thing to claim that a doctor is obligated to assist a patient in dying. The move from the first claim to the second is unwarranted, and therefore the most we can say is that PAS is morally permissible.

Futility

In many instances of critical medical care, the ability to sustain life does not mean that the disease process will be reversed and that the patient will be restored to normal functioning. Technological advances that have enabled many people to survive life-threat-ening conditions have increased the number of patients with chronic persistent illness. The burdens resulting from these inter-ventions can outweigh the benefits. But this judgment is often a source of conflict between doctors and patients or the surrogates or families of incompetent patients. Families may insist that "every-thing" be done to enable the patient to survive. Doctors may insist that continuing treatment is not medically indicated and that do-ing so would not be in the patient's best interests. They may claim that the treatment is "futile," and believe that they are entitled to make a unilateral decision to withdraw the treatment, despite the wishes of the patient, surrogate, or family to the contrary.

A futile action is one that is useless or ineffectual, in the sense that it cannot achieve its goal. The term "futility" derives from Greek mythology, and the idea is implicit in Hippocrates's injunc-tion that physicians should refuse to treat patients for whose dis-eases medicine is powerless. Today, the power of medicine to pro-long life has not resulted in a corresponding power to control many diseases. Yet whether a treatment is futile is open to different and often conflicting interpretations. Doctors usually understand "fu-tility" in quantitative terms, focusing only on the patient's physi-ological functioning. In contrast, families of incompetent patients usually understand the term in qualitative terms. They insist that the value of the patient's life cannot be measured by his or her physiological functioning alone. This second view is problematic as well, however, since the wishes of family members are often mo-tivated by fear, guilt, and other negative emotions influenced by family dynamics. These different interpretations of futility can gen-erate disagreement and conflict between doctors and families con-cerning the goals of treatment and whether they can be achieved. This type of conflict has raised questions about what the goals of medicine are and, indeed, what they should be.

An illustration of this conflict was the *Wanglie* case in Minnesota in 1991. Helga Wanglie was an eighty-seven-year-old patient who had fallen into a PVS and was maintained on a respirator. Her doc-tors argued that continuing life-support would be futile because it could not restore her to consciousness. But Helga's husband pointed out that, while she was competent, she never indicated any preference for or against life-sustaining treatment. He insisted that her doctors not "play God" and that life-support should continue. The hospital sought a court order to have a conservator appointed who might consent to the removal of the respirator on Helga's behalf. Yet the judicial ruling denied the hospital's request and upheld Mr. Wanglie's request that treatment continue. Helga Wanglie died three days after the court ruling despite continued aggressive treatment. In this type of case, it would be difficult to defend continuing life-support because there is no point in sustaining a human organism for its own sake. But in cases where patients are comatose or deteriorating but not in a PVS, the claim that treatment should be discontinued because it serves no beneficial purpose is not such a simple and straightforward matter.

We said that doctors interpret futility in quantitative terms, while patients and families interpret futility in qualitative terms. The first interpretation involves medical facts, while the second involves personal values. But this fact-value distinction is flawed. Many judgments by doctors concerning which treatments should or should not be given to patients are value-laden. This is partly because of the uncertainty in assessing medical information. The same information can lead different doctors to make different assessments of a patient's prognosis. These assessments may involve qualitative judgments about the burdens and benefits of treatment. For instance, while one doctor may interpret the claim that a patient has a 20 percent chance of survival positively, another doctor may interpret it negatively. This disparity can influence decisions about how aggressive treatment should be to sustain life. In addition, there may be disagreement among medical staff about what constitutes a reasonable period of time in trying to reverse or control the disease process. So, many quantitative judgments about a patient's medical conditions may have a qualitative dimension. The value-laden nature of these medical judgments can lead to or exacerbate conflicts between doctors and patients' families concerning whether to continue, increase, or discontinue life-sustaining treatment.

Still, conflicts can be averted through better communication between doctors and families. At the earliest possible time in a case of life-threatening illness, doctors should initiate discussion with families so that they can agree on reasonable goals of treatment for the patient, as well as how these goals can be achieved. There should be some latitude with respect to the duration of the treatment. When doctors believe that treatment should be withdrawn and families believe that it should be continued, a time-limited trial may be the best way to accommodate these conflicting points of view. This sort of compromise is one way of resolving such conflicts. Ideally, greater emphasis on the process of deliberating and deciding about treatment and on involving families and doctors as joint decision makers can avert many instances of conflict.

But when a conflict persists and cannot be resolved through dialogue with families, the case may go through a process of conflict resolution. Here a third party such as an ethics committee makes a recommendation about whether treatment should be continued or withdrawn. If that fails, then the courts will decide. As part of this process, the medical team can argue that withdrawing treatment is justified on the ground that it does not meet a reasonable standard of care and is not consistent with the goals of medicine. Such a decision would be justified when it is obvious that continued treatment could not restore the patient to adequate functioning and would only increase his suffering. The burdens of continuing life-sustaining treatment would clearly outweigh any possible benefits, in which case only palliative care would be justified. If patients are too sick to suffer, then treatment is pointless. Framing the issue in terms of whether a treatment meets a reasonable standard of care is a more constructive way of avoiding or resolving disagreement than using the more controversial "futility."

Many will argue that futility is less about standard of care and more about quality of life. Again, to some extent a doctor's assessment of the patient's condition will be qualitative. Nevertheless, there can be objective agreement on what constitutes reasonable goals of life-sustaining treatment, reasonable means of achieving these goals, and a baseline of quality of life under which no patient should fall. This agreement will involve medical professionals and society as a whole. When a treatment requested by a patient, surrogate, or family fails to meet this standard, it is permissible to stop treatment. Indeed, it may be obligatory to do so if continued treatment causes further suffering and undermines the patient's dignity.

Helga Wanglie's husband and others might argue that the issue here is not futility, but the sanctity of human life. As long as the body is breathing, treatment should continue because the life of the body has intrinsic value. But it sounds counterintuitive to say that the value of a life can be separated from the person whose life it is, or to say that a body can have value when the person who inhabited it has ceased to exist. More importantly, this idea could justify continuing life-sustaining treatment that would increase a patient's pain and suffering. Sanctity of life therefore does not offer a good reason for extending a person's life.

Conclusion

Advances in medical technology have enabled medical professionals to sustain the lives of patients who otherwise would have died from trauma or disease. These advances have raised a number of ethical questions. Some of these questions turn on the more fundamental issue of how we define death. We considered different definitions of death and discussed their implications for procuring organs for transplantation. We also examined the distinction between withdrawing and withholding treatment and found that there is no morally significant difference between them when doing something and allowing something to occur both can cause death. Similarly, we argued that there is no morally significant distinction between intending and foreseeing death when one can cause death both by performing and not performing a certain action. This casts doubt on the DDE as a helpful guide in determining when it is, or is not, permissible to cause a patient's death.

It was argued that sometimes euthanasia and PAS are morally permissible. A doctor can permissibly kill a patient, and permissibly assist a patient in suicide, when death is the lesser evil, continued life the greater evil, and death is in the patient's best interests. With respect to PAS, it was noted that a doctor may prescribe a lethal dose of barbiturates to give the patient a choice between palliative care and terminal sedation and thus greater control over the time and manner of his or her death. Finally, we discussed the concept of futility and noted that better communication between doctors and the families of incompetent patients might help to avoid or resolve conflicts about whether to continue or discontinue treatment.

In too many cases, life-sustaining technology has meant a disproportionate ratio of burdens to benefits for patients. A longer life is not necessarily a better life. Whether a person's life should be sustained, or whether it can permissibly be ended, will depend on the doctor's views on the goals of medicine. But even more so, it will depend on the patient's interests and values. Life is valuable for the person whose life it is. Accordingly, the patient should have at least some control over how that life ends. Dying should be humane and dignified, not a process of prolonged pain, suffering, and indignity. This view reflects the proposals made by the Hastings Center (1997) concerning medical treatment at the end of life. The proposals argue for "the avoidance of premature death" and for the "pursuit of a peaceful death" and maintain that "the struggle against death in many of its manifestations is an important goal of medicine. Yet it should always remain in a healthy tension with medicine's duty to accept death as the destiny of all human beings" (p. 22).

Selected Readings

Brock, D. "A Critique of Three Objections to Physician-Assisted Suicide." *Ethics* 109(1999): 519–47.

Dworkin, G., Frey, R., and Bok, S. *Euthanasia and Physician-Assisted Suicide: For and Against.* New York: Cambridge University Press, 1998.

Dworkin, R., et al. "Assisted Suicide: The Philosophers' Brief." *New York Review of Books* 44(1997): 41–47.

Hastings Center. "The Goals of Medicine: Setting New Priorities." *Hastings Center Report, Special Supplement.* 26(1997): 2–26.

Kamm, F. M. *Morality, Mortality, Volume I: Death and Whom to Save From It.* Oxford: Oxford University Press, 1993.

Kamm, F. M. "A Right to Choose Death?" *Boston Review* 22(1997): 21–23.

McMahan. J. *The Ethics of Killing: Life at the Margins.* Oxford: Oxford University Press, 2001.

Rhodes, R. "Futility and the Goals of Medicine." *Journal of Clinical Ethics* 9(1998): 194–205.

Veatch, R. *Death, Dying, and the Biological Revolution.* 2d ed. New Haven, Conn.: Yale University Press, 1992.

Youngner, S., and Arnold, R. "Philosophical Debates About the Definition of Death: Who Cares?" *Journal of Medicine and Philosophy* 26(2001): 527–37.

CHAPTER 7

Allocating Scarce Medical Resources

Introduction

Providing health care is one thing, but paying for it is quite another. Health care spending has risen dramatically in the United States over the last twenty years. This is due to such factors as an aging population, unnecessary tests and procedures, expensive CT and MRI scans, and expensive drugs to treat various chronic medical conditions. Presently, health care spending constitutes roughly 15 percent of the U.S. gross domestic product, which is well ahead of the percentage in other developed countries. Paradoxically, 43 million Americans (more than 15 percent of the population) have no health insurance.

Rationing is a way of controlling inflation of health care costs. It consists in limiting medical services within predetermined levels, thus resulting in scarcity of medical resources. There is an *economic* sense of scarcity driven by the aim to control costs. This is distinct from a *physical* sense of scarcity, which pertains to such issues as the availability of organs for transplantation. Because there are not enough medical resources to meet the medical needs of all people, we need a system of rationing our resources to meet these needs as best we can. At the same time, however, this system must respect people's claims to have their basic medical needs met. In allocating scarce medical resources, there inevitably will be trade-offs between equality and fairness, on the one hand, and efficiency and efficacy, on the other. Yet any sustainable health care system must incorporate equal access to basic medical services and good health outcomes as complementary rather than competing goals.

Rationing medical care raises the following ethical questions. How much moral weight should be given to the idea of equal access to services and how much to outcomes? Should priority be given to prevention over research and treatment? Is it morally permissible to discriminate on the basis of age, giving priority to the young over the old when they compete for a particular treatment? When we assess the value of a particular treatment in terms of its outcome, how do we weigh additional life-years against the quality of life of those years? Can a person's social worth justify giving him or her higher priority over others for an organ transplant? Can a person's lifestyle justify giving him or her lower priority for a transplant? On what grounds would a two-tiered health care system be justifiable or unjustifiable? We will discuss these and other ethical questions about health resource allocation in this chapter.

Setting Priorities

Any system of priority regarding how medical resources should be distributed presupposes a theory of distributive justice. We briefly discussed justice in Chapter 1; but we need to develop it further here. Justice concerns what is due or owed to persons, especially with respect to benefits and burdens. Distributive justice concerns how social goods like health care should be distributed across persons. There are four main theories of distributive justice. Utilitarian (or consequentialist) theories of justice are based on the principle of utility. These say that a policy is just when it maximizes overall utility. Libertarian theories of justice focus on rights to social and economic liberty, emphasizing fair procedures rather than substantive outcomes. Communitarian theories of justice rely on practices that have evolved through the traditions of a community. Egalitarian theories focus on how some people fare relative to others. They say that a situation is just when there is equal access to certain goods, when access is necessary to meet people's claims of need, and when these claims are given equal weight across people.

Health care in the United States traditionally has been based on the free-market principle that the distribution of medical services is best left to the marketplace. This emphasizes the idea that we should pay for these services, an idea informed by a libertarian conception of justice. We do not have a right to health care. Rather, health care is a good that we can purchase in different forms or different degrees, depending on how we value it. The recent move to make people pay higher deductibles and co-payments for health care is based on libertarian market principles regarding its value. But this means that whether one has health care, or how much of it one has, will depend on one's ability to pay. An unfortunate consequence of this system is the large number of uninsured and underinsured Americans. They either cannot afford the high cost of health care on their own, or their employers refuse to pay for it. Many argue that market principles should not apply to health care because good health is priceless. A communitarian theory of justice offers a possible solution to the main problem with libertarianism, and we will explore this possibility when we address the issue of age-based rationing. Generally, though, the trade-off between equal access to medical services and the outcomes of these services is the main issue in medical rationing. For this reason, egalitarian and consequentialist theories of justice are most germane to our discussion.

The most well-known egalitarian theory of justice is that of John Rawls. He maintains that a situation is just if no changes in the expectations of those who are better off can improve the situation of those who are worse off. Justice is defined in terms of fairness. A fair distribution of a good is one that meets people's claims of need, where the claims of those in greater need are given greater weight. This suggests that the concern is not with equality as such, but with priority. Indeed, in Rawls's second principle of justice, or what he calls the "difference principle," inequalities in the distribution of social goods are admissible only if they benefit the least advantaged members of society. The aim is to give the worse off the same range of normal lifetime opportunities open to better-off members of society. People's basic health care needs must be met in order to have these opportunities. Therefore, those whose medical needs have not been met should be given priority in access to basic medical care. A consequentialist theory of justice is not concerned with equal access to medical services, but with maximizing good outcomes of these services. Such a theory is more concerned with the total amount of a good like health than with the rights and interests of the people who have it. As noted in Chapter 1, consequentialism derives from the utilitarianism of Jeremy Bentham and John Stuart

Mill. It will be instructive to consider various scenarios in which there can be different priorities in the distribution of medical services on the basis of egalitarian and consequentialist reasons.

Genetic research has considerable potential for treatment of many conditions. Most diseases have a genetic component. Research into the genetic mechanisms of these diseases could lead to treatments that could more effectively control or even cure cancer, heart disease, diabetes, and other disorders that afflict large numbers of people. In the future, many people could benefit from this research. Currently, many more people could benefit from such preventive measures as prenatal care, better hygiene, a cleaner environment, diet, and lifestyle. These measures could greatly reduce the incidence of chronic disease and enable many people to be healthy and to have more opportunities over the balance of their lives. Programs designed to prevent disease are less costly than research designed to develop new treatments for disease. Preventive programs can also benefit more people. This suggests that we should give priority in health care spending to prevention rather than to research and treatment.

With prevention, the aim is to meet people's medical needs from the beginning of their lives. With research and treatment, the aim is to meet people's medical needs as they develop over the course of their lives. If more people benefit from prevention than from research and treatment, then it seems that the first should have priority over the second. This does not mean that priority should be absolute, and that the claims of need of the sick should have no weight. Rather, the reasons for prevention are generally stronger than the reasons for research and treatment. These reasons can be egalitarian as well as consequentialist. Preventing disease promotes equal opportunity at the same time that it maximizes benefits and minimizes harms. Similar reasoning applies when the question is whether priority should be given to treatment *or* to research. Because many more people would benefit, priority should be given to treatments that can cure prevalent infectious diseases, like tuberculosis and malaria, over research that might cure rare genetic diseases, like cystic fibrosis or Huntington's. Still, considerable weight should be given to genetic research aimed at controlling or curing infectious diseases because of the number of people they affect.

We can stipulate that the worse off are the sick, and the better off are the healthy. Obviously, these classifications will be matters of degree, because some people will be sicker or healthier than others. On the priority view, the value of a benefit will depend on how sick or healthy one is. A smaller benefit to a sick person has more value than a greater benefit to a healthy person. Yet there is one situation where this claim cannot be defended. When the greater benefit to a healthy person is the avoidance of a condition that would be worse than the condition of a currently sick person, we should give the greater benefit to the healthy person. Thus, priority to the worse off should not be absolute. When benefits to the healthy are significantly greater than benefits to the sick, and when the sick benefit only slightly, we can override priority to the worse off in the distribution of health resources. Moreover, if a sicker person cannot benefit from medical care, and if giving care to him or her means that it will be denied to another person who is not as sick and would benefit from it, then priority to the worse off can be overridden as well.

This last point can be illustrated by the example of how limited resources such as life-sustaining treatment are used in an ICU. Egalitarians would say that each patient with a life-threatening condition has an equal right and an equal claim to have access to the ICU. Those who believe in giving strict priority to the worst off would say that the sickest patient should be treated first. But this can lead to an untenable outcome. If a patient so sick that he or she will not survive regardless of treatment is given priority over another patient who is not as sick and has a better chance of surviving and being restored to normal functioning, then neither patient will benefit and both will die. Leaving aside the question of whether doctors or institutions should be responsible for rationing decisions, limited ICU resources should be used to maximize health benefits for patients. This goal is achieved not simply by enabling patients to survive, but by restoring them to normal functioning. Patients likely to benefit from treatment should receive it, and those unlikely to benefit from it should not. This weakens the force of the claim that any critically ill patient has an absolute right to have access to critical care. When we say that patients should have access to care, we at least implicitly assume that they will benefit to some degree from the care. When two patients differ significantly in the likelihood of benefiting from the same treatment, with the less sick patient more likely to benefit than the sicker patient, this difference can override giving treatment priority to the latter. In Robert Truog's words: "A strategy that seeks to maximize the health benefits available from scarce ICU resources may therefore be justified in overriding the right of individuals to demand unlimited access to resources from which they are very unlikely to benefit" (1992, p. 16).

Admittedly, the ICU involves *acute* care. This is distinct from the *chronic* care in the earlier discussion of priority in prevention versus treatment. These two types of care correspond to two different senses of being worse off. One pertains to being sick *at* a time. The other pertains to being sick *over* time. Some people are worse off for brief periods because of physical trauma or infection. Others are worse off due to conditions such as diabetes, asthma, and heart disease, which affect them for long periods. Accordingly, the care used to meet these two types of medical need will be different, and allocation decisions in each scenario should reflect these differences. In all cases of medical need, though, the aim of providing medical care should be to raise or restore people to a decent minimum level of normal physical and mental functioning. We should give priority to the medically worst off. But this should be contingent on the likelihood that medical care will raise or restore them to the decent minimum. The moral calculus of benefits and burdens depends on where people fall with respect to this baseline. There are egalitarian reasons for this position, in addition to consequentialist ones. Giving resource priority to the sickest patients who are unlikely to benefit from medical care may be a poor use of resources that is unfair to those with less urgent, but still significant, medical needs. It could deny the latter access to care that would maintain them at, or restore them to, a level of normal functioning.

The idea that all people should have access to a decent minimum of care that will enable them to have normal functioning is based on an egalitarian theory of justice. Access to a basic package of immunizations, antibiotics, emergency care, surgical care, and continuity of care with a general practitioner will enable patients to have adequate opportunities for achieving a reasonable level of wellbeing. Yet there are some conditions that prevent people from reaching the decent minimum. Many people with disabilities are unable to achieve what we would call "normal functioning," or a "decent minimum." The very old may not be able to have normal functioning either. Yet both groups can benefit from treatments that reduce pain and suffering resulting from their conditions and thus improve the quality of their lives. They may also benefit from treatments that extend their lives.

The Oregon Basic Health Services Act of 1989 shows the difficulty of setting allocation priorities when diverse groups of people have different medical needs. The aim of the Act was to expand Medicaid coverage to the roughly 16 percent of Oregonians who were uninsured and thus achieve an adequate level of care for all of the state's citizens. To do this, Oregon devised a rationing system in which services were ranked according to seventeen categories that described the expected outcome of treatment. Beyond primary care, medical procedures were ranked in terms of the net improvement that could be expected from a given treatment, compared with non-treatment. This ranking was framed in terms of both life extension and the quality of life that would result from a treatment. Procedures expected to save patients' lives and restore them to a normal level of functioning were ranked higher than those expected to benefit them only marginally. By giving low ranking to and limiting procedures that were costly and not likely to produce a significant benefit, the Oregon plan aimed to reduce costs and use the savings to offer a decent minimum of care for all. In these respects, it incorporated both fairness and efficiency into its allocation of scarce medical resources.

Yet some objected that this proposal was biased against the elderly and the disabled. Because the elderly have lived longer and are more likely to have more comorbid medical conditions than the young, the net benefit of treatments for them would not be as great as the net benefit of other treatments for the young. Generally, the quantity and quality of additional life-years resulting from treatments will be greater for the young than for the old. Similarly, people with disabilities claimed that the Oregon plan was biased against them because, on average, they do not live as long as people without disabilities. More importantly, they argued that the disabled have a different understanding of "benefit" and "quality of life" than healthy people. Some of these concerns influenced U.S. Secretary of Health and Human Services Louis Sullivan, leading him to reject the Oregon plan in 1992. Criticism of the plan was based largely on objections to the use of quality-adjusted life-years (QALYs) as the main criterion for setting allocation priorities.

Quality-Adjusted Life-Years

Economists introduced the concept of QALYs in the 1980s to measure the cost-effectiveness of medical interventions. QALYs measure the value of additional life-years produced by a treatment, adjusted for quality. A QALY regards a year of healthy life expectancy to have a value of 1, but regards a life of unhealthy life expectancy to have a value of less than 1. The value of a QALY will be lower the worse the quality of an unhealthy person's life is. In principle, a QALY could be negative, in the sense that someone's quality of life could be judged worse than being dead. Coronary artery bypass surgery that restores a person who has suffered a heart attack to normal functioning may have a high QALY. It saves the person's life and ensures a considerable number of quality life-years following the procedure. Hip replacement surgery for someone with painful osteoarthritis may have a high QALY as well. In contrast, neurosurgery for a cerebral aneurysm that leaves one with severe cognitive and physical impairment would have a low, perhaps even negative, QALY. The QALY will be higher in the first two cases the younger the patient is, though it would be lower in the third case if the patient is young.

John Harris has argued that QALYs are biased against the old because younger people have more life expectancy to be gained from treatment. People with disabilities raise a similar objection. On average, they have shorter and more painful and restricted lives than younger, healthier people. What QALYs fail to appreciate is that quality-of-life assessments can vary greatly across people. They ignore the fact that there is an essential subjective element to quality of life. These assessments cannot be separated from the point of view of the person who experiences the disability first-hand. A disabled person may say that he or she has good quality of life, even though a healthy person might not agree with that assessment.

This brings us back to the idea of making priority to the worse off contingent on benefit. If a treatment has a low QALY, such that the net benefit of the treatment is low and will not raise a person to the decent minimum, then the treatment should be given low priority. But this may mean that the needs of the elderly and disabled will not be met. Treatments that relieve pain and suffering, but that only marginally improve functioning, will not have much value on the QALY scale. Yet the elderly and disabled may value these treatments highly. Some people who are already badly off because they are well below the baseline of normal functioning will be made even worse off because it will not be cost-effective to treat their conditions.

This leads to what Harris calls the "double jeopardy" objection to QALYs:

> QALYs dictate that because an individual is unfortunate, because she has once become a victim of a disaster, we are required to visit upon her a second and perhaps graver misfortune. The first disaster leaves her with a poor quality of life and QALYs then require that, in virtue of this, she be ruled out as a candidate for life-saving treatment, or at best, that she be given little or no chance of benefiting from what little amelioration her condition admits of. (1987, p. 119)

QALYs can be criticized on the ground that they fail to consider the needs and values of the lives of these two groups of people and therefore are unfair to them. To the extent that the elderly and the disabled value their lives, it seems unfair to give lower priority to treatments that could benefit them because the net benefit of the treatment would be lower than the net benefit of treatments for younger and generally healthier people. Rather than having the highest priority in the allocation of medical resources, the worst off seem to have the lowest priority.

Alternatively, we could use disability-adjusted life-years (DALYs) to measure the value of intervention. Here the aim is not to *increase* the number of quality life-years, but to *decrease* the number of disabled years one would have without an intervention. But DALYs are not obviously any more helpful to those with conditions that would not significantly improve after an intervention.

What should be emphasized is that priority to the worse off is a conditional rather than absolute principle. It depends not only on how much they will benefit (which is what QALYs measure), but also on whether the use of resources for them will limit the use of resources for others who could be raised to the decent minimum. We should differentiate medical resources according to different medical goals and needs and allocate them accordingly. But, given that medical resources are limited, we have to set priorities specifying which of these goals and needs are the most important to achieve and meet. An allocation that gave priority to meeting the basic medical needs of Oregon's more numerous poor over the different but important needs of the less numerous disabled and elderly could be justified. By not receiving a basic package of medical services, the uninsured would not be able to reach the decent minimum and would have a greater likelihood of having chronic disease over the course of their lives. The difference between the benefits and harms to them with and without basic care is significantly greater than the difference between the benefits and harms to the elderly and the disabled with and without the special care they need.

It is important to point out that giving priority to basic care for the uninsured over special care for the elderly and disabled does not mean that services for the latter two groups should be excluded. Each of these groups is worse off than the young and healthy and arguably worse off than the uninsured. This is arguable because young adults and children constitute the majority of the uninsured, and it is not obvious that the elderly fare worse than uninsured children. But there are good reasons for giving priority to those who are badly off but not the worst off if doing so means a greater difference between benefit and harm. The crucial point is to use resources so that the greatest number will be raised to, or remain at, a decent minimum of normal functioning. Ideally, an allocation system could be devised in which we could *both* ensure a decent minimum of health care for all people *and* meet the special needs of the elderly and disabled. Despite its shortcomings, something along the lines of the Oregon plan still appears to be the most promising way of realizing these goals. We must respect people's claims of need and provide access to the care that will meet these needs. But this must be done with a view to maximizing benefits and minimizing harms across all people.

Age-Based Rationing

We have discussed the objection that the criteria of quality of life and life extension in allocating medical resources are biased against the old and in favor of the young. Yet some believe that it is not unfair to give lower priority to the old and higher priority to the young. The idea behind this view is that a younger person should have the opportunity to live as many years as an older person already has lived. Fairness requires that the first individual should have priority over the second in access to medical care so that he or she can complete the same lifespan. This view is based on the belief that people's needs *over* an entire lifetime, rather than *at* particular times or stages of their lives, should provide the temporal framework for allocation decisions.

Norman Daniels has proposed a "prudential lifespan account" in articulating a principle of fair distribution of health resources between the young and the old. For Daniels, the principle of fairness applies not to particular life stages, but to lives as wholes. He asks us to imagine a prudential chooser deciding how to budget resources over her lifetime. She does not know her current age, gender, values, or other particular facts about herself. She asks herself how she should distribute resources over the different stages of her life. Prudence requires that one think of one's life as a temporal whole, and to make that life as good as it can be. The question of how to allocate health resources between different people of different ages reduces to the question of how to allocate resources between different stages of one life. Allocation becomes a question of intergenerational justice.

There are at least two problems with Daniels's account. First, not everyone will reach old age. So an allocation scheme that included all the stages of life might turn out to be imprudent for those who die prematurely. They would not be able to use what they had saved. Second, prudence seeks to maximize total lifetime well-being, and the stages of life are treated equally insofar as they contribute to this goal. This might lead us to discount rather than save for the needs of old age, when declining health can detract from total lifetime well-being. Suppose that one person has been diseased for many years with a low quality of life. Another person has been healthy for the same number of years. Both go to the hospital with an acute condition requiring treatment. On the prudential lifespan account, the fair decision would be to give priority to the person with the lower lifetime quality. Yet it seems objectionable not to focus instead on the present state of need of each patient. The view that we should focus only on medical need at particular times or stages of life has problems of its own, however. The elderly consume a disproportionate amount of health care resources, because they have more medical needs than other age groups. But if we give priority to the old in order to extend and improve the quality of their lives, then the young who are sick and in need of medical care might not receive what they need. As a result, they might not be able to live as many years as the old already have lived. This seems unfair to the young.

Daniel Callahan's proposal for resolving this problem is to distinguish between two general types of medical resources. These correspond to different types of need pertaining to young and old age groups. Like Daniels, Callahan raises the question of how much of a claim different age groups should have to medical resources within a framework of intergenerational justice. This question is motivated in turn by the broader question of how health care can contribute to the good of society. Callahan argues for a revised understanding of aging that will benefit the lives of the old as well as the lives of the young. Our social obligation to the elderly is to help them to live out a natural lifespan of seventy-five to eighty years. Society is obligated only to provide the health care that will enable people to achieve this goal. Beyond that, health care should aim not to extend life, but only to relieve suffering. This could include home care, pain medication, and other treatments that directly address medical needs. By rationing health care among the elderly in this way, the savings gained from what would have been expensive life-extending interventions could be used for medical services that would enable the young to complete the same natural lifespan.

Suppose that each of two people needs an expensive drug to survive, but there is only enough of the drug to save one. One patient is fifty, the other forty-five. We could argue that, because the forty-five-year-old has lived less than the fifty-year-old, he should receive the drug. We could appeal to the "fair innings" argument to support his claim. This argument, which is implicit in Callahan's proposal, says that each person should have an equal claim to complete a natural lifespan. Because a younger person has had fewer innings (years) than an older person, a fair decision is one that gives the first priority over the second. But suppose that the older person has an equally strong desire to go on living. If this desire is not fulfilled, then he suffers the same fate as the forty-five-year-old in not having his desire to go on living fulfilled. Assuming that each patient would have a good outcome from treatment with the drug, that neither has completed a natural lifespan, and that the difference in their age is not significant, the fair innings argument has little force in this case.

The older person's biological age may be significantly greater than his chronological age, which might weigh the balance in favor of the younger person. Yet this would be a consequentialist consideration pertaining to the likely outcome of the treatment. It would not be based on the egalitarian consideration of whether chronological age should be a factor in determining a fair allocation policy. Older people have enjoyed more of life; younger people have enjoyed less. When the difference in age is significant, it may be fair to give priority to the young. The difference in years can mean a significant difference in having opportunities for the projects that enable one to achieve a reasonable level of lifetime well-being. It is not living for seventy-five or eighty years as such that matters, but instead the opportunities that having this many life-years offers to a person. When the difference in age is slight, there will not be a significant difference in opportunities. It is not obvious that one has had more opportunities just because one has lived five more years than another. If two people differ only slightly in age, as in the case at hand, then, other things being equal, there is no decisive reason to favor one over the other for the treatment.

Organ Transplantation

Organ transplantation is perhaps the most obvious example of the need to implement a fair and efficient rationing policy for a scarce medical resource. The reason for rationing organs is obvious. According to the United Network for Organ Sharing (UNOS), 83,472 people were waiting for an organ transplant in the United States as of January 2004. From January to October of 2003, 19,101 transplants were performed. In this same ten-month period, 9,845 organs were recovered from both living and deceased donors. Because of the disparity between supply and need, thousands of Americans continue to die each year waiting for an organ transplant.

To address this problem, UNOS has devised a point system that incorporates considerations of both fairness and efficiency in the allocation of organs. The aim is to respect people's claims of need for organs, while at the same time promoting good outcomes of transplantation. Regarding fairness, those who are the sickest and would die soon without a new organ are given priority because they have the most urgent need. This is consistent with the egalitarian idea of giving priority to the worst off. Even here, though, we need to distinguish between being worse off at a time and being worse off over time. One patient might be sicker and have a more urgent need for a transplant than another patient at a particular time. But the condition of the first patient might not deteriorate as rapidly as the condition of the second patient, who could become the sicker of the two over time. If the deterioration of the second patient means that he or she will not be a candidate for a transplant at a later time because it would not be beneficial, then priority may be given to the second patient. This claim can be sustained even if the first patient has spent more time on the waiting list. Which patient receives a transplant should not be determined by the urgency of need alone. It should also be determined by whether a patient's condition is static or progressive and how this will affect the outcome of a transplant. This requires a careful weighing of need and outcome both *at* times and *over* time.

Blood and tissue type can be important in same-organ transplantation because they can affect the outcome of a transplant. This shows that need is not the only relevant consideration in assigning priority to patients. The estimated outcome of the transplant is just as important. Indeed, considerations of outcome can trump considerations of need. One patient may have a greater need for a transplant, in the sense that he or she will die sooner without it than another patient. But if the first has a greater likelihood of graft rejection of an organ because his or her blood or tissue type does not match that of the donor, and the second patient has a much greater likelihood of a successful transplant, then the second should be given priority in receiving the organ. As noted in Chapter 1, blood and tissue matching are less important now with the newer immunosuppressive drugs, which minimize the risk of a recipient's body rejecting a transplanted organ. But the long-term outcomes of transplants involving donors and recipients who do not have the same human leukocyte antigen (HLA) status are still unknown. Because of this, transplant teams continue to try to match blood and tissue types between donors and recipients, at least with respect to kidneys. Matching is still treated as an important factor in transplantation.

A related factor that may give priority to a patient with a less urgent need over another patient with a more urgent need at a particular time is how likely it is that the first patient will receive an organ at a later time. Difficulty in finding a donor with matching blood and tissue can mean waiting a long time for an organ. This can result in further deterioration of the patient's condition and death. If an appropriately matched donor organ becomes available, then we may justifiably give the organ to this patient. We can say this despite the fact that the patient may not have been waiting as long for an organ as others who also need one. Similarly, a patient who needs two organs may be given priority, even though he or she has not been on a transplant waiting list as long as other patients needing only one organ. A patient who needs both a heart and a liver may jump the queue if he or she will die sooner than two other patients needing only a heart or a liver. Although we could not justify saving one instead of two people on consequentialist grounds, the egalitarian rationale for giving priority to this patient is that without a transplant he or she will die sooner than the other patients. In this regard, the patient has a more urgent need for a transplant.

A scenario similar to the one just described occurred in the case of Governor Robert Casey of Pennsylvania in 1993. The case was fraught with controversy because many believed that Casey unfairly jumped the queue ahead of other patients on account of his social status. Casey suffered from amyloidosis, a hereditary heart disease that causes the liver to produce a protein that weakens other organs and attaches to the walls of the heart, causing heart failure. He had a heart attack in 1991 and had undergone quadruple bypass surgery. By 1993 his condition had deteriorated so much that he was placed on the waiting list for a heart-liver transplant. Six patients were ahead of Casey on the waiting list for a heart and two for a liver in the same geographic region. Yet Casey received the organs ahead of them. Given that the conditions of the others on the waiting list were not as serious as Casey's, and that it was unlikely that Casey would be alive to receive the needed organs the next time they became available, allowing him to jump the queue was not considered unfair to the others.

The diachronic view of need may yield a different judgment about fairness, however, if we compare the claims of people to have a second transplant (because the first was rejected) against the claims of those needing a transplant for the first time. It seems unfair to give one person many opportunities to have an urgent medical need met if it precludes another person or persons from having a single opportunity. One can defend the claim that the first-time transplant candidate and the multitransplant candidate should be on a moral par only if one considers people's medical needs at particular times. On this view, past claims of need and past attempts to meet these needs are not morally relevant. Yet even if we give equal weight to different people's claims of need in such a case, a significant difference in the likelihood of a good versus a bad outcome of a transplant can break a tie between their claims.

Governor Casey was able to jump the queue because priority was based on an allocation system limited to a particular geographic region. The other transplant candidates with whom he competed for the organs were from the same region. If the allocation system has been national rather than regional, then he might not have received the organs so quickly. Similarly, former baseball player Mickey Mantle received a liver transplant soon after he became a candidate in 1995. This was because the liver allocation formula in the Dallas area gave him priority over others who had been waiting longer for a liver. The combination of Mantle's blood type, the severity of his sickness, and the limited number of other candidates for a liver transplant in the same area meant that it was not obviously unfair for him to jump to the top of the list. There was some question about whether the fact that he died from cancer shortly after the transplant should have disqualified him. But this was not the critical moral issue concerning fairness in Mantle's case.

More importantly, both Casey and Mantle received organs sooner than others who had been on the waiting list longer. In both cases, this was because the allocation system was based on a regional rather than a national system of priority. Giving priority to a local patient can be unfair to other patients in other regions who are in greater need of an organ. It seems unfair that whether one receives an organ should be determined on the basis of where they live rather than on their need. Location should not be a factor in determining one's medical status and where one should be placed on a transplant waiting list. Patients should be given higher or lower priority according to medical needs, not geographic location. The only fair system of priority in organ allocation is a national one. Still, fairness might have to be weighed against the likelihood of a successful transplant. This will depend on whether different organs can remain viable while being transported from one region to another.

The *social status* of someone like Governor Casey or Mickey Mantle should not be a factor in determining whether or when he or she should receive an organ. It is not obvious that saving individuals because they are admired or respected can benefit other people. There may be cases, though, in which a person's *social worth* may be a morally relevant consideration in organ allocation. Admittedly, these cases will be rare. Yet they may be morally relevant because they involve situations where the welfare and even the survival of many people depend on the survival of one person.

Suppose that Nelson Mandela needed a liver transplant in 1992.

This was the time when he was leading the transition from apartheid to democracy in South Africa. The transition turned out to be peaceful; but the political situation was potentially volatile. Mandela was essential to maintaining social stability. Suppose further that a younger individual also needed a liver and would have at least as good an outcome with a transplant. In the light of the political and social circumstances, Mandela should have been given priority over the younger patient in receiving a liver. His survival would have ensured the social stability of the country. It would have ensured that many people would not suffer a loss of welfare or life from the social instability that might have resulted otherwise. Mandela's social worth was a function of the dependence of many people's welfare and lives on his survival. That worth would have been a decisive factor in giving the organ to him rather than to another person with the same need.

The consequentialist reasons behind this argument are obvious. But the nonconsequentialist reasons behind it are just as strong. Each of the people whose survival depended on Mandela's survival had an equal need to survive. Giving transplant priority to Mandela over one other person's need to survive at a time would be a more fair decision because it would respect more people's equal need to survive over time. The point is not just to maximize a good outcome, but also to respect the claims of need of as many people as possible. Their need is generated by their dependence on Mandela. As with the other issues discussed in this section, whether one accepts this position will depend on whether one understands medical need in diachronic or synchronic terms.

Another controversial issue in organ transplantation is whether a person should be given lower priority for a transplant if the need results from lifestyle choices for which the person is responsible. If one develops liver failure from alcoholism, for example, and one is responsible for alcoholism, then presumably one is also responsible for one's liver failure. If one is responsible, then one should be given lower priority for a liver transplant than others who are not responsible for their condition because they contracted it through no fault of their own. This idea is consistent with the prudential lifespan account of health care. When we are responsible for planning our medical needs over all the stages of our lives, we can be responsible for later consequences of earlier actions as they pertain to health. End-stage liver disease from alcoholism is a condition for which one could be responsible. If one were responsible for the condition, then one would have a weaker claim to resources needed to treat it, including a liver transplant.

Many egalitarians insist that fairness in allocating scarce resources should be sensitive to people's responsibility for conditions that lead them to make claims on these resources. We should give more weight to the claims of need of the worse off, provided that they are worse off through no fault of their own. The idea is that the strength of people's claims is inversely proportional to their control over and responsibility for their state of need. The more control one has over one's health, the more responsible one is for it and the weaker is one's claim to resources for meeting medical needs. Conversely, the less control over and the less responsible one is for one's health, the stronger is one's claim to receive treatment for a condition. Control and responsibility are not absolute but matters of degree. Thus, if an individual is responsible for organ failure, then the most we could say is that the person should be given lower priority for a transplant. We would not be entitled to say that he or she should be excluded from consideration.

One objection to this position is that our health depends on factors over which we have no control, such as genetics or the social and physical environment. Some people may have a genetic predisposition to alcoholism, while others may become alcoholic in response to an abusive upbringing or poverty. People who are exposed to these factors are more likely to have diseases than people who have a more favorable genetic makeup and better living conditions. It seems to be a matter of luck whether and to what extent these factors play a role in people's health. Still, it is one thing to say that these factors predispose people to behavior that leads to disease. It is quite another thing to say that these factors determine disease-causing behavior. To argue that they do determine behavior implies that people have diseases only because of these factors. This is a causal claim that is difficult to defend. Even if certain factors predispose one to disease, it does not follow that one has no control over one's health. People may be responsible to at least some degree for the diseases they have, and this may be enough to justify giving them lower priority in receiving treatments for these diseases.

Nevertheless, it seems punitive to give people lower priority for medical treatments when they are in a state of medical need. Regardless of how their disease developed, it is morally wrong not to attend to their needs when they arise. Failure to do so results in another version of the "double jeopardy" scenario we described

earlier in the case of people with disabilities. But if we are to uphold the value of personal autonomy in making choices according
to one's own values, then we must also uphold the value of taking responsibility for the consequences of these choices. If people's
health is the result of their autonomous choices, then they can
be responsible for their health. Their responsibility can affect the
strength of their claims on medical resources. This is especially the
case when there is a known causal connection between lifestyle
and disease. Heavy drinking and smoking are two examples.

If medical resources were not scarce and did not have to be rationed, then this argument would have little force. But precisely
because these resources are scarce, we need to use factors such as
control and responsibility in devising a fair system of rationing.
Autonomy is a core principle in medical ethics. This includes not
only the right to refuse medical treatment, but also the ability to
make choices that affect one's health. Autonomy cannot be separated from responsibility. If people can make autonomous choices
about lifestyle that adversely affect their health, then they can be
responsible for their health, even if they become sick as a result of
these choices. This may mean giving some people lower priority
than others in meeting their claims of need for limited medical
resources. It may not be unfair to treat people unequally in this
regard. Extenuating social circumstances may limit people's autonomy. But people often make imprudent choices that are autonomous. The fact that they are imprudent does not justify explaining away responsibility for the consequences of these choices.
To say that people cannot be responsible for choices that affect their
health risks a return to paternalism and the idea that people cannot act in their own best interests. Still, many factors can influence
one's health. Some of these factors are within one's control, while
others are not. There will continue to be disagreement among the
public and health care professionals about what it means to have
control over one's health and whether this should influence how
we assess people's claims to receive different forms of health care.

Two-Tiered Health Care

The right to a decent minimum of care and equal access to this
level of care are based on an egalitarian premise. It is unfair to deny
people basic care and deny them the opportunity to have a nor-

mal, healthy lifespan because it means that their basic needs are not met. But fairness should matter less above the level of adequate care. Fairness consists in giving more weight to stronger claims of need. Yet people's claims of need generally are weaker above the decent minimum. If one accepts this idea, then one will find nothing morally objectionable about allowing people to purchase expedited access to more sophisticated medical services above the decent minimum. Fairness pertains to a decent minimum of care, not to optimal care. Allowing some people access to optimal care is not necessarily unfair to those who only have access to a decent minimum. On this view, a system with lower and higher tiers of health care would not be morally objectionable.

A lower tier would be publicly funded and would include a basic package of benefits providing people with adequate coverage. A higher tier would include forms of diagnosis or treatment that people could purchase at their own expense. The Oregon plan consisted in rationing medical services through a similar sort of tiering. Significantly, this is distinct from a libertarian conception of health care, where even a lower tier of medical benefits is market oriented and not something to which people are entitled.

The main objection to tiering is that some people would have quicker access to better medical services on the basis of their ability to pay for them. Because some people are worse off financially than others through no fault of their own, it is unfair to base access to medical services on the ability to pay. But if those who lack the financial resources to pay for expedited care have access to a decent minimum where their basic needs are met, then any objection they might raise to the idea of others paying for optimal care would not have any moral force. To be sure, a two-tiered health care system would involve inequalities based on the ability to pay. The critical question is whether these inequalities would be unfair to those who cannot afford to pay for expedited or optimal care. We should give priority to the claims of need of the worse off because of how they fare with respect to an absolute decent minimum of health care, not because of how they compare with the better off. Assuming that people have reached this basic level, they would have no moral claim to receive the same care as those who can purchase additional care above that level.

In the United States, health care is rationed by price and ability to pay. Many people who cannot afford to pay do not have adequate primary care (though all receive emergency care). Tiering would be acceptable provided only that everyone had access to a general basic minimum of care. In Canada, health care is rationed in the form of queuing. The limited supply of publicly funded services often requires people to wait considerable periods before they have access to them. One might argue that, if some people were allowed to pay for services and thereby reduce their waiting time, then it would lower the risk that their condition would deteriorate. In addition, it would enable people who could not pay for expedited care to move up in the queue. With waiting times reduced, the quality and outcome of care would improve for all people. On the other hand, one could argue that allowing a higher tier would lead to the gradual erosion of services in the lower tier and thus threaten the very idea of a decent minimum of health care. Attracted by economic incentives, doctors might gravitate to the higher tier. This might occur if the general perception among doctors was that the government was not adequately funding heath care and not paying them their fair share for their services.

If the emergence of a higher private tier undermined access to a decent minimum of care in the lower public tier, then tiering would be unfair and morally objectionable. This is because the basic needs of those in the lower tier would not be met. But tiering would not be unfair because of the inequalities in access to care between them and others who were comparatively better off. Put another way, a two-tiered health care system would be unfair, not because it would make those in the lower tier worse off in *relative* terms compared with the better off who have access to the higher tier. Instead, it would be unfair because the decent minimum itself would erode, and those in the lower tier would be worse off in *absolute* terms regarding the decent minimum.

A scarcity of health care professionals in the public system limits the number of procedures that can be performed. Suppose that some people are allowed to pay for hip-replacement surgery in a private clinic and thereby jump the public queue. This significantly reduces their waiting time for the surgery. Other people who cannot afford to pay take up their places in the queue and reduce their waiting time as well. This is a situation where some benefit and no one is harmed. Some might object to allowing individuals to pay and jump the queue because it creates inequality. Any form of inequality is intrinsically bad and thus morally impermissible. But they will have to respond to the "leveling down" objection to strict egalitarianism. A reduction in inequality can result in a loss for the better off and no gain for the worse off. This implausibly defends a situation where no one benefits and some are harmed. It suggests that, if some people have to wait a long time for hip replacement, then everyone should. On any plausible account of dealing with medical scarcity, allowing some people access to expedited care is preferable to making everyone wait an unreasonably long time for standard care.

Provided that all people are guaranteed timely access to a decent minimum of medical care, inequalities in access to better care above this level need not be unfair. Fairness does not always map perfectly onto equality. In Chapter 5, we said that genetic enhancement might undermine the idea of equality as one of the social bases of self-respect and social stability. This involved raising cognitive or physical functioning above a normal level. Yet now we seem to be saying that inequalities above a certain level of access to medical care do not matter morally. This is not necessarily inconsistent with the earlier point, though. Access to basic care that improves normal functioning should be treated differently from access to expedited care that raises or restores functioning to a normal level. In any case, how one responds to this question will depend on whether one is committed to the value of equality as such, or whether one is committed to giving priority to the worse off so that they can reach a decent minimum level of health.

Conclusion

Because medical resources are scarce, they need to be rationed both fairly and efficiently. We need to respect people's claims to have their medical needs met, while promoting the best outcomes in trying to meet these needs. In this chapter, we examined different ways of rationing and how priorities can be set along egalitarian and consequentialist lines. We discussed different ways in which people can be worse off in terms of their health and how they can have access to a decent minimum level of health care. But we also noted how aiming at this level may lead to a bias against the elderly and the disabled. Specifically, we pointed out that this bias could result from basing allocation decisions on QALYs. However, it was argued that it can be fair to give priority to a younger person over an older one in allocating a resource because one has not lived as long as the other. Regarding the question of who should be given priority in receiving organ transplants, we considered the relative weights of the need for and outcome of transplants. We also considered the respects in which social worth might give one higher priority for a transplant, as well as the respects in which responsibility for organ failure might give one lower priority! Finally, we explained why a two-tiered health care system would not necessarily be unfair or unjust.

As long as medical care in the United States continues to be rationed in terms of price and ability to pay, the percentage of the population that is uninsured and below the decent minimum will continue to grow. Callahan (1992) claims that "rationing is likely the only way in which we can improve care of the poor and manage our health care system in a more efficient manner" (p. 4). To be sure, a fair and efficient health care system must be more sensitive to the needs of the elderly and the disabled. But no health care system can meet everyone's claims of need. Medical rationing that strikes a reasonable balance between fairness and efficiency is the only way for a health care system to be sustainable and to meet people's needs the best it can.

Selected Readings

Brock, D. "Priority to the Worst Off in Health Care Resource Prioritization." In *Medicine and Social Justice: Essays on the Distribution of Health Care*, edited by R. Rhodes, M. Battin, and A. Silvers, 362–72. New York: Oxford University Press, 2002.

Buchanan, A. "The Right to a Decent Minimum of Health Care." *Philosophy and Public Affairs* 13(1984): 55–78.

Callahan, D. *Setting Limits: Medical Goals in an Aging Society.* New York: Simon & Schuster, 1987.

Callahan, D. "Rationing Health Care: Social, Political, and Legal Perspectives." *American Journal of Law and Medicine* 18(1992): 1–16.

Daniels, N. *Am I My Parents' Keeper?* New York: Oxford University Press, 1988.

Harris, J. "QALYfying the Value of Life." *Journal of Medical Ethics* 13(1987): 117–22.

McKerlie, D. "Justice between the Young and the Old." *Philosophy and Public Affairs* 30(2002): 152–177.

Parfit, D. "Equality or Priority." In *The Ideal of Equality*, edited by M. Clayton and A. Williams, 81–125. New York: St. Martin's Press, 2000.

Rawls, J. *A Theory of Justice*. Cambridge, Mass.: Harvard University Press, 1971.

Truog, R. "Triage in the ICU." *Hastings Center Report* 22(1992): 13–17.

Veatch, R. *Transplantation Ethics*. Washington, D.C.: Georgetown University Press, 2000.

Index

IF WE WERE SITTIN' 'cross from each other right now, your ears would be filled with a muddy old voice that sounds somethin' between a preacher's Sunday mornin' sermonizin' and a grizzled seen-it-all coot sittin' at a bar drinkin' and spinnin' some wild bullshit, and you know what?

That voice would belong to me.

Mudbone.

I was born in Tupelo, Mississippi. Long time ago. So long ago it ain't worth rememberin' when exactly, because after a certain while, it's just a long time. Now in that time I met some of the most fascinatin' people ever alive, most of whom you've never heard of. But they was fascinatin'. Trust me. There was a lady I met in St. Louis who liked to . . .

Well, she was fascinatin'. You're just going to have to take my word for it.

The young man who's writin' this book is the most fascinatin' person I ever become acquainted with. He started listenin' to Mudbone back when both of us needed to be reminded that old people weren't no fools.

"Don't get to be old being no fool," I said. "Lot of young wise men deader than a motherfucker."

It tickles my ass just to think Richard Pryor is still around, because he is the motherfucker. Made almost forty movies. Had his name on twenty-five comedy albums, some of which he

actually got paid for. People have gone and wrote books about him. College professors include him in lectures. There was even a television special honoring him for being inspirational and shit. But I know the real shit on the motherfucker. Shit, I know Richard since he was a skinny-ass motherfucker—back in Peoria—shootin' flies off his sweaty face at the slaughterhouse, and dreamin' about having a pension and some pussy. But probably not in that order. And then later on, I still knew Richard better than anyone when he fucked up, which about everyone also knows about. Right?

Remember when he fucked up? That fire got on his ass and it fucked him up upstairs. Fried up what little brains he had.

Course that's nothin' compared to what's happened since then. A while back he had a heart attack. Then he had what doctors called a quadruple bypass, which is an operation rather than what he should've done for some of his wives.

Bypassed 'em.

And nowadays he's got this MS—multiple sclerosis. Which is a very complicated disease. It don't kill you, though.

It just makes you wish you were dead.

Like some of the womens he's been with. Six marriages to five woman. Numerous womens in between. Some at the same time. A revolving door of bitches all come just so he could fuck up their lives and they could fuck up his.

I asked why.

"Because when God makes a fool, he makes a perfect one," he said.

No, seriously.

"Boy, why in the hell don't you just sticks with one pussy? Why you gotta go and marry all them bitches? You even married one of 'em twice."

You know what he said to me?

He said, "Shit, I'm just tryin' to find one that'll fit."

★ ★ ★

THAT'S RICHARD. *Some people fall in love. Others fall in shit. Richard once said they're the same thing. Oh well, no question the boy is funny. Funny like Ali could fight. The heavyweight champ of hilarity. No doubt about that. I remember the motherfucker back when he was young and truly ignorant. Absolutely nobody was funnier. He could make a motherfucker laugh at a funeral on Sunday, Christmas Day.*

Course, that was then. I speak to the boy all the time and I asked him what happened since.

"Monies," he told me. "I got me some monies."

That's what happened to him. He got some monies, and all of a sudden those missed-meal cramps and shit disappeared and he said, "Fuck it."

That's what he told me, anyway.

"Fuck it. I said, 'Fuck it.'"

As for me, I could never afford to say fuck it the way he said it. That's why ol' Mudbone's still hungry. Shit. I've been around so long—long enough that nobody remembers when I started in show business—that I knowed pretty near everybody. Don't mean I liked 'em. I knowed 'em. Big difference. I gave Moms Mabley, who I liked, her break. Moms was an ugly child, and I told her, "Girl, you ought to go into comedy."

Unlike Moms, Richard wasn't ugly. He was just ignorant.

Shit, he didn't even know he was black. Used to call himself Sun. Sun the Secret Prince.

But I told him the same thing as Moms. Go into comedy.

See, I didn't know if he was even listenin'. 'Cause even then you couldn't let him get none of that pot in him. Then it was actually like tryin' to talk to a baboon's ass. I mean, I once talked to him for seven days and seven nights and he was still on the same subject—"Where can I get some more?"

I said, "Boy, why'n't you do something with yourself."

"Like what?"

"Since religion ain't your thing, maybe you can try ballet. You're gonna be black a long time. So you might as well enjoy

yourself. Because there ain't many black motherfuckers doing the ballet."

And then he said, "What about comedy?"

This, of course, reminded me of Moms. For here was another opportunity to start another career.

"What's that like?" he asked.

NOT EASY.

See, I was honest with the motherfucker. I told him comedy—real comedy—wasn't only tellin' jokes. It was about telling the truth. Talking about life. Makin' light of the hard times.

"Definitely not as funny as it looks," I said. "You start telling the truth to people and people gonna look at you like you was askin' to fuck their mama or somethin'. The truth is gonna be funny, but it's gonna scare the shit outta folks.

"And maybe you, too."

In any event, the boy was still interested. I could see that much. So I went on. Told him the truth about how I'd lived through hard times.

I said, "People talk about how these are hard times. But hard times was way back. They didn't even have a year for it. Just called it Hard Times.

"And it was dark all the time. I think the sun came out on Wednesday, and if you didn't have your ass up early, you missed it.

"So I happened to be out there one Wednesday and the sun hit me right in the face. I grabbed a bunch of it and rubbed it all over myself. Shit, I didn't have nothing else. And I said, 'Shit, I might as well have some sun on my face.'

"Time went on and I remembered it was Thursday, and because there was no one else around, I said to myself, 'Damn, that sun was a bitch. That's why they didn't want us to have any of it. 'Cuz it'll cheer you up inside.'"

Needless to say, this made quite a bit of sense to young Rich, who didn't have no sunshine in his life back in Peoria but, in fact, recognized that he might be able to grab some if he went into comedy. Steppin' on stage, bein' in front of the hot spotlight, hearin' the applause and whatnot. The whatnot, of course, bein' all the pussy he knew he'd get as well. It was a risk, a big risk, which he knew.

That sun can get so hot it'll fry your ass like two eggs in a skillet.

But . . .

But I'm getting ahead of the story, and there's plenty of that to go around.

SEE, *not too long ago, I asked him,* "After all this, why you want to go and write a book, and especially a book about you? Ain't livin' enough? Ain't survivin' been hard enough? You're the motherfucker. You did it all and it all ain't pretty."

He said, "I know."

So I said, "Then why you want to tell it all again. What good do you think that'll do?"

"Besides make me some monies?" *he asked.*

"Shit. Of course, besides that."

He said, "It's like this. You didn't have to come to this motherfucker, and you sure can't choose how to leave. You don't even know when you're going to go. So don't take this shit serious. All you can do is have fun and you better have plenty of it, which I did."

"No question about that," *I said.* "But do you remember it?"

He said, "I remember what's mine."

Shit, you can't argue with that. And what the motherfucker don't remember, I might.

Then I said, "Now what all are you gonna write about? Where you gonna start?"

He laughed. You know how he laughs. Then he lit a cigarette and took a long puff, and that's when I know'd that he'd learned somethin' through all the shit he'd been through. Acquired wisdom. Done become a philosopher.

He said, "There ain't but two pieces of pussy you gonna get in your life. That's your first and your last. All that shit in between—that's just the extra gravy. And that's what I'm gonna write about. The gravy."

Yes, sir. Sounded good to me.

But since I've knowed the motherfucker for so long, and I also know the story, I had but one piece of advice for him.

He asked, "What?"

And I said, "Keep some sunshine on your face."

"I'll try," he said. "I'll try."

ONE

To everyone from fans to wives, I would always be a dark comic genius, the Bard of Self-Destruction, but in the summer of 1986 I literally saw the light, and if that didn't change who I was, it certainly transformed my life. It was the middle of the night. Lying in bed beside my ex-wife Deboragh in my house at Hana, on the island of Maui, Hawaii, I watched shards of light explode across my field of vision as if I was standing in an empty field during a lightning storm.

I didn't know what to make of it. I stared at the lights a long time. They didn't entertain me. Nor did they scare me. I thought I was onto something unique. Then I woke up Deboragh to tell her about it.

"What are you talking about, your theory of light?" she said, unamused and tired.

"Can't you see it?" I said.

"No," she said.

"There!" I exclaimed, pointing at another bolt spearing the darkness. "There! Right there, goddamn it."

Two months later I sat on an airplane, heading for the Mayo Clinic in Rochester, Minnesota. Deboragh sat beside me, as if to prevent my escape. Not that I could've gone anywhere at thirty-five thousand feet, though, I admit, the thought did cross my mind. Death had knocked on my door before. Bullets had just missed me. Womens had gone for my heart, and worse—my

balls. I had even set myself on fire and suffered third-degree burns over 50 percent of my body in 1980.

But the stuff that'd been happening lately scared the shit out of me.

It was as if Death had returned for a visit.

"Hey, Rich, remember me?"

"No."

"Rich, why you want to hurt my feelings like that?"

"Get the fuck away, motherfucker."

"HA-HA-HA-HA-HA-HA!"

After seeing the flashing lights in Hawaii, weird shit snuck up on me without warning. My feet went numb. My hands went numb. My fingers didn't do what I told them. My neck went stiff. (Needless to say, if some part of my body was going to stiffen, I preferred it to be my dick.) Suddenly, I couldn't move. Shit would last for a moment or two and then I'd go, "What the fuck was that about?"

Then I'd hear the laughter.

"HA-HA-HA-HA-HA-HA!"

"What was that?"

"Hey, Rich, you remember me now?"

As soon as I began worrying for real that my body was becoming more unreliable than my mind, I saw a doctor at UCLA. The UCLA doc put me through tests and then sent my ass to the Mayo Clinic, where I was poked and prodded as if I was an experiment in Dr. Frankenstein's lab. I mean, shit, they X-rayed me, they tested my reflexes, they put me on a contraption that turned me around like a piece of meat on a rotisserie and shot me and stuck me and drew things out of my poor, confused body.

And they were so casual about it.

"Good morning, Mr. Pryor, and how are you? Today we're going to be taking samples of your blood, shit, and piss. Have a good one."

You ever try to piss in them bottles? There's something too clean about pissing in those bottles. Your dick don't want to do

*it. I mean, your dick looks at it and says, "Why I gotta piss in
this? Well, I ain't gonna do it. You take me over to the toilet
where I used to piss. I don't want to piss in the sink."*

*You say, "Piss, man, please. I'll never be able to leave if you
don't."*

Finally, if you do start, you can't stop.

"Nurse! I need another bottle! Quick!"

You lose your pride real quick in hospitals. During one test,
a doctor stuck a long tube down my ass. No matter what you do
to an asshole, it's still an asshole. Ain't going to get any prettier.
So there I was, having an intimate relationship with this damn
machine, when I turned my head to the side and saw a handful
of doctors in the doorway, looking at me. Nothing I could do
but turn back to the business.

"Please, Doc, back there," I said. "Them faces."

Nobody stirred.

I asked, "What am I? The treat for the day?"

I'm sure they went home that night and when their wives
asked if anything exciting happened at work, they said, "Yeah,
I looked up Richard Pryor's asshole."

After a week of intensive, scary, and sometimes humiliating tests, the doctors finished. Seated in one of the main docs'
diploma-filled office, I was told the diagnosis. It turned out to be
worse than all the tests.

"Mr. Pryor, you have multiple sclerosis."

"Hey, Rich, remember me?"

*Oh, shit. I knew who it was this time. No use pretending.
Death was back. He sounded like Jim Brown on steroids.*

"Am I gonna die?"

*"Naw, not yet. I'm just gonna fuck with you for a while.
HA-HA-HA-HA!"*

You know how sometimes you're too stupid to be frightened
when that's really the way you should be acting? Well, I was

both stupid and frightened. I didn't know what the fuck the doctor meant when he informed me that I had multiple sclerosis. Nor did I want to know. Deboragh and I went straight back to the hotel, packed, and caught the first available plane back to L.A. I don't think we mentioned MS once.

But eight years have passed since that fateful day in Rochester, and now I know more about MS than some doctors. MS is a strange and, thus far, incurable, degenerative disease that attacks the protective sheath around the nerve fibers. They say it affects motor skills, balance, and simple involuntary acts such as swallowing. But it doesn't merely affect them, it takes them the fuck away.

People call me all the time and say, "Richard, I heard you were dead."

"What do you think?" I reply. "You're talking to me. Does that help?"

I know what they're talking about, though. MS makes you feel like a decoy in a shooting gallery for self-pity and depression. In my mind, I've written the obituary countless newspapermen have had waiting for years. RICHARD PRYOR DIES. But instead of the cause being drugs or a heart attack or an angry woman, as most would've expected, MS has added a punch line.

"Pryor died when he fell down and couldn't get up."

I'd be lying if I didn't admit there've been many days when I wanted to pick up the .357 beside my bed and drop the curtain. Call it a show. But I've never taken the easy way. Even when it seemed easy, it wasn't easy. Why, I don't know. That's just the way it's been. Black man's fate, I suppose.

So rather than surrender to forces beyond my control, I've decided to hang on till the end of the ride. See where the motherfucker takes me. I've had similar experiences with women. I mean, you know the bitch is going to be trouble, but you still can't help yourself.

The brain says, "Get the pussy, get the pussy," and you can't do nothing else.

⋆　⋆　⋆

I've found that my life, instead of ending because of MS, has only changed. Perhaps it was God's way of telling me to chill, slow down, look at the trees, sniff the flowers rather than the coke, and take time for myself and see what it's like to be a human being. See what it's like being human.

I lived big for a time, but never appreciated life. I never realized that people really liked me.

Me, Richard Pryor, a human being.

But like I said, that's all changed since I became ill. I've been surprised and deeply touched by people in more ways than I could've imagined. We're still years away from any sort of cure for multiple sclerosis, but I'm able to make do. I look in the mirror. I know that's me looking back at me.

"Hey, Rich, how you doin'?"

"Above ground."

This is my life. I know the truth. If you ain't here, you're nowhere. So, I go on, because it ain't over. Only stranger.

Shit.

Who would've ever guessed I'd make it this far?

TWO

never thought I had a self-destruct mechanism working inside of me, but considering the way things worked out, I see I caused most of the problems myself. It was always plain to other people, I suppose. When I was a kid, my grandfather and uncle bet that I wouldn't make it to fourteen. Even I figured the chances of me making it to twenty were slim.

That's sad, betting against yourself.

Why didn't you see that then, Rich?

Sometimes survival depends on blindness. After living on this planet for fifty-four years, I realize that my entire life might've been decided when I was five years old. Imagine that. Going about business for forty-nine years, searching for the key that'll unlock all the answers, and then finding out it happened way back.

That's what people mean when they say life is funny.

I wasn't much taller than my daddy's shin when I found that I could make my family laugh. It happened outside the house at 313 North Washington, in Peoria, Illinois, where I lived among an assortment of relatives, neighbors, whores, and winos—the people who inspired a lifetime of comedic material.

I was a skinny little black kid, with big eyes that took in the whole world and a wide, bright smile that begged for more attention than anybody had time to give. Dressed in a cowboy outfit—the only range rustler in all of Peoria—I sat on a railing

of bricks and found that when I fell off on purpose everyone laughed, including my grandmother, who made it her job to scare the shit out of people.

From that first pratfall, I liked being the source of making people laugh. After a few more minutes of falling, a little dog wandered by and poo-pooed in our yard. I got up, ran to my grandmother, and slipped in the dog poop. It made Mama and the rest laugh again. Shit, I was really onto something then. So I did it a second time.

"Look at that boy! He's crazy!"

That was my first joke.

All in shit.

And I been covered in it ever since.

I spent the first twenty-one years of my life in Peoria.

They called Peoria the model city. That meant they had the niggers under control.

Black people didn't have it so good in Peoria. If they worked at all, they were probably employed at one of the nearby slaughterhouses. My family dodged that fate. They ran whorehouses, bars, drove trucks, and shit. But the fact was, almost half the black people living in Peoria's ghetto didn't have any job whatsoever. Only two restaurants and two movie theaters in town served people of color, and if a black man wanted a hotel room for the night, he had to find it elsewhere.

We had a curfew in my neighborhood. Niggers home by eleven. Negroes by midnight.

That was the reality. But childhood is colored by ignorance, a good ignorance, one that leads you around in a blindness necessary for survival. Even the best of days in Peoria were tainted

by gloom, a murky darkness that hung over people the same way smog lays flat over a city as pretty as L.A. It just fucks up the picture. I saw shit that would cause an adult nightmares. Heard tales about hangings and murders that happened just because a man happened to be black. Strange shit.

I didn't understand it.

"Didn't you know you were black?"

"Shit, I didn't even know I had a color."

I never wanted to be white. I always wanted to be something different than a nigger, because niggers had it so rough. I tried to be a black cat with neat hair. I thought that was the problem—the hair.

In my imagination, I gave myself a new identity. I called myself Sun the Secret Prince. As Sun the Secret Prince, I was colorless. I was just light and energy, caroming off the planets. No boundaries. Simply alive.

Then one day my grandmother brought me down to earth. Told me I was black.

Said, "Boy, you're black."

Okay, Grandma. I see that. But I still didn't understand the things that went with being black. That came later.

I was being prepared, though. The movies fucked me up. So did television. I watched shows like "Father Knows Best" and believed that was how everybody in America lived. But my family didn't resemble them one bit.

White folks do things a lot different than niggers. They eat quieter. "Pass the potatoes. Thank you, darling. Could I have a bit of that sauce? How are the kids coming along in their studies? Think we'll be having sexual intercourse this evening? We're not? Well, what the heck."

Black families be different. When my father ate, he made noise. "Hey, bitch, where's the food? Goddamn, Mama, come

on. *Shit. Come on, motherfucker, can't you make that meat stick to the bone."*

White folks fuck quiet, too. I've seen it in the movies. "Ou, boop, eh, boo."

Niggers make noise. "Oh, you motherfucker. Oh, goddamn, baby. Oh, don't lose that thing."

So if I wasn't like those people on TV, what did that make me?

Where did I fit in?

Those were the questions I often asked myself, and continued to do so my entire life. But there were others I never got a chance to ask. Like those concerning my family's background. As far as I could tell, my people had been around since the beginning of time, like Adam and Eve. They just were. Despite a natural curiosity about those origins, I didn't want to upset anyone by asking questions they'd consider nonsense—not to mention a waste of time.

I didn't want to hear that familiar refrain, "Child, can't you see I'm busy!"

No one was busier than my grandmother, Marie Carter. She reminded me of a large sunflower—big, strong, bright, appealing. But Mama, as I also called her, was also a mean, tough, controlling bitch. One of twenty-one children, she was born in Decatur, Illinois, and grew up knowing terrible prejudice. The kind of shit that adults didn't have to speak about because they all knew. It was in their eyes. Rage, fear, wariness. Once I overheard her talking about a black man who was lynched by the Ku Klux Klan.

"Why, Mama?" I asked.

" 'Cuz he was a nigger."

I thought about that hard. Tried to understand why something like that happened.

You don't forget that shit.

"Am I gonna get hanged, Mama?"

"Go and play, boy."

LeRoy Pryor must've been some specimen. It's impossible to know whether or not Marie ever married him, but they had four children together. After the last child was born in the late 1920s, LeRoy went off to work on the railroad. Though he planned on being gone only a short time, he got buckled between two trains. The collision should've killed him instantly. But when the trains parted, he stepped out and walked to a nearby tavern.

Man wanted a drink. And then he died.

Bless his soul.

I hope I have some of that strength inside me.

In 1929, Marie packed up her children and belongings and moved to Peoria, where she met Thomas Bryant. I would call him Pops. Like Marie, he was a hodgepodge of heritage, including part Native American. In fact, he was raised on a reservation, but left at age nine, preferring the road over family.

"Why'd you leave the reservation, Pops?" I asked.

As a boy, I was fascinated by cowboys and Indians and couldn't imagine leaving an actual reservation.

"'Cuz people used to squat and shit," he said. "Right there in the dirt. It wasn't nice."

Pops and Marie made quite a picture. He was a conservative Democrat who believed in America and the law. Marie was a beautiful young woman with hustle in her bloodstream. Pops was ten years older than her, a man with itchy britches. He roamed. Marie had four kids who anchored her in one place. But instead of running the other way, Pops told Marie that he liked her so much he'd take care of her family.

"That's strange for a young man," I once remarked.

"It's different," he replied.

So were they. Although married for something like forty or fifty years, Pops and Marie barely exchanged a single word. They quit speaking after she caught him fucking one of her whores. Rather than throw his ass out of the house, Marie did worse. She defied Pops to ever have another woman. Any woman other than her. Know what I mean? She fucked his head up good.

From what I could tell, Pops didn't mind not talking to Marie for most of their married life. He swore that his real punishment was having to sleep with me after Marie threw him out of their room. I used to roll and toss all over the bed. Pops said I was the kickingest motherfucker he'd ever met in his life. Couldn't sleep with either Marie or me. Bless his heart.

Then there was LeRoy Jr., my father. He was better known as Buck Carter. Big and strong, he was a Golden Gloves boxing champion as a teenager. Later, he traveled from Chicago to East St. Louis, working odd jobs until he got the urge to move on again. The girl he finally took up with, Gertrude Thomas, lived in the same neighborhood as Marie and Pops. Gertrude was a bookkeeper. Not to mention trouble.

I know that Buck loved her. For real. He felt that deep kind of love that doesn't ever do a person good, that ends up kicking you in the ass, leaving you crying and tormented. Years later, Buck admitted that he was glad Gertrude had gone. He loved her so much, he said he probably would've killed her.

Buck and Gertrude were involved—as were some of the other Carters, Bryants, Pryors, and Thomases in Peoria—in operating the whorehouses and bars that gave the Washington Street area its reputation. I know my mother didn't expect to get pregnant. Nor did she want the baby who arrived on December 1, 1940.

Or so they told me.

But the circumstances surrounding my birth seem obvious. My dad wanted the pussy. My mother had the pussy. Nine months later, my Uncle Franklin had a premonition about seeing a baby in a manger. And then I arrived.

At least Gertrude didn't flush me down the toilet as some did. When I was a kid, I found a baby in a shoe box—dead. An accident to some, I was luckier than others, and that was just the way it was.

I don't know where my mother got the name Richard. Franklin, though, was my uncle's.

Richard Franklin.

The next one, Lennox, was one of my aunt's boyfriends.

Richard Franklin Lennox.

Thomas was her maiden name, and Pryor was my maiden name.

Richard Franklin Lennox Thomas Pryor.

I wish I would've asked my mother more about how I came to be, but I didn't. Why didn't you, Richard?

Gertrude drank a lot. She'd be home for six months or so, and then one day she'd leave the house as if she was going to the store, say goodbye and be gone for six months. How did that make you feel, Rich?

My dad always seemed to know when Gertrude was about to take off and it didn't bother him any that I could tell. But I just thought it was nice to see her whenever she was at home. I didn't want to upset her by asking any questions.

You know?

She was my mom.

I didn't want to shake up shit.

THREE

From my earliest days, I learned that expectations had to be balanced against reality. Take the first Christmas I remember clearly. I was two years old, standing up in my crib, staring at the multicolored lights on the Christmas tree. I realized it was a special time of year. The decorations on the tree added a brightness that wasn't normally part of the house, and the presents under it were even better because some of them belonged to me.

As I plotted my escape from behind bars, my cousin Martha came in the room. She was my Aunt Dee's daughter. She was also my chance to fly out of that crib.

"Hey, bitch, lift my ass out of here," I wanted to say, but at that age the only thing I managed to do was lean against the railing of the crib, making funny sounds, and look at her with my friendly wide eyes. Maybe Martha would help me out. Let me get at those presents. I could only hope.

But you know what happened?

Martha vomited on me.

She did. Bless her heart. She was drunk.

Family is a mixed blessing. You're glad to have one, but it's also like receiving a life sentence for a crime you didn't commit. My people had a variety of last names—Carter, Bryant, Thomas, and Pryor. They were an industrious, busy group. My grandma

and mother ran houses. My father and uncle helped at Pop's bar, the Famous Door. There was also a trucking business, a beauty parlor, and so on. Anything to stay afloat.

My Aunt Dee and Uncle Dickie were prime examples. She came to Peoria from Mississippi and nabbed Dickie in his youth, married him, and then turned him out. Made him a pimp. I don't blame him, though. He didn't know nothing.

Later, Dickie took over tending bar at the Famous Door when my dad went in the service, but it always seemed to me his main occupation—the one he preferred—was getting me in trouble. One time my grandma called down to 317 North Washington. I picked up the phone. She wanted Dickie, but he squatted in the background and put words in my head as if he was a bad conscience.

"Tell her she ain't the fat hen's ass," he whispered and then laughed.

"Hey, Grandma, you ain't the fat hen's ass."

She said, "I'll be right there, son," and then a few minutes later, she showed up and whacked me with a belt. Made me holler and tell the truth.

"I promise. I ain't ever gonna say you ain't the fat hen's ass no more."

Whack! Whomp! Whack!

"Damn right you aren't."

What she should've done is beat the crap out of Dickie. But he'd disappeared, leaving me to catch her wrath.

The house where I grew up at 317 North Washington had a strange, dark, big feel. It stood amid whole blocks of such places. In between were various businesses—a trucking office across the street; further down was a parking lot of semitrailers; a garage; liquor stores.

I lived in a neighborhood with a lot of whorehouses. Not many candy stores or banks. Liquor stores and whorehouses.

Niggers love to drink. They say. White people have banks and shit. But you guys have to go four miles to get some liquor. A nigger can get liquor by walking out the door.

My grandmother's house was at 313. Between hers and ours was China Bee's, where the pretty whores lived. That says something about the whores who worked for my grandma. Didn't seem to matter either way, though. Both places did pretty good.

There was a little vacant patch of dirt down the block from our home, just to the left. A little patch of dirt and grass looking for the countryside. Asking, "Why I got to be in the city? Why can't I have no trees and grass?" For some reason, these giant sunflowers grew in the middle of that patch. I don't know how they got started or who watered them, but every summer they headed up toward the sky as if they were trying to escape the ghetto. After realizing they couldn't get out, they bloomed. Big. Like giant sunbursts. I loved those flowers, man. Looking at them made me feel good.

One day in 1944, a strange person wearing a soldier's uniform walked into our home as if he owned the place. A little frightened by his sudden appearance, I watched him come inside and puzzled over what he was doing there. Like who the fuck was he? I was used to strangers coming and going, but all of them had business to do. Getting the pussy.

But this guy didn't seem to have anything on his mind except lingering. I watched him go upstairs. A few minutes later, he returned in a different set of clothes and then I recognized him as my father. He'd come back from the Army.

Everyone celebrated, and I had the impression that for those few hours none of the usual hustle and worry mattered. Daddy slipped back into his old job bartending at the Famous Door, where my mom also waitressed in a tight, white dress. I loved how it looked against her velvet tan skin. I thought it made Gertrude look very sexy.

The Famous Door was where I hung out. It was a wild, colorful place for a kid to spend most of his time, but everybody in my family congregated there. The news you picked up there was better than what you got in the paper. I remember Uncle Dickie running in and informing everybody that his friend Shoeshine had murdered his two women in a chicken shack after discovering that they were fucking each other rather than him.

"He took that for real," Dickie said. "Absolutely."

As a comedian, I couldn't have asked for better material. My eyes and ears absorbed everything. People came in to exchange news, blow steam, or have their say. Everybody had an opinion about something. Even if they didn't know shit about sports, politics, women, the war. In fact, the less people knew, the louder they got.

Some niggers used to drink and want to fight. Some drank and had a seizure. Everybody knows some nigger who drinks and every weekend gets his ass whooped. He never wins, but he always wants to fight. Nice guy during the week. "Hi, how ya doing?" But the weekend comes and he's "Motherfucker, get out of my face."

You see him in the bar and he's fucked up. Starts in, "Man, leave me alone, nigger. Shit, you ain't gonna start fucking with me. Give me some money . . .

"Nigger, give me my whiskey. What? I'm drunk? What you mean I'm drunk, motherfucker? You crazy. Shit, you didn't say that an hour ago. When you were serving me that shit and I was buying everybody in here . . . something. Give me a beer. For everybody. One motherfucking beer."

One night some guy came in and cussed my grandmother. Buck heard it, grabbed a pistol, and shot the man full of bullets. Emptied the magazine. Blam! Blam! Blam! Scared the shit out of everyone in the place. But liquor makes you do strange things. Like not die when you're supposed to. The man was pissed, and

he managed to crawl across the floor and cut Buck on his leg. My father was crippled the rest of his life. The other guy showed up for drinks a few months later.

Another night a marine came in and raised hell. Like it was in the movies. Yelling. Throwing shit. Grabbing the women's titties and ass. Dickie and Buck grabbed him and started throwing punches. That marine got pissed, turned around, and kicked their ass. The three of them fought for a good half hour. But when it was all over, they laughed and drank together.

"Daddy, what's going on?" I asked after some similarly crazy incident in the bar.

He turned around and smacked me.

"Shut up. Don't ask questions."

When you're a little guy watching all this weird shit happen and no one explains it, you formulate your own thoughts. Once I saw some guy who was fighting get knifed in the stomach. With his guts hanging out, he wanted to get to the liquor store down the street. I didn't understand. The dude was screaming for someone to help him down the block. His eyes locked on me.

"Come on, man," I said bravely. "The ambulance is coming. Why don't you just lay there."

He looked at me like I was the crazy one and said, "Shit, I'm going to get me a half pint."

I wondered where he was going to put that half pint. If he drank it, I thought he'd die instantly.

Of course, that's what I thought. But I found out different. Assholes don't die. They multiply.

FOUR

On Sundays, my grandmother made me go with her to the Morning Star Baptist Church. I didn't want to go, but you didn't fuck around with Marie. You did what she said. After a while, though, I drifted to the Salvation Army Church where I got to beat the collection drum. And when it was somebody's birthday, I got to beat it a few extra times. Made me feel special.

There was lots of talk in my house about God. "Help me, God." "Please, God." "Why you doin' this to me, God?" "Goddamn it." Shit like that. And then there were all them Bible stories, which scared the motherfucking crap out of me. They were all horrible stories in which God always managed to do something spectacular at the last minute. Kind of like Superman.

As a result, I learned early on not to fuck with this God guy, this God person.

Every wino knew Jesus. "You know Jesus Christ?"

"Jesus Christ? Shit, lives over there in the projects. Runs the elevator in the Jefferson Hotel. Nigger ain't shit. Neither is his mama."

The only person scarier than God was my mother. Gertrude was a trip. My dad understood this, but I guess he couldn't help himself. One time Buck hit Gertrude, and she turned blue with

anger and said, "Okay, motherfucker, don't hit me no more."

She said that. I give her that.

But I guess Buck didn't care. Standing in his underwear and T-shirt, decked out like an inebriated bedroom heavyweight, he whomped her again.

Mistake.

"Oh no, don't do that," she said, coiling like a rattlesnake about to strike. "Don't stand in front of me with fucking undershorts on and hit me, motherfucker."

Quick as lightning, she reached out with her finger claws and swiped at my father's dick. Ripped his nutsack off.

I was just a kid when I saw this.

My father ran down the street to 313 hollering, "Mama! Mama! Mama!"

A grown man.

I stood outside and saw him running up the block. His shorts were all red with blood.

"What happened, Daddy?"

"She cut my nuts open!"

"Who did?"

"Your bitch-ass mother! Gertrude!"

Traumatized, I wandered back home. Mama stood in the doorway, looking satisfied with herself. She seemed happy to see me.

"Hi, baby," she said, and then she hugged me. Rubbed my head. Confused my ass just by being so nice to me.

But she wasn't nice to my dad that night. Ended his pimpship right then.

The Pryor men know about pain. One afternoon I crawled under the front porch so I could play in the soft dirt. My grandma caught me, gave me a scolding, and then hauled my ass to the bathtub. She washed me off and put on clean clothes. So what did I do next? Went back outside and crawled under the porch.

I was happy as a dick in pussy digging in that soft, cool dirt when she stepped out and found me again.

"Oh, so you don't believe fat meat's greasy, do you?" Marie said.

She snatched me up, threw me back into the bath, cleaned me up again, threw on another set of clean clothes, and let me go back outside. Didn't bother me any. I went under the porch just like before and played in the soft dirt, until she busted me again.

"I'm going to beat your ass this time," she said.

Bless her heart. And she beat my ass.

That's just the way it was. As much as I wanted love and attention, I couldn't help but feel that I was a source of hardship for my parents, something they'd as soon forget as let me intrude on their lives. Summer was the worst time. All the men and women went to the Cardinals baseball games in St. Louis. I wanted to go, too. Each time, I got ready and waited by the front door as they came downstairs.

"Look at that boy," my mama said. "Where does he think he's going?"

There was laughter.

"You ain't going," my dad said with finality.

"Oh," I said, lowering my eyes.

After they left, I cried. Not in front of them. Only after they were gone. Only after I pressed my nose to the window and watched their car swing around the corner and out of sight. I knew they didn't hate me. So why didn't they want to take me?

"Why, Grandma?" I once asked.

She looked at me. Then slapped me upside my head.

Growing up was a minefield. I had to watch every step, but it was hard to remember all the time. I was something like six years old when a sick pedophile turned me into a pincushion for his perverted urges. What did I know, though?

I was playing by myself in the alley behind our house, throw-

ing stones at trash cans and scaring rats out from their hiding places and pretending to hunt them.

Suddenly, this older guy appeared from around the corner. He stepped in from the shadows. His name was Hoss. He was in his late teens, probably around sixteen or seventeen. Right away, I knew he was trouble. I saw it in his bloodshot eyes. In no uncertain terms, he said, "I'm gonna fuck with you, you little chickenshit pussy."

I should've run. But I didn't. Because he was right about me in that sense—I was a little chickenshit. It was as if the terror I felt paralyzed me. Glued me in place and made me easy prey. Hoss threw me against the wall in a darkened corner shielded from the view of anyone passing by. Then he unzipped his pants and put his dick into my mouth.

"Suck it," he ordered.

Relieved he didn't want no asshole, I did as told. Afterward, Hoss walked off happy and left me trembling in the chilly darkness. I cried and shook and tried to make sense of what had happened. I knew something horrible had happened to me. I felt violated, humiliated, dirty, fearful, and, most of all, ashamed. But I couldn't sort that shit out. Fuck.

I carried that secret around for most of my life.

I told no one. Ever.

Hoss quit bothering me after a partner of his told him he couldn't do that to me anymore. The same guy also came up to me and said, "Hey, man, you can't suck no dick."

Aw, shit. Somebody else knew. I was humiliated and shamed even more.

Several nights later, I sat at the supper table with my dad and grandmother. In the middle of eating, my dad started singing the song "I'm Forever Blowing Bubbles." I felt a shiver of embarrassment and mortification run up and down my spine like rats in a wall. What the fuck? Did he know, too?

And if he knew, I wondered, why didn't he do something? Why didn't he cut off Hoss's dick?

Then again, maybe it was a coincidence that he sang that song. I don't know why he sang it. I never asked. He never said anything, either. But it sure upset me.

For the rest of my life, I cursed Hoss like no motherfucker's ever been cursed. I even invented new cuss words. Chickenlicking-motherfuckingdickfucker. I beat his ass a million times. I re-played the rape, but in my revamped version I bit his dick off rather than do as he told. I laughed at him. I did everything short of murder him. Because I hated what he did more than anything that had ever happened to me.

The man put his dick in my mouth!

Many years later I went back to Peoria to make *Jo Jo Dancer, Your Life Is Calling* and heard that Hoss was look-ing for me. Oddly, even though I was a famous and success-ful comedian, surrounded by big, menacing bodyguards who would've killed at the snap of my fingers, I was seized by that old sense of fear of Hoss telling me to suck his dick.

I thought I'd shaken the memory.

Guess not.

Motherfucker.

Had me a ghost rattling in the attic. It didn't matter that I lived in a big house behind a gate in Los Angeles, some half a country from the bricks and bars of the old neighborhood. My ass was haunted by the image of Hoss's dick.

As I waited for him, I imagined him winking, asking me to go outside and then to suck his dick.

I wondered how to respond.

I thought about killing the motherfucker. Getting even after all these years. But I'm too much of a chickenshit, and I knew, given my luck, that he'd live to testify against me and send my ass to jail. And I knew the kind of dick I'd get there.

Finally, one afternoon Hoss showed up at my trailer. I was curious how he'd look after all these years, but I was more con-

cerned with how I'd respond to him. I didn't know what the fuck to do. I opened the door. Hoss stood there looking older but otherwise not much different than I remembered him. He had a small boy with him. His arm was on the boy's shoulder.

"This is my son," he said, extending his hand toward me as if we were old friends.

I couldn't believe it. After preparing a lifetime for this moment, I suddenly had nothing to say. Nor did Hoss. What was done was done. What was there to do?

"He's a real big fan of yours," Hoss said of his little boy. "I told him I'd bring him down and ask for an autograph."

"Okay," I said.

The boy was about the same age I'd been when his father raped me. I never could forget. I hoped the boy fared better.

FIVE

M y dad loved my mom so much that he was forever asking himself the question "Why?" That happened to me at the end of several marriages. Sometimes you can't help yourself.

Buck and Gertrude were like that. They had a strange relationship. He was rough, but she talked nasty, disappeared for long, mysterious spells, and when she was around, she drank and argued.

One night Gertrude, as she did so often, said goodbye to my dad and walked out of the house. Only this time she wasn't planning on coming back. She went to her family's farm in Springfield.

Soon after, my grandma had me dress in clothes I only wore to church and then I went with her and my dad to court.

I was ten years old. Not too wise, but savvy enough to know my mom and dad were getting a divorce and that I had to deliver certain lines at the custody hearing. My grandmother said, "Don't be nervous now. When the judge asks you who you want to live with, you say me. All right?"

I wanted to know more about why my mother wasn't coming back to stay with us, but I also knew to shrug off what I couldn't understand.

"Yes, Mama," I whispered.

Then the judge did his thing and asked where I wanted to live.

"With her," I said, pointing to Marie. "I'd like to be with my grandma, please."

The judge nodded. There was more discussion. I didn't know if I'd done good or bad. Then my grandmother was made my legal guardian. I still didn't know if I'd done good or bad.

That I remember. I also remember thinking that I broke my mother's heart by denying her that right.

But Ma, I thought they were going to kill me if I said that I wanted to live with you.

Oh, well.

Gertrude stayed a part of my life. Every so often, I packed my suitcase and took the train to Springfield. Half an hour before I arrived, I began staring out the window, looking for her. I was always relieved to see Gertrude standing on the platform. Then she took me back to the farm in her father's car. Once I spent an entire summer on the farm, and recall that time as the happiest of my life.

The farm was paradise, a playground where my imagination could go wild. At night, I listened to crickets instead of creaking beds and moans, and in the morning, I woke to the sound of roosters crowing and the smell of hot biscuits and fresh-brewed coffee. My grandpa, Bob Thomas, allowed me to help with the chores, which gave me a sense of purpose I didn't have at home.

In addition to farming, he drove a garbage truck. He hauled rubbish to the dump he owned next to the farm. That dump was the site of numerous adventures. At night, for instance, I took a .22, wandered down to the dump, pretending that I was a cowboy or soldier, and waited for some big motherfucking rats to come out. Then I opened fire.

Ka-chu! Ka-chu!

Yes, sir, I fucked up some rats.

★　★　★

My mother didn't stay single for long. After she remarried, she asked me why I didn't call her new husband "Daddy."

"He's your father," she said. "You call him that or I'll beat your ass."

"But he ain't my daddy," I argued.

That pissed her off even more.

"Well, you call that other woman 'Mom.'"

The other woman was Viola Hurst, and my mother was right about the fact I called her Mom. I don't know why I did that, but my daddy and I were going to see Sugar Ray Robinson fight in Chicago, and on the way he surprised me by stopping next door at China Bee's house to pick up Viola. I watched her get into the car and thought she was very sexy.

"This is my son, Richard," he said.

"Hello there," Viola smiled.

"Hi, Mom," I said.

It's strange I called her that. But the night before, I'd overheard Gertrude tell my dad that she thought I was nuts. I didn't know why she said that. Nor did I ask anyone for an explanation. So many things were impossible to understand that after a certain point you just quit trying. You dealt with the facts with survival. You didn't trust anybody. You watched your back. You covered your ass. You said whatever you had to to stay out of trouble.

On television, people talked about having happy lives, but in the world in which I grew up, happiness was a moment rather than a state of being. It buzzed around, just out of reach, like Tinkerbell, flirting and teasing and laughing at your ass. It never stayed long enough for you to get to know it good. Just a taste here and there. A kiss, a sniff, a stroke, a snort.

Yet those were the moments I learned to chase.

I remember the first time I had an orgasm. Because when you first started jacking off, you didn't come. You just had that funny feeling.

In fact, the first time I came I thought something was wrong with me.

Said to my dick, "Oh, shit, look what you've done to me."

An hour later, I was back, Jack. Asked my dick, "Can you do it again?"

It's only natural for a young boy of ten to think about sex, but living in a whorehouse gave me special access to those mysteries of the flesh that elude most people until they're older. I spied through the keyholes, putting my eye to the little opening every chance I got. I bumped my head a lot, but I also got an education you couldn't get in school.

Once I saw my own mother in bed with a man. White dude. She didn't seem to mind. But it fucked me up.

Tricks used to come through our neighborhood. That's where I first met white people. They came down to our neighborhood and helped the economy. I could've been a bigot, you know what I mean? I could've been prejudiced. I met nice white men. They said, "Hello, little boy. Is your mother home? I'd like a blow job."

I wonder what would happen if niggers went to white neighborhoods doing that shit. "Hey, man, your mama home? Tell the bitch we want to fuck!"

The prostitutes sat in the big picture window and waved to customers. All sorts. Whites and blacks. Businessmen. Politicians. Junkies. I spent a lot of time sitting with them, yakking, laughing, and bullshitting.

God, there were some characters. Like Mary. She was a real, honest-to-goodness hermaphrodite. Had a pussy *and* a dick. That shit fucked me up. But she didn't mind. People asked what her name was and she said, "They call me Coffee, 'cuz I grind so fine."

I never had nothing to do with her, other than laughing a hell of a lot. She was a funny lady.

But as soon as some guy entered, those womens kicked me out, closed the door and went to work.

It was weird. I remember a white dude used to come down and ask, "Do you have any girls who'll cover you with ice cream? And little boys that'll lick it off?"
And he was the mayor.

They had me run to the store to get them tampons. I cleaned up in the bathrooms and stuff and found all their women shit around. You know? That's when I decided women are nasty motherfuckers. Then my dick came to life. Started thinking for itself. Bossing me around.

I discovered masturbating when I was about nine or ten. I was in the tub and said, "Hey, I'm onto something here. Shit, I bet Dad don't know about this." After that, they couldn't keep my ass out of the tub.

I never got to scootch any of the whores, but they sure made my dick hard. Swear to God.

One time I crawled up into a vent that looked into one of the upstairs rooms, where one of Mama's whores had brought a john. Shit, they attacked each other, humping and pumping with a furiousness I'd never imagined. I got so involved watching him suck her pussy that I took the vent out and stuck my head out into the room.

Tricks would be fucking, right. They'd be, "Oh, oh, God. Golly, ma'am. Is it really good? Is it really good?"
And the whores be going, "Oh, it's good, baby. Oh, god-damnit. Oh, shit. Damn, there ain't nobody like you, baby. Oh, goddamn."

Years later, I got to be with the same prostitute and I told her the story.

"No, I didn't see you, baby," she said.

"I saw you," I smiled mischievously. Then I pointed to the vent. "I was right up there."

She didn't even open her eyes.

"Go ahead, tell me about it, baby, as you suck on my pussy."

Girls mystified me, man. Scared the crap out of me. I don't know, maybe I thought I was ugly or stupid or something.

When I was a teenager, I didn't get nothing from the girls. Some of the cool guys could get something all the time. Remember those guys? They could say "Bitch," and all the girls would melt. I said that and got an ass whoopin'.

I lost my virginity courtesy of Mr. Spinks. Spinks was a local player, a pimp and dealer. He defined the word *jive*. He lived with this beautiful lady named Penny, who reminded me of Ava Gardner and often crept into my horny imagination.

One day I ventured over to their place, knowing that Spinks was out doing his things and that I could have Penny all to myself. I didn't expect to do anything more than talk and do weird, disgusting things to her in my mind. I wasn't alone with her for ten minutes before Penny asked me to do some of that stuff I was thinking about. Feel her titties, grab her ass. As I complied, my dick showed its appreciation. But I didn't know what to do once I got to that point, which was embarrassing.

"You never fucked anyone before, honey?" she asked. "Did you?"

I shook my head no.

Never mind getting into a girl's panties. I'd never been in one's house.

Fathers kicked ass in my neighborhood. They talked to us on the porch. "Say, boy, what's your name? Jenkins? Let me tell

*you something, boy. You stay away from my house. See, I
workst too hard to send my girls to school to get an education,
and not the kind you wants to give them. Now if I catch you
around here, I'm gonna take this bad leg off and wear your ass
out with it."*

"Come on over here," Penny said. "I'm gonna show you
what they do when the doors are shut."

And she did.

She said, "Just put it in there. Yeah, right there. Now up and
down, you now."

I did what she said.

"Yeah, baby," she continued. "Go up and down. Up and
down. Don't stop."

She fucked me good.

Afterward, I understood why that man had been on top of
my mother.

Getting the pussy just like me.

Then Spinks came home. I was in the bathroom when I
heard the door open and close. Then I heard him say hi to
Penny. Oh, shit. He wanted to make small talk. He asked what
was going on. I listened, my ear to the door as I pulled on
the rest of my clothes and wondered how I was going to *get the
fuck out.*

But I couldn't move. I was too scared.

"Come on out of there," Spinks said.

Was he talking to me?

Then I heard pounding on the bathroom door.

"Rich, get the hell out of there!"

I didn't say a word.

"Listen, boy. Get the fuck out."

I prepared to get clobbered, maybe even killed. Then I
opened the door and braced for the worst. After nothing hit me,
I slowly opened my eyes. Spinks and Penny were on the sofa,
staring at me. Their grins were the size of Chevys.

The embarrassment I felt then was even worse than not knowing what to do with my boner.

"Hi," I said sheepishly. "Uh, thanks. Uh, I gotta go. See ya."

Thinking about it now, I can see that Spinks probably told her to do that to me. Not that I'm complaining, you know.

SIX

My folks gave me a chance at something better by putting me in Catholic school, where I thrived. I made friends. I got straight A's. I showed promise. The teachers were impressed. They thought I was smart and encouraged me to aim high. Then someone found out about the family business and that blew my chance. They gave me the boot. Kicked my ass out into the cold.

I was crushed by this inexplicable rejection by people who professed love and forgiveness.

"Why'd they kick me out of school?" I asked my grandma. "What did I do?"

"Nothing, baby," she said. "Some people just don't know right from wrong, even though they think they wrote the book."

Mama left it to me to discover that the world overflowed with hypocrisy, and it didn't take long. Despite being expelled from Catholic school, I was forced by my stepmother to continue going to catechism on weekends. One Saturday a priest came on to me like a girlfriend. He snuck up on me and gave me a smooch on the lips. I ran home, bawling and heaving the whole way but especially hard as I told and retold the story.

"See, I was in church," I explained. "And the guy there gave me some smooches."

"Where?" my daddy asked.

"On the lips."

"Where were you?" my Uncle Dickie asked.

"In the church."

"Now who kissed you, baby?" my grandma wanted to know. "You said a man kissed you."

"Yeah. The priest."

Black preachers know God personally. Say, "You know, I first met God in 1929. Outside a little hotel in Baltimore. I was walking down the street, eating a tuna fish sandwich. In 1929, you ate anything you could get. And I heard this voice call unto me and the voice had power and majesty. And the voice said, 'Psst.' And I walked up to the voice and said, 'What?' And the voice got magnificent and holy and it resounded, 'Give me some of that sandwich.'"

I knew it was serious when everyone gasped after I identified the molester as a priest.

"What else, honey?"

"Well, Mama, after he kissed me, he said that he'd like to call me someday."

I saw my dad and Uncle Dickie past the point of being angry. Both held back laughter.

"And what'd you say?"

"I said, 'Call me tonight, later tonight,' and then I ran like hell," I said.

The next move was debated. My grandma and some aunties wanted to let it blow over, but my dad and uncle realized that they could probably get some money by blackmailing the priest. They hatched a plan. If the priest called, they told me to goad him into making incriminating comments. They'd listen on another extension. They also told me to arrange a meeting, at which they would surprise the priest and demand money.

"We'll collar him," my dad punned.

I was excited by the scam, but more so by suddenly being the

center of attention. I also liked thinking about the monies my dad and uncle said we'd get. I thought that I might also get a cut and use it to go to the baseball games or the movies. Buy my way into the big time.

Later that night, the phone rang. My dad and uncle ran for the extensions. I nervously did my thing.

"Hi, baby," I purred in the soft, seductive voice they told me to use.

"Oh, my little doll," the priest said.

I heard the excitement in his voice. We cooed sweet nothings back and forth like that for a few minutes. I sensed my dad and uncle's scheme working. Suddenly my grandmother heard what was going on and called a halt to the charade from her bedroom.

"Don't do that to the boy!" she hollered.

Her loud, booming, angry voice threw me off the script and ended my lovey-dovey conversation with the priest before the crucial meeting was set. My dad and uncle scrambled into the kitchen. They made me promise to call him back. But then Grandma Marie yelled for us to get our ass into her bedroom and asked what the hell we were up to.

My father and Dickie denied everything. But I caved.

"Mama, I don't want to do this," I said.

Mama shook her head in disgust and ordered us to put an end to the scheming. It was disappointing. We had the priest hooked; however, she wanted us to throw him back as if he was a small bass. Then she urged forgiveness.

"Richard," my grandmother said, "you've got to understand that everybody's human."

"Yes, Mama."

"Don't ever forget it," she continued. "No matter what they are. Everybody's human."

For a young black boy, that statement was hard to believe. It was clear that some people believed that they were more human

than others. At my new school, Irving Elementary, I developed a crush on a little girl. She happened to be white. But she could've been any color, it didn't matter to me. I just liked her.

One day, as a token of my affection, I gave her a scratch board—the kind on which you scribble pictures and then lift up the plastic paper to erase the drawing. She promised to take it home and make it her favorite toy. I was pleased.

The next day her father showed up at school holding the toy. He looked mean. You weren't supposed to look at fourth-graders like that. He asked the teacher which "little nigger" had given his daughter the scratch pad. She pointed to me, and he ran straight up to me.

"Nigger, don't you ever give my daughter anything," he yelled.

That really put me back.

What the fuck had I done? Why was he calling me a nigger? Why did he hate me?

I mean I knew. I knew it was because I was black. But still, I didn't know why.

That shit is stuff that people like my grandmother warned me about. I also overheard others telling stories, nervously ex-changing anecdotes, and such, but you don't believe it until you're actually confronted by it. Like a holdup or attack. You see it on the news every night, figuring it's always going to hap-pen to someone else. Never you. But then some dude steps in your face and calls you a nigger.

If I was four and a half feet tall then, the girl's daddy cut six inches off. Zap. Six inches of self-esteem gone.

That was my indoctrination to the black experience in Amer-ica. They don't teach that shit in school. But I'd learn, as every African American does to some degree, that such degradation and assault to one's dignity has gone on since the slave ships brought black people from Africa to this land of equality and opportunity.

I couldn't figure out why the teacher didn't defend me. She didn't say a word. My dad went to school the next day and

confronted her. I'd never seen him so angry. I loved that he was defending me.

"How could you do that?" he asked. "How could you not say anything to that man?"

The teacher looked down. She shook her head, showing that she, too, was disgusted. At the man. At herself. My daddy gently patted her on the back. They reached some kind of understanding.

Then he turned to the little girl I'd tried to befriend.

"Did you get his present?" he asked.

"Yes," she sniffled. "But he wouldn't let me keep it."

"That's okay," I chimed in.

Or so I said.

But I didn't mean it.

My brain didn't segregate people by race. My eyes didn't see any one color. One of my favorite activities was going to the movies, where I lost myself in the fantasy projected on-screen. My heroes included Tarzan, Rhonda Fleming, Milton Berle, Kirk Douglas, Sid Caesar, and Boris Karloff. I loved Jerry Lewis. I wanted to be John Wayne. I saw the *Red Ryder* cowboy serials over and over, and one time I went in the back to look for Robert Blake's Little Beaver character. I thought I'd be able to find him behind the screen. But the crew chased me out.

There were only a couple theaters in Peoria that allowed black people inside. But then, having paid for tickets and popcorn the same as white people, we were restricted to sitting in the balcony. It was the same as public buses and washrooms. Except the odd thing was, nobody I knew seemed to mind at the theater. They liked the balcony. The view was good, it was like a party, nobody threw shit on you.

But I wanted to sit up close, in the front row. You know how kids are? I wanted to feel as if I could jump into the screen.

However, one afternoon the manager grabbed my arm, yanked me from my chair, and told me I had to sit upstairs.

"In the 'Colored Section,'" he said. "Up where all you people are supposed to be."

"No, I ain't gonna do that," I said.

"Well, then you'll have to leave."

Niggers be holding their dicks. Some white people go, "Why you guys hold your things?"

Say, "You done took everything else, motherfucker."

I loved the movies, but the manager didn't give me a choice. I knew what was what.

So I left.

SEVEN

At twelve years old, I transferred to Blaine Sumner, a primarily white school. By then, I'd given up on acquiring an education. After all, I'd been raped, expelled, abused, and victimized by the sting of racism. What more was there to learn?

I couldn't lie to my old man because he could hypnotize me. He heard my mind. Checked me right out.
"Say, man, are you fucking up in school?" he asked.
Huh?
"Yes. I. Am."

In class, I let my motor idle. Between bells, I wondered if my teachers were good fucks. Stuff like that.
I also jacked off.

A lot of people didn't jack off. I used to jack off so much I knew pussy couldn't be as good as my hand.

My friend Andy and I had secret jack-off contests at our desks, though one time in art class our X-rated antic wasn't as private as I thought. After the bell, someone pointed out that all the desks had a front, except for mine. Everyone in the class had watched.
"Ain't this a bitch," I said. "And here I thought I was being slick."

★   ★   ★

I witnessed salvation come to people in a number of ways—
drugs, gambling, women, and alcohol—and though I wouldn't
say I was saved by Marguerite Yingst Parker, one of my teachers at Blaine, she did give me a shove in the right direction. Miss
Parker was an attractive woman who had a pretty daughter
about my age. I joked that I wanted to get together with her.

"Maybe we'll get married," I told my teacher. "Then you
and I will be family."

"Oh, Richard," Miss Parker said sweetly.

What set Miss Parker apart from the rest was her ability to
handle me. She did it with kindness and patience, a combination
that's always slayed me. Ordinarily, I acted dumb in front of my
teachers, but Miss Parker refused to believe my performances,
no matter how convincing.

"I guess I'm too retarded for that," I whined.

Miss Parker always laughed at my silliness. Then she sat me
down, assured me that I wasn't as dumb as I said, and in a gentle, sweet, reassuring voice she goaded me into at least trying to
learn something.

In truth, she blackmailed me. If I would make an attempt at
working, she said, then she would permit me to stand in front of
the class each morning and tell jokes.

The deal was irresistible.

My routine was always something I'd picked up from a TV
show. Red Skelton, Jerry Lewis, Sid Caesar. Sometimes I imi-
tated friends; other times I risked impressions of the school's
teachers and bullies, who all of us knew were assholes. I never
thought of myself as having a gift, but I made my classmates
laugh, and when I heard their laughter, I felt good about myself,
which was a pretty rare feeling. But nice. Real nice.

By high school, I'd tried running with gangs. But I was tough for
about half a minute. That was it.

I was in every gang in Peoria. They had about five. I was in all of them. Whichever one was winning.

"That's my side!"

The real tough guys hung out at Proctor, a recreation center where they spent all day practicing how to be criminals. Fighting, rolling dice, drinking. Guys showed up at noon and hung around all day, waiting for the cops to come.

The scared pootbutts like me went to Carver Center, a safe haven thanks to the effort, vision, and devotion of Juliette Whittaker. A tiny young lady, she might've been the toughest soul in Peoria. She didn't take shit from anybody, and people who didn't even know her respected her for having something most others didn't—an education.

She was a black woman who came from good parents and had gone to college. That was something downright inspirational.

More so, instead of leaving for better neighborhoods that had higher-paying jobs, Miss Whittaker stayed in Peoria. She had beliefs about doing good, a conviction that she could help kids like me realize their dreams—if they dared to dream in the first place. She was good.

I picked up on that. Although Miss Whittaker reminded me of a toad, I saw the beauty inside her. Her smile made you forget about things. That's beauty. I proposed to her a couple of times, but I guess I was too young for her.

She'd just started at Carver when we met in 1951. She was in the midst of staging the play *Rumpelstiltskin* and had cast all the parts except a small role of a guy who goes onstage and sneezes. It wasn't a walk-on as much as it was a walk-off. But I got it and was thrilled, especially when she gave me a script to take home and learn, though there was nothing in it for me to memorize.

I learned all the parts anyway, and when the kid who played the king came down with the flu, Miss Whittaker turned to me.

No one in the history of the theater was more prepared to move up than I was, though my performance was unique. I modeled my portrayal of the king after my Uncle Dickie and turned the fairy tale into a black comedy.

"Hey, baby," I said to the miller's daughter, "you keep on spinning that straw into gold for me and I'll get you a car. Something fine. Something for your mama. I'll make you my woman . . ."

Miss Whittaker noticed my talent, quick wit, ambition, and need—especially my need. She began centering skits and revues around me. I had no trouble being the center of attention and generating laughs. The spotlight suited me. In fact, I once pasted my name over Marlon Brando's on a photo of a movie marquee I cut out of the newspaper.

I spent all day making up shit. Practicing. It was like some kids stood on the corner and sang. I talked.

My father was one of those eleven o'clock men.
"Say, where you going? Nigger, you ain't asked nobody if you could go no place. What, you're a man now. Okay, then get a job. I don't give a fuck where you're going. Be home by eleven. You understand eleven, don't you, nigger? You can tell time, can't you? Eleven o'clock, you bring your ass home. I don't mean down the street singing with them niggers, either . . . And bring me back a paper."
But nothing starts happening till eleven-thirty. Dudes be standing around. You ask, "What you waiting on, nigger?"
"Eleven-thirty. We gonna pitch a bitch at eleven-thirty."
I'd have to go home with my blue nuts.
"I thought I told you to be home at eleven," my dad yelled. "I don't want to hear that shit. I'm gonna kick your ass."
"Can I jack off first?"

Most of the shit I said was true. I just reported on what I saw and heard, adding a twist here and there.

"Your shoes are run over so much, looks like your ankles is broke."

Shit like that.

I did a character called the Rummage Sale Ranger. The Rummage Sale Ranger was a black superhero, but he was too poor to have his own shit. He had to go to the rummage sale. Find some woman's tights. Steal a fucking cape because he was out of change. Shoes that were too big. Nothing fit right.

Kids at the center loved the shit. The material flowed from my mouth without stop, which was a problem for some.

Like Mr. Fink, my science teacher. But I gave him reason.

Mr. Fink was serious about teaching. I sat in the back row and entertained my neighbors as if I was at the Comedy Store working out a new routine. One day he got so fed up, he grabbed me by the scruff of the neck and took me downstairs. Just to show I had a sense of humor, I took a swing at him.

That was it.

He opened the front door to the school and literally threw my ass on the ground. Out of school.

"Don't come back," he said.

The door slammed shut with a loud bang. I knew there was no use arguing my way back inside. It was as if school was a train ride and the conductor was talking to me.

"Eighth grade. End of the line!"

"Aw, shit," I said out loud.

Then I thought about my folks. What were they going to say?

"Fuck!" I said. "Now I've got to go home and deal with those people."

EIGHT

Everybody listened to what happened. My grandmother. My dad. Viola. My aunts and uncles. They then taught me the lesson you learn after leaving school.

"It's okay," my dad said. "But I'll tell you this. If you don't put nothing in the pot, you don't get nothing out."

Dinner that night was my last free meal. The next day I began looking for a job.

As a fourteen-year-old high school dropout, I had low expectations. I begged local shop owners, and eventually I got a job cleaning a strip club. Sweeping and mopping. My problem was that I liked the show more than I did the work. The club's owner complained to Uncle Dickie, who confronted me.

"He says the girls lay down on the stage and get all dirty," Dickie explained to me. "What's the matter, boy?"

"I can do the sweeping," I said. "But I can't do no mopping. My arms too skinny."

Next, I shined shoes at the Pierre Marquette Hotel. I enjoyed that. I thought I was Numero Uno. I made the shine cloth crack like a bullwhip. Told jokes. The money was easy and the conversation good.

But I fell in with some bad guys who persuaded me there was an easier way to make money. By stealing it. One afternoon, we targeted a small grocery store in the neighborhood. As one guy went in and distracted the owner, another guy and I opened the

cash register and grabbed the coins from the box. Nothing fancy. Plain old till-tapping. Except I dropped the coins. My friends ran. The owner calmly walked toward me, shaking his head in disgust.

"Boy, what the hell are you doing?" he yelled.

I froze and saw my future.

"We've got your son down here at headquarters. What about it?"

"Fuck him."

I'd be praying something would happen to him on the way down to the station. But he always showed up.

"I'm going to get you out, nigger. But then I'm gonna kick your ass."

My hands went straight up. There was nothing in them. I did one of those looks that said, "Who? Me?"

"Yes, nigger. I'm talking to you. Put that money back."

I put the coins back real nice, as if that would make it like nothing ever happened.

"I'm gonna tell your daddy," he threatened.

My so-called friends stood outside, looking through the window and laughing.

"And don't come back here no more," the owner added.

That hurt. Because that was my local store. I went there all the time.

About then Dickie was picked up for dope and went to jail. I remember when the cops got him: he was holding a big box of counterfeit money. Right before they cuffed him, he set it on top of a garbage can. Real calm. They never bothered to check it.

He went to prison in Michigan. He did about three years and came out a changed man.

He said to me, "Richard, I can only tell you one thing about prison."

"What's that?"

"Don't ever go."

After racking balls at Pop's Pool Hall and driving a truck for my dad's carting business, I finally got my first serious job at one of the local packing companies. I shook and folded hides and loaded them on the trains that took them to Chicago, where they were turned into shoes, coats, bags, and shit. It was nasty work. All the shit that got on me during the day, the rock salt, water and whatnot, froze in the cold. By quitting time, my pants were as stiff as a board.

But the job was mine. I made monies. I had the jingle-jangle of possibilities in my pocket.

One day I heard about a better-paying position cutting beef. I went upstairs to where they did that shit to investigate. However, as soon as I saw guys hitting the fucking bulls in the head with sledgehammers, I knew I couldn't handle it. Neither could I handle dealing with those bulls while they were alive. As I stood there, one of them escaped.

Guess he had other ideas.

I saw him look at that sledgehammer and say, "What? Excuse me, what's going on?"

Suddenly, he charged out of his stall, ran through the shop, upstairs and downstairs, snorting and kicking and butting everything in his path. Then he got outside. The police finally had to shoot this motherfucker because he was running down the street with one thing on his mind: What motherfucker ordered steak?

I spent about half my pay at Yakov's Liquor Store, where I ate pickled pig's feet, drank ice-cold beer, and bullshitted about the

future. I didn't expect to stay employed at the packing company forever. Eventually, I figured on buying a pair of steel-toed shoes and punching a clock at the Caterpillar tractor company. Work, pension, die. In between, I'd get fucked up and watch TV and chase pussy.

Getting some pussy beats anything. I ain't lying. Coming is a lot of fun. I never got no pussy when I was a legal teenager. You had to sing to get pussy. Be one of those niggers on the corner who sang. I couldn't sing.

Besides, the girls weren't giving no pussy in the fifties. It was very seldom you got any parts of pussy. You'd be tongue kissing and your dick got harder than the times in '29. Nuts would go up into your stomach and you said, "Oh, baby, you gotta give me something now."

"I'm not giving anything," she said. "I'm on my period."

"You're on your period again? You gonna bleed to death, bitch."

At seventeen, I started fucking regularly. One was an attractive little package.

She and I used to hide out in the garage of a house my family owned on Goodwin. It wasn't the Playboy mansion, but it was kind of our private place.

It was pure fun.

I used to wrestle with her for two hours. That's when those rubber panties came out—those long rubber panties. And every time I'd get a grip, she'd move and I'd lose my grip and have to wrestle two more hours. And by the time I'd got them, I was too tired. "I'll see you tomorrow."

Then her father would catch us. There'd be a knock at the door. "What are you doing here, Mr. Pryor?"

"Oh, nothing. Just sitting here on the couch with my pants off."

I fell in love with that girl. Fell hard.

But then I loved falling in love.

Looking back, that turned out to be my curse. Falling in love, you know. It was never enough.

In late 1956, she took all the fun out of what we had going. She said she was pregnant.

For a moment, I thought the baby was mine. But she had slept with lots of people, including my dad. Nine months later she gave birth to a little girl. My Aunt Maxine reassured me that the baby wasn't mine.

This was revelatory, a weight off my back.

I was like "Oh, somebody else claimed it?"

She said, "Yeah. I was out in the chicken shack and someone else said it was his baby."

Well, that was all the excuse I needed. The little girl grew up with her mother and grandmother in Peoria. I saw her occasionally, and eventually we got to know each other. Not an ideal relationship. Just a fact of life.

In 1958, I volunteered for the Army. I ask myself why I did something like that, a chickenshit like me.

I was serving my country. It was either that or six months.

I wanted out of Peoria. I wanted to see something different. No place in particular. Just beyond, you know.

I took the train to Chicago, went to the induction office, and spent the day taking tests. I must've done okay, because right after, I was sworn in. They gave me a free round-trip train ticket that got me home and back to Chicago.

To me, that was exciting shit.

Basic training was at Fort Leonard Wood, in Missouri. I received eight weeks of plumbing school.

Once again I was covered in shit.

I went to kill class. Turned me around. I thought the Army was like hunting, camping, a little fishing. But I learned to kill from a guy who killed in World War Two, and then they couldn't stop him. So they gave him a job.

"Can't let him on the streets, so we'll let him train these guys for World War Three."

Then my papers come in, and I was transferred to Idar-Oberstein in Germany. For an eighteen-year-old who'd never been farther than Springfield or Bloomington, it was exciting. Idar-Oberstein sounded like an exotic woman.

Then reality. I called my sergeant and told him I was on my way to the base.

"I'm so happy you're coming," he said.

"Thank you, sir," I said.

"Yeah," he laughed, "I've been working with a nigger for the last three years."

Uh-oh, I thought.

"Yes, sir," I said. "Well, I'm glad I'm here, too, sir. Yes, sir."

I expected Germany to be a little freer, but the *Fräuleins* were skinny rather than fat, and when I ventured to the section where all the bars were located, I found that out of like 150 bars only three let in blacks. Why should you have been surprised, Rich? Well, I was, because I thought all that shit was behind me.

Unfortunately, I met a woman whose boyfriend was a bartender in one of the white bars, and one night I went there. Her boyfriend, who usually called the MPs on me, wasn't working that night, so I had a chance. But before I ordered my first beer, a fight broke out between two U.S. soldiers, and before I knew it, I heard someone cry out, "Nigger!"

I glanced around. There was no one else of any color there but me. I ran upstairs, where the strippers changed clothes, beg-

ging the first girl I saw to help. She gave me a look of hate that I knew too well from back home.

"Get out of here," she said in a heavily accented voice.

"You don't understand. They're fighting down there."

"Get out of here. I call police."

The MPs arrived at the same time I snuck outside and ran back to the barracks. I never forgot that stripper, though.

Of course, you never forget the cruel ones.

But there were other, kinder women, thank God.

My kind of women. The kind who liked to fuck. This one woman let me give her head, which was a revelation, something that changed my life, because until then, my family only fucked in one position—up and down.

My uncle had said, "Boy, don't you ever kiss no pussy. I mean that. Whatever you do in life, don't kiss no pussy."

I couldn't wait to kiss the pussy. He'd been wrong about everything else. Woman had to beat me off.

"It's enough! It's enough. Two days!"

Eventually, the Army turned me into a vicious killing machine. The transformation occurred in full one weekend night as our unit watched the movie *Imitation of Life*. This white soldier laughed at the wrong spots. Several of us finally took exception, including a big black soldier, who got into a slugfest with the white guy.

But my guy was a dumb motherfucker in terms of fighting. The white boy seriously hurt my guy's ass.

A crowd gathered. People wanted blood. We'd spent months training for combat, but this turned into the biggest battle anyone had come close to, and I knew my guy was going down if something didn't happen.

From within the crowd of soldiers, I reached into my pocket and drew out a switchblade. Pushed the button.

Flifft!

No one but me suspected anything. I waited for the right moment. Then I stabbed the white motherfucker in the back six or seven times. He didn't stop, though. You know? He kept throwing punches. As soon as I realized he wasn't going down, I ran the opposite direction, tossing the knife into the bushes on my way to the barracks.

A while later, the white dude came in accompanied by an angry-looking MP. I peeked at the white guy's back. His T-shirt was shredded from my stabbing and soaked with blood. I thought, Goddamn, I did that and he didn't even stop. Didn't even feel it. Why didn't he feel it?

He stared at me like that bull from the packing plant where I'd worked. Then he tore off his shirt.

"See what you did to me, chickenshit?" he said.

"Wasn't me."

He said, "Yes, it was. You're the one. See all these holes? You're the asshole nigger who did this."

"No, I didn't do it."

My denials meant shit. An MP threw my ass in jail. There wasn't anything in that cell except for me, the cement floor, and a single, annoying lightbulb. I fell onto the cot and began to think seriously about getting the fuck out of jail and the Army.

The base commander agreed. He was on the verge of retirement, and the last thing he wanted to deal with was a silly enlisted man fucking up regulations.

I was lucky. Lucky I didn't kill that white guy and luckier still that they didn't kill me.

Because back then, the way things were, few people outside of Peoria would've missed one more dead black man.

NINE

I returned to Peoria speaking enough broken German to impress the local girls, but I was disappointed that I hadn't connected with the service. I had hoped to start a new career, something with more future and security than working at the packing plant or Caterpillar.

Instead, I settled into the most popular career path among young uneducated black men—unemployment.

I allowed plenty of free time for inspiration to find me.

I remember seeing Redd Foxx and Dick Gregory on television and thinking that I could do something similar. I had no trouble making people laugh. I made a fool out of myself as good as the next guy. Did it all the time. The guys I hung out with said I was a funny motherfucker. Shit, I might as well get paid for it.

I knew where to go, and one day I walked into Harold's Club and asked Harold Parker, the club's owner, for work. Harold's was a black and tan club, meaning both whites and blacks went there. Harold himself was like that. We used to say he was too light to be bright.

"What do you do?" he asked.

"I sing and play piano."

Okay, I lied. I didn't do either. But Harold was a friend of my father's.

"How much you expecting to make?" he asked.

I answered, "Not much."

"That's good," he said. " 'Cuz you won't."

For my nightclub debut, I sat at the piano and improvised using the three or four chords I knew. I sang whatever words popped into my head. I saw that people didn't know whether I was putting them on or weird. But I put in enough time for the waitresses to serve their drinks and collect their tips.

Afterward, I tried to look cool, but when Harold came up to me backstage, I still had sweat pouring off me.

"You've got more nerve than anybody I've ever seen," he said. "Would you like to keep coming?"

"Yes, sir," I said. "I would like to do that."

Harold also hired Sonny Stinson, a real singer, who brought his own band. He was the main attraction. I did my thing during their breaks. After a while, I realized that the audience responded better to my jokes than to my singing, and so, shit, I wasn't stupid. Talking was easier than making up songs. I told jokes, did impressions of Dean Martin, Jerry Lewis, and Sammy Davis, Jr., and sometimes I simply picked up a book or the newspaper and read the shit in a strange voice while adding funny asides.

One of my earliest bits was a takeoff on "Person to Person," the TV show, on which host Edward R. Murrow interviewed famous people in their homes. In my act, I wondered what might happen if instead of talking to a celebrity, Murrow walked in on a dirt-poor black family in Mississippi.

"Hi, Mistah Murrah. Just step over the chickens. Yes, that's it. We're going to have one for dinner if you want to stay.

"Yes, sir, that's our chair. And our TV. And our sofa. The wallpaper is newspaper. Put it up ourselves.

"That house in the back?

"No, that ain't no guesthouse. We piss in there. Go ahead, if you need to. We'll keep the chickens back."

★   ★   ★

I was desperate to matter. I wanted to grow and bloom like the patch of sunflowers I admired as a boy. The laughter and attention I got on stage fed that desire.

Then I received an additional boost. Sonny Stinson introduced me to marijuana and uppers. I'd never tried either. I drank, but drugs were new to me.

"It's part of show business," said Sonny.

Whether or not that was true didn't matter once I tried the shit. I liked the buzz. It eased my pain and insecurity, erased the fear, turned me into a whole new man. Sometimes I stayed up two or three days straight, feeling so cool and jive. Eventually, Sonny tired of me always asking for freebies.

"You want more, it's gonna cost you," he said.

Shit, I didn't care. I loved the high, hated the crash. Said I'll take two instead. Stayed awake forever. Then at two in the morning on the second or third day of being awake, I'd be screaming for help.

"Please, God, there's an Indian playing a drum inside me. Tell him to stop."

"That's your heart."

"Well, tell it to stop. Let me sleep."

"HA-HA-HA!"

I was as easily hooked on women, too. My next love, Patricia, was a nice, tender little thing, who reminded me of the Patricia Neal character in the movie *Hud*. Same name, same situation. She probably shouldn't have gotten involved with a confused young comedian who didn't have a plan. But, hey, I made about $50 a week and I thought that was good, you know?

For us, it was.

But in 1960 I didn't know certain stuff. Patricia got pregnant. I felt responsible, which might've been the first and last

time I did. But my dad told me flat out I didn't have to marry her.

"You don't have to do this, son," he said.

Yes, I did. Just to spite him I did.

Geez, I was a sick puppy.

Patricia and I married in the little corner house on Goodwin. My grandmother, dad, and Viola were among those who attended the event. They came when Richard Jr. was born, too. At the hospital, I stared at him for the longest time. He looked like a little ape, and when I told my dad that, he laughed.

"So did you," he said. "Like a little gorilla. That's what Mama said about you."

"Yeah?" I muttered. "Then I guess he's mine."

But that was about all. After Richard Jr. was born, Pat and I quit living together.

Why'd I split?

Because I could.

TEN

B y 1962, I also started performing at Collins' Corner, another black and tan nightclub, though it was actually more black than tan. The club's owner, Bris Collins, promoted me from opening act to emcee, which paid between $70 and $100 a week and gave me an excuse to hang out with the headliner, a pretty girl from St. Louis who could sing her ass off.

She had a big act that included dancers and backup singers, most of whom, I discovered, were transvestites. Men dressing up as girls. I was greatly relieved to find a few real females. One sang, one danced, and one had a sister who looked more like a brother. I always thought she was a man. Then one night she gave me some pussy. I swear I thought she was going to pull out some kind of dick.

But she didn't. She liked me.

I listened to them tell stories of playing the different black-owned clubs in the Midwest that formed the Blackbelt circuit and dreamed of hitting the road just as they did. It was my way out.

"Maybe one day I'll emcee a rock 'n' roll show," I said to Bris Collins.

That day came sooner than I imagined.

One day my woman—this whore who'd been given to me by my dad—told me to beat her. I didn't know what she was talking about, but she screamed, "Hit me. Hit me." Well, I didn't

know that when a woman told you to hit her you weren't supposed to go crazy. But I went crazy. I started fighting as if it was a real fight. Bruised and hurt, she ran to my father. It looked as if he might beat me.

"What the fuck are you doing?" he yelled. "You don't know how to beat a whore."

"But she said to hit her," I explained.

"Get out of here," he said.

"What?" I asked, realizing he was serious about kicking me out of the house. "What'd you say?"

"Get your ass outta here!"

I hadn't planned on such a hasty departure, but I had no choice. I grabbed some clothes, some cash, and a little alto saxophone, which I later pawned to buy groceries, and walked in a swirl of confusion over to Collins' Corner. I didn't know what I was going to do or where I was going to go, only that I wasn't going to stick around Peoria, and as I slammed the door behind me, I said, "You'll see, motherfucker. Someday, you'll see."

At Collins' Corner, I told both the guys who were girls and the real girls what had happened. They invited me to travel with them to East St. Louis, where they were booked into the Faust Club, a club on the Blackbelt circuit. I couldn't believe my luck. One minute kicked out of the house, no prospects. The next I was on the road in show business.

I was too raw for the Faust Club, whose acts were all experienced. But the club's emcee watched me work a few times and tried to help. My routines weren't bad, he said, but my delivery was.

"You've got to talk to the people," he said. "You always look like you want to kill them. Persuade 'em."

"Okay."

When my friends moved on, I was left to fend for myself. But I had picked up on how the system worked from other

performers, particularly from one dancer. She had given me the mystery eye and led me into her dressing room. I mentioned that I'd been in the Army, in Germany. She was impressed and asked what I'd done there.

"I learned to eat pussy," I said.

Smiling, she eased back on the tattered dressing-room sofa and told me that if I ate her pussy, she'd speak to the club owner at her next job and get me hired as the emcee. And that was how things operated. You worked a little on stage and a little off it. I also realized why they called the Army "the service."

On the Blackbelt, there were no booking agents or managers who got you jobs. Instead, the performers traded information among themselves—strippers, musicians, dancers. They told the club owners who was good, bad, and indifferent, who liked to drink, fight, gamble, do drugs, and shit like that.

There weren't a lot of options, so basically you went wherever you were wanted and hoped it worked out.

Towns flew by in a blur. Cleveland, Chicago, Buffalo, and so on. I took cars, buses, trains, hitchhiked. It was hard times, but exciting times. I was going someplace else. Every day was different, a surprise, an adventure through uncharted territory, and it forced me to sharpen my skills and learn my craft just as Redd Foxx, Dick Gregory, Godfrey Cambridge, and other black comics had done before me.

It was like going to school, especially this one funky club in Youngstown, Ohio. That's where I discovered God blessed me to be stupid enough not to know better. Everybody, it seemed, but me knew the place was owned by shady characters. Tough guys. People who settled arguments by throwing guys off bridges and such.

For real.

None of these stories bothered Satin Doll, the beautiful singer who headlined the club. Then toward the end of our run,

I heard her crying in her dressing room. I walked in and asked what was wrong. I expected to hear that her lover had been fitted with concrete shoes. It was worse.

"They aren't going to pay us," she sobbed.

"Not going to pay who?" I asked. "Motherfuckers aren't going to pay me. I was raised better than that shit."

Back then, I carried a blank pistol with me. For protection, of course. Shows how ignorant I was.

So I got the gun, busted into the club's office, and ordered the motherfuckers to give me the money they owed me.

I talked my best black shit. That usually scared the average white motherfucker. But you know how it is when you do something and the motherfucker don't react and you can feel there's something wrong?—and you got the gun!

You think there's something wrong. There's some look missing in this motherfucker's face.

I'm sure those men are there today, laughing. Because he just started laughing.

"This fucking kid," he said. "Ah-ha-ha-ha-ha."

Then he called his partner Tony.

"Hey, do it again, Rich. Put the gun away and do it again. Say 'Stick 'em up.' Ha-ha-ha-ha! You fucking kid. I like you. Fucking stick 'em up. Hey, Tony, was you scared? Ha-ha-ha . . ."

It got worse in Pittsburgh, where I met a singer. She liked me a lot. Why, I don't know. But it was nice. Except I didn't know enough to keep my mouth shut.

Thinking I was a big shot, I told people we were going out and that she was giving me money and shit. Someone told her and she came looking for me, seeking revenge. At the confrontation, backstage, I thought she was going to do serious damage to me, so I beat her ass first. I didn't think about hitting a woman as much as I thought about my own survival.

But shit.

Pittsburgh was like a small town. Her father knew some cops, and one night, as I was about to go to sleep, they busted in the rooming house where I lived, fixing to turn me inside out. Once they saw me, though, all 150 pounds of skin and bones and no muscle, they must've felt as if she should've taken me, or that at least it was a fair fight.

Instead of beating me up, they let me get dressed and we shot the shit as they took me to jail.

Still, it wasn't a good situation. Skinny black kid. Broke. In jail. My lawyer told me to keep quiet in court.

I tried, but . . .

"Ninety days," the judge said.

Shit.

I remembered what Uncle Dickie had said about going to jail, which was don't. I also remembered that Spinks, the player from Peoria who'd helped me lose my virginity, had always sworn he wasn't going to ever go to jail, and when they finally sent him off, he stayed true to his word by dropping dead of a heart attack as soon as he heard the clink of his cell door being shut.

But it wasn't so bad. In jail, I met a guy on his way out who knew my Aunt Maxine. Through him, I got her to send me twenty bucks, which I used to play the numbers. I put a dime on 313 and it came up. I won $70 and after doing thirty-five days, I used my winnings to buy myself out of the pokey.

It was freezing the day I got out of jail. On my way back to the club, I heard Sammy Davis, Jr., had performed the night before and was still in town. For some reason, I decided that I had to meet Sammy, who would become a friend years later, so I walked to his hotel, found out his room, and sat in a chair at the end of the hall. Just sat there.

For hours, nothing happened. Every now and then, a policeman shuffled through and gave me the once-over, but in my suit

I appeared to be part of Sammy's entourage. Or at least someone who had reason to be there.

A few times, Sammy peeked out his door and saw me. Once,
one of his guys brought me a plate of food, which I devoured.
He probably figured I was some bum hoping for a handout, but
in all honesty I think I just wanted to shake his hand and hope
some luck rubbed off on me.

The next day, Sammy finally came out of the room. I stood
up, grinned like a fool with nothing to say.

But it was Sammy Davis, Jr.!

"What's happening?" he said.

"Well, I was working in town," I stammered, "and I thought
I'd see you and maybe get a job with you or something."

Sammy nodded. He let me bum a cigarette and gave me a bit
of hope. But he was so jive. He had the walk, the talk, the attitude. Didn't mind being a star one bit. It was a beautiful thing
to see. Made me envious.

From there, I went to Buffalo, where I met Donnie Simpson, a
struggling comic like myself, though he talked more shit than
anybody I knew, including me. He dragged me to Windsor,
Canada, and then to Toronto, always promising we'd meet
more beautiful women and earn bigger paychecks. Finally, up in
Toronto, we ran out of clubs.

It was 1963. I remember opening a copy of *Newsweek* magazine and seeing an article on Bill Cosby. It devastated me. I told
Donnie, and later reiterated to others, "Goddamn it, this nigger's doing what I'm fixing to do. I want to be the only nigger.
Ain't no room for two niggers."

"Then why's your ass here, Rich?" he said. "You got to go to
New York. That's where all them bit cats are."

ELEVEN

looked as good as could be when I arrived in New York. I wore a ragamuffin suit, a pencil-thin tie, and patent leather shoes. Although I had only $10 in my pocket, I looked like $50.

At the train station, I paid 50 cents to shower, slapped on some Canoe cologne, walked outside, and breathed in Manhattan. Skyscrapers, taxis, crowds racing along the sidewalks. It was a lot to take in for someone with no place to go. I heard alarms go off in my head and wondered what the hell I'd done.

The only place I knew in Manhattan was the Apollo Theater, in Harlem. I caught a bus uptown, got off at 125th Street, and wandered around. I didn't know a soul, but seeing all those black people made me feel better.

At the Apollo, I met the guy who was in charge of booking acts. He looked and sounded like someone who'd seen and heard everything and was just waiting till sometime later.

"I'd like to work here," I said. "I'm a comedian."

"Yeah, right," he answered. "Why don't you try down at the Village."

This was my first time in New York, and perhaps I was dumber than dog shit, but wasn't this a city? A big city?

Why was he talking about a village?

He gestured.

"Downtown," he said.

I caught a bus and sat down next to a guy who listened to me ramble about how I'd come to town to be a comedian and didn't know anyone. I told him I planned to stay at the YMCA nearest the clubs and asked if he knew where that was. He insisted that I stay with him at his rooming house on Thirty-sixth Street.

The guy was gay, which scared me, but he turned out to be nice and helpful. He introduced me to the landlady, got me a room, and then gave me a talk on who was naughty and nice in the area.

In 1963, the Village was alive. Full of cats similar to me. A bunch of hobos looking for work. I met talented young comics like J. J. Barry, Martin Harvey Freeberg, and Ron Carey. They educated me about the club scene. Someone told me to introduce myself to Manny Roth, the owner of Cafe Wha?, and before long, I was opening for Superman Victor Brady and his Trinidadian steel band, telling jokes such as:

"I watch a lot of television, and so I see those commercials, like the one where the woman says, 'Honey, I got a giant in my washer.'

"And her husband says, 'Yeah, well he better be gone before I get home.'"

Once I decided I was going to be in New York for a while, I took a small apartment on Fourteenth Street. It was a strange place. You could lock the door, but any key opened it. One night a thief broke in just after I'd gone to bed. I heard the door open. Then somebody walked in. He began rummaging through my stuff when he felt the burn of my gaze like a flashlight beam and turned around.

"Um, I think you've got the wrong room," I said calmly.

The dude played it just as cool and said, "I guess you're right," and then left.

He wasn't the only strange character I met. No, not in New York.

Once, I was in a restaurant with a group of people, including a beautiful lady who flirted with me. She was white, and her advances really upset the guy next to me. As soon as I picked up

on this, I added grease to the frying pan, suggesting that she change seats so she could sit beside me. A few minutes later, we left for a nearby hotel.

But then the joke turned on me. As we sat on the bed in the hotel room, I put my arm around her and started rubbing her sumptuous body. We worked up to that magic point, and just as I was about to ask her to give me head, my hand touched her arm. It was like no other arm that I'd ever felt.

In fact, it was wooden. I checked it out with my fingernail. Hard as a tree. Could've used the motherfucker for kindling. Right away, my dick said adios, retreating into my stomach, and I guess she sensed my discovery.

"Does that bother you?" she asked.

"No," I squeaked. "But it scares the hell out of my dick."

Before long, I became a regular at the Bitter End, the Living Room, Papa Hud's, and all the other clubs. The scene reminded me of Harold's and Collins' Corner back in Peoria, but instead of Sonny Stinson, the performers were Bob Dylan, Richie Havens, and Bill Cosby. I met George Carlin at the Café Au Go Go and introduced myself to Woody Allen at the Bitter End. Woody said, "Stick around, watch me, and you'll learn something."

But oddly, I learned more from a hooker in Baltimore. I was working the Playboy Club when I met her, and after the show she took me to her place and said, "I want you to hear something." Then she put on a green-colored record album, something that I'd never seen.

"What's that?" I asked.

"Listen," she said.

Then I heard Lenny Bruce for the first time.

"Lima, Ohio."

I'd never heard anything like him before, especially his bit about the kid who went to the hobby shop to buy some airplane glue but was afraid to ask for it. Instead, he asked for everything

else, all sort of crap, one item after another. Finally, after he'd gotten everything else, he blurted out that he also wanted something like two thousand tubes of glue.

That destroyed me. I went fucking crazy.

One night at the Wha? I got offstage just as a guy ran in all excited because Lenny Bruce was outside taking pictures. Lenny! My God. I raced outside to see the brightest and bravest of all.

Outside, I saw a crowd gathered around a mounted policeman and his horse—this big brown thing that had crapped in the street—and through the mass of laughing people, I spotted Lenny. Scuttling about, he held a camera and, as near as I could tell, was snapping pictures of the horse's dick.

That was strange, you know. Unfortunately, that's as close as I ever came to seeing him perform.

Bill Cosby was the guy who was most envied. I remember seeing a picture of Bill on the cover of *Time* magazine. Every comedian I knew had seen it and was jealous as an ugly whore. But damn, Bill was good. Once when I played the Wha?, I heard Bill was at the Cellar, and so between sets I went over to see his work for myself.

"Noah?"

"Who's that?"

"God."

"Yeah, right."

The man was amazing. Truly amazing. Do you hear me? I was amazed.

On my way back to the Wha?, I decided that's who I was going to be from then on.

Bill Cosby.

Richard Cosby.

*I grabbed the crook. It was the wrong move. He threw
me down. I got up again. He knocked me down. I got up. He
kicked me down. I got up. He said, "Get up."*

I said, "Ha, haaaaa!"

*Then my wife threw him across the furniture. She slapped
me. The police came. She beat them up. They took her away.*

Me and the crook livin' happily ever after.

If the material wasn't exactly Bill's, the delivery was. So
much so that I should've informed people.

But the other comics caught on and asked, "What the fuck
happened?"

I said, "I'm going for the bucks."

I finally met Bill Cosby at Papa Hud's. There was no doubt in
anyone's mind, he was on his way. Like a fucking rocket ship,
Cosby was going to the top. You could've put every dollar you
had on that number. But he was still nice to me. He advised me
to "find my own thing." Then one day I told Bill that I was
booked at the Apollo, my first big show there.

"I'm opening for Billy Eckstine," I said. "My name's even on
the marquee."

I convinced Bill to jump in a cab and go uptown with me so
I could show him my name on the Apollo's marquee. On the
way, he told me to be careful. Not to cuss. Not to talk foul. Not
to act no fool.

"But I'm being paid to be a fool," I said.

"You know what I mean," he replied.

At West 125th Street, the cab pulled up in front of the leg-
endary theater. Bill and I got out and stared at the marquee.

BILLY ECKSTINE

AND

OPENING ACTS

Bill scratched his head and looked at me, puzzled.

"Where's your name, Rich?" he asked. "I see Billy Eckstine's. But not yours."

"Right there," I said, pointing. "Underneath."

"I don't see it."

"What do you mean? Right there. 'Opening Acts.'"

"That isn't your name."

"But it's me," I insisted. "I'm one of the opening acts."

On August 31, 1964, I made my TV debut on Rudy Vallee's summer variety show "On Broadway Tonight." Rudy himself, over his producer's objections, insisted on putting me on the show. I considered it a stroke of luck, my first opportunity at nationwide exposure. Back then, Cosby, Dick Gregory, and Nipsey Russell were among the few black comics who appeared on TV. I was happy to join them.

Nervous and stiff as I stared into the camera, I began my set with an introduction.

"I'm gonna tell you folks a few things about myself, because a lot of you probably don't know me," I said.

"I'm not a New Yorker. My home is Peoria, Illinois. I had a wild neighborhood, I gotta tell you. Because my mother's Puerto Rican, my father's a Negro, and we lived in a big Jewish tenement building—in an Italian neighborhood.

"So everytime I went outside, they'd yell, 'Get him! He's all of them!'"

I continued:

"When I was young I used to think my people didn't like me. Because they used to send me to the store for bread and then they'd move."

After the show, my family called to congratulate me. My dad, in particular, was tickled.

He said, "We're proud of you, son. At least you aren't sticking nobody up."

TWELVE

By the mid-1960s, my reputation as a comic had spread beyond the downtown nightclubs, where I was as well known for acting strange as I was for getting laughs. Thanks to appearances on television variety shows like "Merv Griffin" and the "Kraft Music Hall," I entered the mainstream.

My personal life remained less conventional. I caught women as if they were taxis. But you know how sometimes you'll get a driver who's strange? That happened to me when I became involved with Tia Maria, a prostitute.

She took me back to her apartment. Introduced me to cocaine. Her friend, the white lady.

"Come on, everybody's doing it," she said.

"Okay. I'll try some."

I started snorting little tiny pinches, saying, "I know I ain't gonna get hooked. Not on coke. My friends have been snorting fifteen years and they aren't hooked.

She set out nice little piles the size of small pearls. Real pretty. And I liked it.

Yes, I did. From the first snort. It made me feel cool. Got me brave.

I started snorting little teeny things. Didn't even make any noise. Coke etiquette, Jack. "Pass the album, please. Oh, no

more for me." Six months later. Oink. Snarf. Licking the al-
bum. Trying to get a freeze.

Tia Maria was nice for a liar. We would be laying in bed and
she'd suddenly announce that I had to leave. Immediately.

"Why, baby?"

"My uncle is coming over. I don't want him to know you're
here."

She never wanted me to meet him, and for some reason I
never asked why. I'd do as she say.

I got dressed and left. Then I pleaded to come back. Wanted
the pussy.

"Oh, God, are you calling again? God, Richard, please,
don't do this to yourself. I mean, why don't you go home and
bathe or something."

Then I heard her on the phone. Say, "Just a minute, John."

One night Tia Maria had a big party at her house. Everybody
got smashed on something. I asked where she got a piece of furniture that I admired. She said it was a present from her uncle.
Someone else asked his name. One of her girlfriends heard the
question and chimed in, "It came from John."

"John?" I asked.

"You know, John," she said with a wink.

Everyone laughed. Finally, I got the joke. Tia Maria had a
sugar daddy. Her uncle.

"You're a whore?"

"I'm whatever you want me to be, baby."

Tia Maria turned into a wild, crazy creature when she got high.
She liked to take off all her clothes, climb out the apartment
window and walk on to the ledge of her building. With her tit-

ties blowing in the wind, she yelled at people on the street. Put on one of the most exciting shows in town.

Part of me enjoyed watching.

You think up some weird sexual fantasies when you be on coke. You say shit like, "Baby, I got a great idea. I want you to get up on the roof. I'm gonna run around the house three times. On the third time I want you to jump off on my face."

Part of me also hated it. Maybe she got off on that shit, but it scared the hell out of me. I yelled for her to get back inside, come to her senses—like I had any myself.

"Leave the bitch alone," a friend of mine said.

"But she's going to jump," I said. "One of these days she's going to jump."

"So. That's her business."

After several more of those episodes, I knew our days were numbered. I couldn't take that much excitement. There were other womens around, including Sonya, a friend of Tia's, who was a beautiful girl. I fucked her a few times, and then I got the guilties so bad that I confessed to Tia.

She freaked out. I thought she might throw me off the damned balcony. But not because of the obvious. See, Sonya was Tia's lady. They were lesbians. I didn't know until then, and once it was in the open my ass was the one shoved out the door.

Then I met Maxine Silverman. She dated my friend Frank. One night I got a girl and the four of us went out on a double date. By the end of the evening, I liked Maxine better than my date. I spent the next couple days charming my way into her life.

Maxine was a phenomenal chick, the cutest white girl I'd ever seen. She zoomed along in the fast lane. She knew things, sophisticated things that I'd never learned, like which forks to

use at a nice restaurant and shit like that, and she grooved right along with me in treating life like a party.

Somebody told me if you put coke on your dick you could fuck all night. Shouldn't have told me. My dick had a Jones. Six hundred dollars a day just to get my dick hard.

We were kids. If Maxine and I had really gotten to know each other, we would've discovered we were mismatched. We had fun together, but we didn't belong as a couple. It didn't stop me from putting her on a pedestal. That's what I did with womens. Raised them high. Treated them like royalty. Until I got them up high. Once that was accomplished, I didn't care anymore, you know?

But what do you say?

Nothing. You just feel bad. Let that weirdness gnaw at you like termites.

"Hey, Rich, what's wrong?" my conscience asked.

"Nothing."

"I know you lying. You can tell me."

"Fuck you."

The trouble starts when that shit visits you. One night after several days of nonstop snorting and drinking and snorting, I succumbed to a paranoid flittamajitter. My whole life dropped in uninvited. Broke into my room like thugs collecting money. I didn't know what the hell was happening, but it scared the fuck out of me, no doubt about that.

Locked in my bedroom, I saw myself being stalked by people who wanted to kill me. Family members. Guys I knew. Dealers. Women I'd fucked and promised shit to. The womens wanted me dead most of all.

I kept checking the locks on my apartment door. I had about twelve of them. I kept turning them. Click-click. I was so fucked up that I missed a booking on "The Ed Sullivan Show." My agent called the next day as I was finally returning to normal and asked what happened.

"I have no idea," I said. "I'm just lucky to be here, you know?"

"I'll smooth it over, Rich," he said. "But listen: In this business, people talk. Don't blow it."

I made the next "Ed Sullivan Show." Got paid something like $500, which was a lot of money then. Maxine and I walked down Fifth Avenue feeling like we owned the world. We met up with musicians Dion and Kenny Rankin. In the Village, we bought some LSD. What did I know about acid? The guy who sold it to me said it was a cool high.

White dude gave me some shit. Talking 'bout how I'm gonna be trippin'.
Shit, I ain't goin' no place without my luggage.

Neither Maxine nor I had tried LSD before, so we didn't know what to expect. We started out at a rock show, but by the time that shit kicked in we had made it back to the safety of our home. Thank God.

I can't imagine what it would've been like had we stayed out, because once I started tripping, I got into a thing with our kitty. Ordinarily, me and the cat didn't have much to do with each other. We put up with each other.

"Hi, kitty. How ya doin'?"

"Don't talk to me, asshole. I see how you treat women."

Suddenly, this cat follows me around as if we were attached, as if the cat was my shadow. Real close. Too close. Particularly, for somebody on LSD. Wherever I went the cat crept right beside me, rubbing, touching, meowing. I thought the cat was fucking with me, you know?

"Get the fuck away."

"Fuck you, Rich."

I swear me and that cat got into an argument.

Hey, man, look at this. I can catch my hand.
Waaaaaaaaaaaaaa!

At one point, Maxine and I achieved a meeting of the minds, a perfect intersection of thought and awareness, something that happens only during an acid trip. Laughing hysterically, we stared deep into each other and shared a simultaneous thought: Our relationship was wrong. Then we laughed some more, and I said, "This ain't right, is it?" We should've quit right then. But we didn't.

Ohhhhhhhhhh, shiiiiiiiit.
I've got to get the fuck outta here.
Waaaaaaaaaaaaaaaaaaaaa!

It's amazing we survived the shit that happened. One day I gave our last $200 to some actor who wanted to fly to L.A. to audition for a movie. Over Maxine's objections, I wrote him a check. Late that night he broke into our apartment and stormed into the bedroom holding the check.

"Rich, they couldn't read your signature at the bank. You have to write me another one."

"I don't have to do anything now," I said. "I'm sleeping."

"Rich, please, man."

"Ask Maxine."

He woke her up. She got pissed all over again. She stormed out of the bedroom. I got angry at her for getting angry while this actor was angry at both of us for fucking up his big chance. Maxine ran onto the balcony and starting screaming shit. Shades of Tia Maria. Very high drama.

I said, "Max, take it easy."

We fought like truly mad people. We didn't even know what we were fighting about. We just fought.

Then she picked up a knife.

"I'm gonna cut you, motherfucker," she screamed.

"Go ahead, bitch."

You might say shit like that, but if you thought about it for a second, you'd know you don't mean it.

She kind of lunged. I kind of danced into the blade with my left arm. There was a slight collision. But the knife was extremely sharp. Sharp enough to cut through flesh with only the mildest of swipes.

I saw red.

Blood.

My blood!

I can't breathe. I don't remember how to breathe. Something's wrong. I'm gonna die. I don't even know where the fuck I am. Shit. I'm gonna die. I'm gonna die . . .

I rushed to the emergency room, where the admissions nurse gave me one of those ho-hum looks, handed me a clipboard with forms attached, and asked me to sit down and fill them out.

"With what? Blood? Look at my arm!"

"Here, use a pen."

Finally, someone recognized me from TV and took care of me. I got a shot of something that numbed my arm. Then a doctor stitched me up. As he sewed, he asked me how I'd gotten the gash.

"I was trying out a knife trick," I said.

"And so you stabbed yourself in the upper part of your arm?" he asked, not buying my explanation.

"Yeah. I don't have it down yet."

"Well, don't try it anymore. Please. For your own sake."

"Okay, Doc, I won't."

I lived the kind of drama and tragedy that made for great comedy, but I let only bits and pieces creep into my act. Instinct told me to do more, except the pressure was to go with the flow.

"Don't offend, Rich."

It was a politically charged time. Martin Luther King fought for equality and dignity. Malcolm clamored. But in terms of entertainment white America wanted their black comedians colorless.

Negro.

Colored.

Those were okay.

But as comedy writer Murray Roman, a nice man who didn't know any better than to reflect prevailing opinion, advised me, "Now I'd introduce Bill to my mother. But a guy like you . . . Don't mention the fact that you're a nigger. Don't go into such bad taste."

Don't say . . .

You can fuck white women and if they don't come, they say, "It's all right. I'll just lay here for a while and use a vibrator."

Black women, they'll talk about you. "Nigger, well, is that it? Hell, you got to grind my pussy. Oh, nigger, fuck me. Shit. Don't put my legs down, motherfucker."

The trouble was, I didn't know any better than to listen to Murray Roman and people like that. I didn't have a view of the big picture. I didn't know myself well enough. Charlie Chaplin had the Little Tramp, but I hadn't yet discovered my character, and that was because I tried so hard to be someone else. I didn't think about artistry as much as I did making monies.

Monies. That was the goal, the dream. The more the better. I figured the more distance I put between me and poverty, the happier I'd be.

Just tell jokes, Rich.

Tell stories.

Tell 'em like Bill would.

And so my routine included harmless spoofs of life in the ghetto such as when I pretended to be a doofus saying, "I heard

a knock on the door. I said to my wife, 'There's a knock on the door.' And my wife said, 'That's peculiar. We ain't got no door.'"

But see, I didn't know any better.

Like Cosby, I got a shot at playing Las Vegas. Bobby Darin, a fan of mine from the clubs, signed me as the opening act for his three-week stint at the Flamingo Hotel. Bobby was cool. He could sing his ass off, and he was married to that pretty little girl Sandra Dee. And the $2,400 a week he offered to pay me was more monies than I'd ever made.

Maxine went with me, and once I arrived in Sin City, I fell in love with the bright lights, party-time atmosphere, and around-the-clock hustle of the Strip. Seeing my name on the Flamingo's marquee, in the same air as Sinatra and Sammy, was as big a thrill as I'd had up to that time. But the shows were something else. I knew I wasn't as good as the reviews said I was, and I knew why. I just didn't want to say it.

I didn't have to. One night Don Rickles came backstage and praised my act.

"It's uncanny," he said. "You sound just like Bill Cosby."

Shit.

Why'd he have to remind me?

THIRTEEN

n Los Angeles, Bobby Darin threw a party in my honor at a chi-chi Beverly Hills restaurant. The place was so fancy it made me nervous. I was even more uncomfortable being the center of attention, especially among all the famous people he'd invited. I sat across from Groucho Marx, who told me that he'd seen me on "The Merv Griffin Show" a few weeks earlier, when I'd guested with Jerry Lewis.

It hadn't been one of my better moments—Jerry and I had gotten laughs by spitting on each other, and Groucho, it turned out, had a few things to say about that.

"Young man, you're a comic?" he asked.

"Yes," I nodded. "Yes, I am."

"So how do you want to end up? Have you thought about that? Do you want a career you're proud of? Or do you want to end up a spitting wad like Jerry Lewis?"

The man was right. I wondered how he knew I was so unsure of myself.

"Huh?" I mumbled.

"Do you ever see plays?" he repeated.

"No," I answered.

"Do you ever read books?"

"No."

I could feel the stirrings of an identity crisis. It was coming on like the beginning of an acid trip. Groucho's comments

spoke to me. "Wake up, Richard. Yes, you are an ignorant jerk, pimping your talent like a cheap whore. But you don't have to stay that way. You have a brain. Use it."

The thing was, I didn't have to. Sid Caesar eased me into movies. I met him at the Chateau Marmont Hotel in Hollywood. He interviewed me about being in *The Busy Body,* a loopy cops-and-gangsters picture he was about to start filming. Having grown up watching "Your Show of Shows," I was intimidated meeting Caesar, and also by having to keep up with his quick mind.

"I can do German," he said. "What about you?"

I stared at him and said to myself, "Goddamn, Sid Caesar's talking to me."

But apparently I said something good. Outside the hotel, my agent said, "You're going to play a detective."

The movie zipped by before I learned what I was supposed to do. On the set, I met fellow comics Dom DeLuise, Jan Murray, and Godfrey Cambridge, but otherwise I tiptoed around the cameras, lights, and shit while asking myself, "What the fuck am I doing here?"

As for acting, I faked it. Tried a little of this, a little of that. Some Steve McQueen, some Humphrey Bogart. Bless my confused heart. But it was hard because I didn't have my own thing to do.

Why, Richard? Why's that?

Because I didn't know shit about myself.

As soon as I finished, I went on a nightclub tour of the Midwest and dropped in on my family in Peoria in October. It was my first trip back home since leaving five years earlier. Nothing had changed. The places and people were the same.

Going home's nice. Some of the brothers still want to break my face. "Nigger, you ain't shit. You wasn't shit when you were

*here. I seen you do that shit on TV. That's the same shit you
were doing around the poolroom. It ain't nothing."* Then a moment later: *"Let me have a dollar."*

I fell into the old routines. Playing cards. Fishing. Drinking.
Scootching whores. Slipping in shit and getting laughs.

"This will always be your home, baby," my grandma said.

Yet I'd changed. Or so I thought. I'd seen more. Seen possibilities. Played for bigger pots.

When I'd left town originally nobody'd noticed. Now the
Peoria Journal Star wrote a story about me coming back and
quoted my dad saying that my success had done the family
proud and even "brought a tear or two."

That was nice, Dad.

How come we never talked like that in person?

Questions like that were probably what'd brought me back
home in the first place. Over the past five years, I'd become
more successful than I'd ever imagined. I'd also forgotten who
the person was who'd left Peoria. I'd lost my way when I decided to go for the bucks.

I had to rediscover Richard Pryor, the Richard Pryor whom
club owner Harold Parker had allowed to pretend he could play
the piano and tell jokes, and then described as "having more
nerve than anybody I've ever seen."

But how?

By April 1967, Maxine was nine months pregnant and due almost any time. She wanted a commitment from me, something
I had no intention of giving her.

I gambled. I stayed out all night at clubs. I could barely commit to being me. How could I give her more? But the more I said
no, the more adamant she became. The only reason we stayed
together was because neither of us had any other place to go.

We were stuck, and it wasn't fun.

One night, unable to stand the pressure any longer, I walked outside and stared up at the moon. It was like a big orange balloon. A big orange titty talking to me. "Hey, Rich, what's going on? Why don't you come and get me?" There was just something about it—the air, the vibes, the moon, the way it beckoned. I said, "Damn, this moon's got something to do with me."

So I went with it.

I jumped in my car and followed the moon.

I drove as if I was holding on to a rope, and when I finally let go I was in Tijuana, Mexico. For the next few days, I rested, drank, and partied with several pretty little whores, who showered me with loving attention and for a while had me forgetting Maxine.

The guards at the border weren't as nice. On my way back into the United States, they pulled me over and searched my car. I didn't look guilty, but I was black and I'm convinced that was the reason I got stopped. They searched me and said that they found an ounce of pot.

Bullshit.

There wasn't even enough to roll a joint.

But.

They busted me anyway.

So there I was. A black man going to jail for drugs as he tries crossing the U.S. border. It didn't look good for Richard, no, it didn't.

I was fucking terrified for my life, you know?

I was in jail in California. When they arrest you, they be serious. They'd look all in your asshole. You talk about degrading a nigger. That degrades you immediately. "Take off your clothes." I didn't know what they be looking for. "What you be looking for, man, in my ass?" There ain't be nothing in my asshole. If I had a pussy, I might dig it. You can hide something in

your pussy. But in my ass? What am I gonna hide in my ass-hole? A pistol?"

They threw me in a cell by myself, which was something of a relief. I laid down on the top bunk. Then they brought in another guy. Another black man. Unlike me, however, this dude was big and scary. I don't want to accuse nobody of being guilty of anything before they're tried, but I knew from looking at him that the world was a little safer with him behind bars.

But was I?

Without saying a word to me, without even acknowledging me, he stripped off all his clothes and walked around buck naked. He reminded me of an angry bull, brooding, snorting, grinding. I feared what was going to happen when he caught sight of my skinny ass. I thought, Christ, I'm going to have to knock this motherfucker out. God, please give me the strength or else I'm probably going to have to get fucked.

Eventually, he laid down on the bottom bunk and didn't bother me, and I didn't say shit to the man, either. Honest. I didn't even get off that top bunk. Not a peep from Rich.

Many hours later, a deputy looked in the cell and asked with genuine surprise what I was doing there.

Was he more ignorant than me?

"I was arrested," I said.

"Why are you still in here, though?" he asked.

Several possible responses came to mind, before I said, "They won't let me out."

"But you've got all this money."

In the panic and confusion of getting arrested and going to jail, I'd forgotten there was $7,500 in my pocket.

"You can get your ass out of here," he continued.

"Well, let me out, then," I said.

After posting bail, I got in my car and drove home and found out my daughter Elizabeth had been born. Congratulations, Rich. But you didn't care, did you?

Well, to be honest, not that much.

You know, my attitude about kids and fatherhood was something stupid, something selfish, something that put all of them after my own momentary concerns.

As she should have, Maxine resented me to the point where I was unable to take it anymore. I had a hard time thinking about anything but my own needs, and no matter how much she screamed or fought with me, I simply wasn't going to change.

It's nothing to be proud of. It's just the way it was.

Finally, the day came when it was just all-out war between us, and I said, "You know what? I could leave here."

Maxine didn't argue.

I remember that day. It was clear.

As I left, I felt like I could see all the way to tomorrow and the next day, you know?

FOURTEEN

I don't remember how the summer of 1967 was for the rest of the country, but my ass landed at the Sunset Tower Motel in Hollywood, home for a hodgepodge of Hollywood dreamers, schemers, and hustlers. For about $100 a month, I not only got a place to sleep but also an interesting social life.

For starters, the girl I dated lived there. Brandi worked as a phone operator, but moonlighted as a dancer at the Whiskey A Go-Go. Another dancer friend of hers, Carol, also lived in the Tower. The first time Brandi took me to Carol's apartment, I walked in and saw another guy in there. I said the first thing that came to mind, "Let's take off our clothes and have an orgy."

How was I supposed to know the other guy was Carol's brother? Paul Mooney, a large black man who loved to talk and talk and talk, would become a comedian, my lifelong friend, collaborator, comic foil, alter ego, antagonist, and so on.

But as soon as Mooney heard me suggest having a sex party, he exploded. He threw my ass out in the hall.

"Get the fuck out, nigger," he said as the door closed behind me.

Mooney and I began seeing each other at comedy clubs, and we became friends anyway. He was fascinated by me. He always said he'd never known anyone who didn't give a shit about rules or propriety. Someone who didn't care about anything except what he wanted at the moment.

That was me—especially once I discovered instant gratification through a drug dealer I called Dirty Dick. He was a
funny-looking black dude who talked in bullshit rhymes.
Handled top-of-the line cocaine. I used the motherfucker as
if he was an automatic teller machine, snorting up $100–$200
a day. And I didn't even realize how much I liked to snort
coke.

After one night with Dick, I came home fairly well fucked
up. Not a great idea in the building where I lived because it was
a strange place if you weren't careful. For instance, the elevator
had a mind of its own. If you pushed 3, you ended up in the
basement. If you pushed basement, you were fucked.

So while I was attempting to navigate a path to my apartment, something happened between me and the motherfucker
working the late shift at the front desk. I don't know what, but
it was loud and nasty.

"You can't say that crap to me," he said.

"If I want, I can say it to you *and* your mama," I snapped.

In a blur, this motherfucker turned into Bruce Lee with a bad
attitude. He snapped his shoes off, crouched in a karate stance,
started waving his fists and snarled, "Come on, nigger. Come on
and try it."

I thought the motherfucker was funny. He moved way too
much to know something. Police records indicated that I hit the
motherfucker in the face and broke his glasses.

I don't remember shit about that.

But then the cops arrived, only I didn't know they were cops,
and when they slapped some handcuffs on me, I thought something strange was going down. I thought maybe I might be going for a swim with the fishies. Held in front of the hotel, I
shouted toward the building and passing cars, "Hey, y'all, help
me! They're taking me someplace. Help me!"

I was high, crazy.

I went to jail. Then the fucker sued and won $75,000.

What could I do?

I just said, "Fuck it."

★   ★   ★

Then Maxine sued me for child support and assorted bullshit. She claimed that we'd lived together like husband and wife. I didn't contest it, and the court sided with her. I tried to avoid the mess by shuffling from one club to the next.

In a way, I used that to my advantage. I saw myself as a victim of the system, an outsider for whom justice was out of reach, a dream, and then I saw how closely my situation mirrored the black man's larger struggle for dignity and equality and justice in white society.

That was me.

I was that character.

That was the person to whom I had to give voice.

I decided to drop out of the whole damn thing altogether. Got rid of my driver's license. Quit carrying identification of any kind. Stopped using banks, paying traffic tickets, income taxes, and all that shit.

Why not?

I couldn't win. It didn't seem as if any of us could win.

I saw the judge give one nigger forty years. He said, "That's right, fella. Forty years. You want more time, buddy?"

Dude had a court-appointed lawyer, right. Copping a plea. "Your Honor, this man is not a heroin dealer per se. He's being manipulated by these people. He was merely trying to get enough monies together to help his dear mom. She had a spinal condition. She needed an operation, and she didn't have the funds to do this. He was merely trying to raise the money. He tried every odd job he could, and he couldn't have raised the money. When the officers caught him with the 280 kilos, he was trying to purchase a hospital in the Bahamas."

Judge said, "Motion denied."

Nigger was so fucked up when they laid him away, he said, "Thank you, Your Honor."

At our last meeting, my agent sounded like one of my grand-mother's whores singing to a john. "You're great, baby. Oh, you're the best. No one else like you, baby." The money was getting bigger. Checks piled up around my place like litter on the highway. I didn't have to worry about work.

My agent booked me at the Aladdin in Las Vegas. It was a big deal. I was nonplussed. In fact, as we shook hands, I had the feeling that I was making a pact with someone who just wanted to suck my blood.

Hey, man! Say, nigger. You with the cape. What you doing peeking in them people's window? What's your name, boy?

Dracula?

What kind of name is that for a nigger? Where you from, fool?

Transylvania?

I know where that is, nigger. Yeah. You ain't the smartest motherfucker in the world, you know. Even though you is the ugliest. Oh, yeah. Why don't you get your teeth fixed, nigger?

I couldn't explain the transformation taking place. I don't understand it myself. I only know my days of pretending to be as slick and colorless as Cosby were numbered. There was a world of junkies and winos, pool hustlers and prostitutes, women and family screaming inside my head, trying to be heard. The longer I kept them bottled up, the harder they tried to escape. The pressure built till I went nuts.

Better get home before the sun come up. See your ass in the day, you're liable to get arrested!

By the time I rolled into Vegas in September, I was com-pletely fucked up, okay on the outside but I felt as if my legs were going to give out any minute. I was sandwiched between the headliner, Pat the "Hip Hypnotist" Collins, and the Brasilia

Jazz Review. Or so people have told me, because I don't remember shit.

Only that it was opening night.

"Now, please welcome a very funny gentleman. You've seen him on a number of TV shows. Mr. Richard Pryor.

I came out. Nice applause.

I looked out at the audience. The first person I saw was Dean Martin, seated at one of the front tables. He was staring right back at me.

At me!

I asked myself, Who's he looking at, Rich?

I checked out the rest of the audience. They were staring at me as intently as Dean, waiting for that first laugh.

Again, I asked myself, Who're they looking at, Rich?

I didn't know.

I couldn't say, They're looking at you, Richard, because I didn't know who Richard Pryor was. And in that flash of introspection when I was unable to find an answer, I crashed. I had a nervous breakdown.

I looked back at Dean, who was still looking at me, waiting for something, you know?

You want to suck what? Nigger, are you some kind of pre-vert? An ugly pre-vert. You ain't sucking nothing here, junior. You want to suck some blood, go down to the blood bank, nigger. Hope you get sickle cell.

I imagined what I looked like and got disgusted. I gasped for clarity as if it was oxygen. The fog rolled in. In a burst of inspiration, I finally spoke to the sold-out crowd: "What the fuck am I doing here?"

Then I turned and walked off the stage.

God was much funnier than me that night.

Instead of guiding me offstage to my dressing room, He pointed me in the wrong direction. I found myself standing on a narrow ledge behind the curtain. I couldn't turn around. Nor would I. So in my tux, I inched and clawed my way along the tiny lip of wood, toward the faint glow of an exit sign, scraping my nose until it bled and muttering, "Fuck, fuck, fuck . . ."

Backstage, I gathered my clothes and left the hotel, climbed into my '65 Mustang, and drove to L.A.

My agent was hysterical, incredulous. How could I have walked off? What the fuck was going on?

"Do you know what you did?" my agent screamed. "Do you know what this means?"

"No, you're the agent. You tell me."

Then I heard those famous words.

"You'll never work in this town again. Did you hear me? You will never work in this town again!"

I have a thing for nudity. I always like to get naked. I did that in Vegas. Got naked and ran through the casino nude. Jumped up on the table and said, "Blackjack!"

I can still hear him saying that.

YOU WILL NEVER WORK IN THIS TOWN AGAIN!

FIFTEEN

C ontrary to rumor, my Las Vegas flameout wasn't in front of a Mafia audience. It didn't cause the mob to put out a contract on me, lead to a ban from ever performing at the hotels, or serve as my ticket to the loony bin.

The only fact was the inevitability. The breakdown was the only way I could shed the phony image I'd created and start rebuilding my self-respect.

I was a Negro for twenty-three years. I gave that shit up. No room for advancement.

In the weeks after, I continued to hear the threat: "You'll never work in this town again."

So.

It would've been a different story if my agent had said, "You'll never fuck in this town again."

Then I would've listened.

As it happened, after returning to L.A., I fell hard in love with Shelley Bonus, a rich hippie girl who would become my second wife. We met at a nightclub. Shelley noticed me looking at her, strolled over to where I sat, and then kicked up her leg as if finishing a dance step.

That was so goddamn cute. I was hooked immediately.

There's nothing better or more exciting than falling in love,

and, if I do say so, I do it well. However, it's like jumping in a pool when you don't know how to swim.

I hear myself screaming, "Edge! Rich, get to the edge!"

And so it was with Shelley.

We didn't waste any time getting together. She moved into my rustic cabinlike place above Laurel Canyon, and we fell passionately, madly, silly in love. She walked around barefoot, wore love beads, lighted incense, knew things, and at a time when I was struggling, she made me feel free.

Her simplicity was charming. We could do absolutely nothing and be happy. We used to walk around, picking up rocks and giving them names. We kissed them. We gave them to each other as presents. Stupid shit that made us laugh.

Then we got married. It was really fun, man. All those funny things we used to do together. I'd bring her a rock. She'd go, "Oh, a rock. For me?"

She got me to marry her while we was balling and I was coming.

"Will you marry me?"

"Yes! Yeah! Oh, yeah!"

At the end of December, my dad called with bad news. My stepmother Viola had died. I told him I was sorry and hoped that was enough. But he wanted me at the funeral.

"Dad, I ain't going," I said.

I couldn't imagine dealing with all the family shit.

"That's all right, son," he said. "You don't have to come. But the next time you be on 'Ed Sullivan,' it'll be a duo."

"What do you mean?"

He said, "It'll be you telling jokes and me kicking your ass."

That made me laugh. But I knew he meant it.

A few hours later, my Aunt Dee called to check on whether or not I had any sense at all.

I said, "Yes, tell Dad I'm coming home, but only because I don't want him kicking my ass on 'Ed Sullivan.'"

My dad was very broken up when I got there. Everybody else talked about the weather.

We was going to my stepmother's funeral. It was one of the coldest days in the history of Peoria, Illinois. Like twenty below zero. I'm sitting in the backseat with my father, crying and shit, and I say, "Pop, it's all right. Hey, man, it's gonna be okay."

He said, "Man, it get any colder, I'm gonna have to bury the bitch myself."

That's my father. I'm not lying. He'd be at the graveyard, talking to the preacher. "Say, man, when's the shit over? God-damn. Get to the part about the date. Shit, I love you, baby. But shit, goddamn, it's cold out here."

Paul Mooney started taking me to Redd Foxx's club located in Central Los Angeles. It was the right place for me at the right time. With a black audience, I was free to experiment with material that was more natural. It was frightening, since I didn't know myself and had to learn who I was. It was like I was there but I wasn't there, you know.

Yet it was also lovely, comfortable. I talked about the black man's struggle to make it in a white world, which was also my struggle. For the first time since I began to perform at Harold's Club, I saw black people laughing—and not just at cute shit. They laughed at the people I knew. The people they knew. It was enlightening.

None more so than Redd Foxx himself. Redd was a player, a hard player from the old school. He carried a switchblade. Sometimes a gun. He ran the club like a gangster, treating friends like relatives and enemies with scorn. People were beat up regularly. Redd also liked the cocaine, too. I spent many nights when I felt as if we were in the coke Olympics.

But Redd was a mesmerizing storyteller—the best ones al-

ways concerned his friend Malcolm X. Not only did listening to that shit fascinate me, it sparked a fire inside my brain. It was an awakening. Malcolm was a bad motherfucker, Redd said, but he also took care of business. He was proud, brilliant, sincere, passionate, dedicated to teaching about human beings, about being human.

"In the early days, Malcolm hated what he called the white devil," Redd explained. "Then he realized that we were all different shades of the same stick. The motherfucker got killed for it."

It was the same evolution that I'd go through. Strangely, I hadn't been affected by Malcolm X's death when it occurred. However, after Redd introduced me to him as a person and what he stood for, I missed him terribly.

A few months later, Martin Luther King, Jr., was assassinated outside his Memphis motel room. I was in Chicago that day. I watched the news on the TV in my hotel room and tried to understand the loss. I couldn't.

Neither could I make any sense of Robert Kennedy's murder two months later in Los Angeles. At the time, I was walking down a hotel corridor in Washington, D.C. It must've been right after the shooting. Ed Sullivan passed me rushing the opposite direction. Something seemed wrong. He didn't stop or say hi. He seemed in a daze. Moments later, after I turned on the TV, I was overtaken by that same glassy confusion.

The good good ones were being bumped off.

John, Malcolm, Martin and Bobby.

What to make of it?

I wanted to understand why that shit had happened. But there was no way. It was part of a whole collage of shit that I couldn't get a grip on. I probably wasn't alone in that respect, though I sure felt like it.

In early 1968, I worked at the Village Gate in New York, one of the few clubs that didn't object to the new material I was performing, which the more conservative bookers consid-

ered inflammatory, crude, and in some cases obscene. (And to think, I was just starting to find myself.) Going there gave me the opportunity to meet actress Shelley Winters, who came backstage and asked if I'd be in her next movie, *Wild in the Streets*.

"I don't know," I said. "But I'll try."

The money aspect interested me, but far more important at the time was meeting jazz great Miles Davis, who was the club's headliner. Though our paths hadn't crossed, Miles and I were brothers waiting to meet. Kindred spirits. Before we even spoke, he did something that no one else would've done, because no one would've understood the shit I was going through without a detailed explanation.

But Miles' radar picked me up like a lost plane. About half an hour before the show, he had one of his guys come to my dressing room and tell me the lineup had been changed.

"Miles is gonna play first," he said.

"What?" I asked, wondering what the fuck was going on.

"Miles is going to open. Then you follow."

The gesture was pure Miles—intuitive, supportive, generous, and in sync with the moment. By trading places, he was giving me a vote of support. Beyond that, he was leading me to the edge of the diving board. He knew that I was frightened, and he knew I thought the jump was hard. But he also knew that I could do it if given a nudge. I just had to believe in myself.

Be brave, he was telling me.

Be true to your own self.

Listen to the music inside your head, Rich. Play with your heart.

After the show Miles invited me to his dressing room. When I entered he was kissing Dizzy Gillespie, with tongue and shit, which made me wonder what kind of shit he had planned for me.

But Miles played a different tune with me. We got in a cab and went to a midtown apartment where he introduced me to a woman I called the Gypsy Lady. She was dark and mysterious, with eyes as hot as fire, and she had the best cocaine I ever tried. It was a big motherfucking rock. Like the Hope Diamond. We chopped and snorted until the sun crept through the windows and then we disappeared like vampires.

"From now on, you get your coke from her," Miles said as we left. "She's got the best."

After that evening, our lives became intertwined, my Miles' and mine. I played his music, collected his art, admired his independence, understood his rudeness, and loved the way he talked. That was probably the best thing about Miles. That voice. It fascinated me like nothing else. No matter what he said, Miles sounded cool.

Those shows marked the beginning of my transformation into Richard Pryor again, though change was not without its price. I didn't act as if I was married. I hung out till all hours at nightclubs. I indulged my appetite for drugs and booze and jive. I let temptation serve as my muse.

I wasn't close to being normal. I couldn't stop drinking till the bartender said, "We got no more fucking liquor."

I had no conscience. One night Mooney brought April, a beautiful sportswriter, to Shelley's and my little cabin in the hills, and as with any attractive female, I wanted her, chased her, I got down on my hands and knees and begged and then I went off with her. Shit, did Shelley ever want to strangle me.

I couldn't stop myself even after Shelley became pregnant in the fall of 1968, but then I didn't see myself as clearly as others did. I remember Redd Foxx and I spent an entire night and most of the next morning at a little table in his club, battling each

other for the attention of a sexy waitress, listening to jazz, and snorting cocaine by the spoonful. I kept asking for more, more, more, and Redd kept giving it to me, until finally I was too tired to inhale.

"Hey, Redd, why do I always want more?" I asked.

He laughed as if to emphasize my ignorance.

"Because you're a junkie."

Then it was my turn to laugh.

"Bullshit."

I just didn't see it.

Later, when I finally went home, Shelley was waiting for me and she wasn't happy.

"You don't love anybody, do you?" she asked.

"I love Miles," I said.

That wasn't exactly true.

At the end of September, while I was working on the movie *Wild in the Streets,* my father died. I was still in bed when the phone rang. Shelley and I ignored it. But the ringing continued as if that phone was screaming, "Get the fuck up and answer me, motherfucker." Shelley got it.

"Richard, it's your grandmother," she said.

"Hello, Marie . . ."

He'd been with five women. Five!

At the same time.

In the midst of it, his heart gave out.

Shit.

I want to die like my father. He died fucking. He was fifty-seven. The woman was eighteen. He came and went at the same time.

Didn't nobody cry at his funeral. Everybody just said,
"Lucky motherfucker."

And nobody else would fuck the woman for two years. "I
don't want none of that pussy. No, thank you."

I hugged Shelley for a long time. Needed her strength as tears
ran from my eyes.

"The king is dead," I finally muttered. "Long live the king."

Shelley traveled with me to Peoria, where I was immediately
overwhelmed by the pull of family.

"You can never escape, can you?" I asked myself. "Not even
when you die."

My dad lived in a nice house that he'd bought several years
earlier with twenty grand in cash that I'd handed him one night
following a Chicago club date. A lot of shit went down inside
me when I walked through that door and he wasn't there.

My whole family was gathered there. The place was packed.
Still, I felt an unmistakable absence.

Daddy.

"Your father fucked everything," my Aunt Maxine said.
"Just be glad he didn't fuck you."

Okay.

Tender thought.

My grandmother, who had already taken over his house,
chose me to go to the funeral parlor and pick out the casket. I
didn't want to do it. I was his child, his baby. Inside, I cried,
"Why, Mama? I don't want to."

But who else was there?

I was the only son.

I was the only one with monies.

Well, I picked out something that seemed like him. Nothing
fancy. Nothing crazy. Just a casket.

And when I got back home, they gave me the worst shit.

Why'd you get that? What kind of casket is that? Did you try to save money? Didn't they have anything fancier? This is your father, after all. Shit, I didn't know what to say. It was as if they were beating me up because they didn't know what else to do.

Thank God for Shelley. She came to my defense.

"Damn it, you all shouldn't have done that to him," she yelled. "He went down there. He went through the pain. He did his best. None of you offered to help."

There was silence. Stunned motherfucking silence. Because no one dared talk back to Marie. But Shelley did. And everybody knew she was right. Because of her outburst, that day became very important to me. It didn't mean I loved anybody less, but in a way it freed me some. Loosened those chains.

Shelley flew home before the funeral. Since my father wasn't Catholic, the service was held in St. Patrick's gymnasium on October 4, 1968. He was buried in St. Joseph's Cemetery later that day. I didn't think it would hit me as hard as it did.

White people love their dearly departed, but their funerals be different. They don't give it up easy. They hold that shit in until they get home. Then they cry softly. "Ah-hoo, boo-hoo, ah!"

But black people let it hang out. "Whaaaaaaaaaaaaaaaaaa!" Then they fall on your ass. They don't ever faint. They just lean on your ass. You have to carry them to the car. "Say, bitch, get up. Damn, you got to get on me 'cuz that motherfucker's dead?"

My grandmother yelled like that. Scared the shit out of you at a funeral. "Whaaaaaaaaaaaa!"

I said, "What's the matter, Mama?" I thought maybe my dad had raised up or something.

Naw, he was dead. The odd thing was, now that he lay dead, I couldn't stop talking to him. You know, inside my head. Conversation flowed, man. But when he was alive, I don't think we ever really talked. No "Hey, dad, can I ask you," shit. No pass-

ing on stories or advice. Most of the time, he'd come into the room, say some stuff, and I'd go, "Yes, sir." Even as a man.

One time I got tired of my dad kicking my ass. I had a fight with him in the front yard. Well, it wasn't exactly a fight. I did the best I could. I said, "Man, I'm tired of taking these ass whippings. I ain't taking no fucking more. And that's it."
"What're you a man now, motherfucker?"
"Yeah, okay."
And he hit me in the chest so hard that my chest just caved in and wrapped around his fist and held it there.

I looked at my dad one last time. Wearing his best suit. I put a little money in his pocket.

Hey, Dad, just in case there's any action up there.

SIXTEEN

Watching television, which supposedly puts your brain to sleep, has always had the opposite effect on me. Paul Mooney and I used to yell at the shows as if the actors could hear us. The shit was so stupid that it was funny. I knew I could write much better.

I always wondered why they never have a black hero on any of the shows. I always wanted to go to the movies and see a black hero. I figured maybe someday they'll have it on television, man. (Some funky music plays and then):
"Look! Up in the sky!"
"It's a crow!"
"It's a bat!"
"No, it's Super Nigger!"

As with so many ideas hatched in living rooms beneath clouds of dope smoke, mine sounded crazy but brilliant. Instead of a television show, I was going to make a movie. I'd write, direct, produce, and star. Since Hollywood wasn't overflowing with opportunities for black actors, Paul and I would create our own opportunity.

It sounded so simple that it seemed possible.

"We'll get our friends together and do it," I said.

"Where we gettin' the money?" he asked.

"Me," I said. "I'll put it up. I'll produce."

"Who's gonna direct?"

"Me."

"Who's gonna be in it?"

"Everybody we know."

"Oh, shit."

We began shooting *Bon Appétit* in March 1969. Penelope Spheeris, a successful director now, was the camera operator because she had gone to film school. But that's as much legitimacy as the film had.

The picture opened with a black maid having her pussy eaten at the breakfast table by the wealthy white man who owned the house where she worked. Then, a gang of Black Panther types burst into the house and took him prisoner. As he was led away, the maid fixed her dress and called, "*Bon appétit,* baby!"

The rest of the movie, which was retitled *The Trial*, was a silly stab at a political statement. The Panthers held the guy in a basement and put him on trial for all the racial crimes in U.S. history. *Black Caesar, Superfly,* and *Cleopatra Jones* hadn't come out. I thought we were breaking new ground.

But halfway through the editing process, we ran out of money. To keep the dream alive, I borrowed money from a shady character I knew. Eventually I brought in a few more people like him. Then there was a falling-out. The unfinished print was stolen. I brought it back. And then it disappeared again.

It was a better story than the film itself.

One day Paul saw the film advertised as a coming attraction at a downtown art house. After some investigation, I managed to reacquire the print, which still wasn't completed. In a last-ditch effort, I persuaded Bill Cosby to put up money for a final edit. Then he and I watched the final print. He said only one thing: "Hey, this shit is weird."

I agreed. The movie was strange. Too strange. Even for me. Despite the effort, I shelved the print and learned a lesson. To

make a movie from start to finish, you need a good reason.

I just ran out of them.

There was one successful production that summer. On July 16, 1969, the day the Apollo 11 astronauts lifted off, Shelley gave birth to our daughter Rain. She was the first of my three children to arrive when I was in a state where I could welcome her. I just wasn't sure about the rest of the world. After Rain was born, a nurse told me she had to fill out a birth record and asked what she was.

"A human being," I said.

The nurse, irritated, asked the question again, this time adding, "Is she black or white?"

"I already told you," I responded. "She's a human being. Just write that on your goddamn form."

I didn't know anyone more aware of their image than Billy Dee Williams, who I met on the TV pilot "Carter's Army." Suave and handsome, he was also very serious about his career and what people thought of him. Mooney and I played poker at his house, but he didn't like hanging out with us anywhere else. He worried that we were going to get him in trouble.

I didn't remotely identify with that worrywart shit. My life was populated by characters. There was Prophet, a moody but talented painter. Dirty Dick. A whole circus of hustlers, whores, winos, and hangers-on. I thought they were people who knew stuff worth knowing. But then I've never claimed to be a great judge of character, you know?

I did slightly better with pets. Shelley and I, renting Redd Foxx's house at the time, filled it with a menagerie of creatures, including a couple of Afghan hounds, some lovebirds, and fish. Mooney gave me a squirrel monkey, who I named Boyfriend.

We got along okay. I even thought he kinda liked me more than was normal for a monkey.

I called it Friend. Because the first time I opened the cage, he ran up my arm and stuck his dick in my ear. It felt like a wet Q-tip. And when there wasn't no action for him, he got mad and pissed all over my cheek. I grabbed the motherfucker and threw him up to the ceiling. He grabbed the chandelier and laughed.

"Thought you had me, didn't ya?"

I felt sorry for Boyfriend. As I watched him swing through his cage, he seemed lonely. So I bought him a friend, a female squirrel monkey who I called Girlfriend.

I got him a beautiful little woman. I called her Sister. And he did the same thing to her. He ran right in the cage and stuck his dick in her ear. She said, "Freeze. First thing I gotta do is show you where the pussy's at."

And then he got some monkey pussy and went crazy.

Mooney, who begrudgingly watched the animals whenever Shelley and I went out of town, resigned his caretaker post once I added Girlfriend to the mix. In need of a new babysitter for several weeks, I pressed Dirty Dick into service. He was my only option. Still, I should've known better.

When I got back, both of the monkeys were dead.

"They killed themselves," he said. "Committed suicide."

"What?" I asked, shocked.

"Yeah," he said, pointing to a gas burner on the old stove in the middle of his kitchen. "They accidentally turned it on and suffocated."

I thought he killed them on purpose. Distraught, I went home and cried. Shelley didn't understand why I was taking it so hard and asked me to cry outside. As I sat grieving, the mean

German shepherd from next door hopped the fence. Normally, he terrorized the monkeys, but he seemed forlorn too and put his head in my lap.

I felt something pushing my hand. I looked down and he said, "Hey, Rich, what's the matter?"

"My monkeys is dead. They died."

He said, "What? Your monkeys is dead? You mean the ones that used to be in the trees? Damn, I was going to eat them, too."

Then he said, "Life's a bitch, ain't it? One day you're here, the next day you're gone. Well, don't linger on it. You know, that shit can get to you."

"Thank you."

He went away, walked to the fence, and got ready to jump over. He turned around and said, "You know I'm gonna be chasing you tomorrow."

The monkeys weren't the only casualty. Shelley and I weren't going to make it much longer. The sparks were gone. We fought constantly. Mooney referred to our place as "the House of Pain." Instead of giving each other pet rocks, now we threw them at each other.

My wife and I had a lot of fun for a long time. But she had this girlfriend. With big titties. You know the type I'm talking about. You try to ignore them for six months. Then she'd come into the house and you say, "Hello, there. How're you doing? No, I don't really notice your tits."

One day my wife came home and said she left her wallet over at her house. I ran. "I'll get it!"

Then I got the guilties. I had to tell her. 'Cause I thought she knew when she asked, "Have you seen Ethel?"

"I did it!"

"Did what?"

"Fucked Ethel."
"You fucked Ethel?"
She went and kicked Ethel's ass.

As Shelley's and my fighting became fiercer and more frequent, I took increasing refuge at Dirty Dick's. In good times I had spent much of my time buying cocaine and shooting the shit with the lowlifes, whores, and addicts who were always at Dirty Dick's. Now I spent even more in his den of debauchery.

Shelley knew what went on up there. She hated Dick, and she hated how much time I spent hiding out with him. Periodically, she threatened to follow me to his house. Go there with me. Participate in the games. But I kept it off limits. The place was too nasty for her. It was also mine.

"I don't want you up there," I once said. "It's no place for you."

"Well, then come home," she said. "Spend more time with your family."

What did you think, Rich?

Yeah, right.

That's why I was up there, you know? I didn't want to spend time with my family. Didn't want to spend time with myself. Didn't want to spend time.

Wanted to buy me some time.

"I will," I said. "Just give me one more night. I need one more night."

Good, Rich. Why'd she believe you?

You think she did?

No.

Because one more night turned into dozens more. Couldn't help myself.

Like Redd Foxx said, I was a junkie.

No matter what I promised, once was never enough.

Shelley was smart. She knew that.

One night she went up to Dirty Dick's to find me and drag

my doped-out ass back home, where I had promised to leave it. Only I wasn't at Dirty Dick's that night. I was getting high someplace else. Hanging with some other characters of ill-repute, I'm sure. But the fact that Shelley had crossed into Dirty Dick's shadowy world made me crazy with anger and paranoia and jealousy.

Knowing the sordid shit she would be exposed to at Dirty Dick's, I should've been concerned about Shelley. Worried. Protective. Ready to apologize and admit my wrongdoing. Instead, I thought, Why is she doing this to me?

What right does the bitch have? Telling me what to do?

What the hell was she doing anyway?

I got pissed, you know.

You be in love you don't want nobody in your puss. Especially when you find one that fits. I don't want no motherfucker stretching your pussy out.

The trouble was this: I didn't want to admit the truth. Shelley and I were history. We just hadn't reached the finish line yet. We still had to limp down the final stretch, shouting at each other and fighting as if that would help.

Heartache is like an education for a man. We don't really grow up until a woman breaks your fucking heart. That's your diploma. If you come through that, Jack, you're a man.

My first comedy album, recorded live at the Troubadour, didn't quite measure up to my favorites. I had loved Bob Newhart's first recording so much that I'd pilfered it from a little store in Peoria. Bill Cosby's debut album was perfect, perfectly hilarious. And in my mind, nobody, to this day, has made an album as brilliantly funny as Lenny Bruce's *Lima, Ohio*.

Mine was a good, though uneven, effort. Routines like "Su-

per Nigger" revealed the voice that was trying to break through. A point of view was percolating beneath the surface. I just didn't know enough to put all the pieces together.

For the cover, I took off my clothes and parodied the cover of *National Geographic,* though when I think back on the day I was photographed I don't remember going native as much as I do the way Shelley went after me. During the shoot, Sonny Stinson, my old friend from Harold's Club, showed up. Shelley saw us hugging and went ballistic. Worse, she beat the shit out of me.

"What the fuck is wrong?" I yelled.

But I knew. I was affectionate to everyone but her. She was right. I deserved the beating.

I just didn't want to take it, you know.

And that was it. The end.

We find Super Nigger, with his X-ray vision that enables him to see through everything except Whitey, disguised as Clark Washington, mild-mannered custodian for the Daily Planet. *He's shuffling into Perry White's office.*

"Hey, man, I'm quitting, baby."

"Great Caesar's Ghost! I can't talk to you now."

"Talk to me, Jack. 'Cuz I'm ready to quit, man. You dig? I'm tired of doing them halls. Every time I finish, Lois Lane and them come slipping and sliding down through there and I got to do them over again. You dig it, baby? I'm through."

With an arrest warrant issued against me for failure to pay child support to Maxine and with Shelley wanting to kill me, I had more than enough motivation to get the hell out of Dodge. My life was a mess. It was as if I was stuck to a funnel cloud that was tearing a path of destruction everywhere I went. I sensed catastrophe around the corner and knew I had to get out.

One day Mooney and I got in my car and aimed the mother-

fucker north. I wanted to go to Berkeley. I don't know why there, except I had it in my head.

For eight hours we drove up Interstate 5, drinking cheap wine and singing Motown songs at the top of our voices. When we ran out of songs, we made up new ones.

Obnoxious, loud, drunk, and exhausted, we rolled into the red-hot center of the counterculture as if late for a party.

I didn't have a single notion of what I was going to do, but being there felt right.

"I can't talk to you now," Perry White says to janitor Clark Washington. *"The warehouse is on fire!"*
"What warehouse?"
"Warehouse 86."
"Damn. That's where I got my stash. This looks like a job for Super Nigger!"

SEVENTEEN

I settled into a life that was drastically different from the comfortable but miserable one I'd fled. I rented a small, one-bedroom house for $110 a month. I bought a bed, threw it on the floor, and stuck a TV by it.

Don't tell Martha Stewart, but that was it. I was done with the furnishings.

I thought it was nice, though. Ghetto chic.

Such austerity was necessary. If I was going to find my lost soul, I needed to cast off everything but the bare essentials. I had to renounce the past in order to discover the future. House, car, clothes, women, friends—I tossed them all away. No one knew where I was, and no one got in unless I wanted them to.

It was the freest time of my life. Berkeley was a circus of exciting, extreme, colorful, militant ideas. Drugs. Hippies. Black Panthers. Antiwar protests. Experimentation. Music, theater, poetry. I was like a lightning rod. I absorbed bits of everything while forging my own uncharted path.

I indulged every thought that popped into my sick head. I read and reread a copy of Malcolm X's collected speeches. I put Marvin Gaye's song "What's Going On" on my stereo and played it so often it became the soundtrack for my life up there.

"What's goin' on?" Marvin would sing.

"Fuck if I know," I'd answer.

In a city of spectacles, I became one myself. I shambled in

and out of coffeehouses in an old kimono, sandals, and a tall, cone-shaped hat that made me look like a deranged wizard. My sense of humor was equally bizarre. Some nights at clubs such as Basin Street West, Mandrake's, and the Showcase, I just made strange animal noises. Other nights I repeated a single word like "bitch" or "motherfucker," but gave it fifty-seven different inflections.

Each outing was like playing jazz, searching for that one perfect note that would carry me into a higher state of bliss. I never thought about what I was going to do until I did it. Sometimes I stunk. Sometimes I surprised myself. But I went with whatever happened, you know.

As a result, I became braver, more confident, and willing to tap into whatever provocative or controversial thoughts I had. During one such performance, I repeated the most offensive, humiliating, disgraceful, distasteful, ugly, and nasty word ever used in the context of black people. The word embodied the hatred of racism as well as a legacy of self-hate.

Nigger.

And so this one night I decided to make it my own.

Nigger.

I decided to take the sting out of it.

Nigger.

As if saying it over and over again would numb me and everybody else to its wretchedness.

Nigger.

Said it over and over like a preacher singing hallelujah.

Hello, I'm Richard Pryor. I'm a nigger.

Nigger. Nigger. Nigger.
Niggerniggerniggerniggerniggernigger.

Maybe you didn't notice, you know. Because they didn't tell me till I was eight years old.

Saying it changed me, yes it did. It gave me strength, let me rise above shit.

Faster than a bowl of chitlins. Able to leap slums in a single bound.

Honest. It made me feel free to say it.
Clean.
It was the truth.
That's all I was looking to say. The truth.

I'm glad I'm black. I'd hate to be white. 'Cuz y'all got to go to the moon.

Ain't no niggers going to the moon, you know that. First of all, there ain't no niggers qualified. Or so you all tell us.

If niggers was hip, they'd help y'all get to the moon.

"Hey, let's organize and help them white motherfuckers get to the moon."

"So they leave us alone!"

Among my discoveries in Berkeley was an extremely passionate, highly charged, supersophisticated renaissance of black intellectual, artistic, and political activity. It was fueled by the minds and fervor of stars like activist Angela Davis and novelist Ishmael Reed, who were smart, proud, committed . . . and uncompromisingly black.

The bunch I knew could also party their ass off. Cecil Brown, who wrote the novel *The Life and Loves of Mr. Jiveass Nigger,* told some of the earthiest, most entertaining stories ever around 3 A.M. Through Cecil, I met Claude Brown, the author of *Manchild in the Promised Land,* and Reed, who impressed me as one of the most honest people I've met.

By comparison, I was uneducated and ignorant, though listening to their ideas inspired me just as Malcolm X's writings

had. I wanted to do something. One night I served as the disc jockey on a radio station, playing Miles and rambling on about Nixon, the Vietnam War, the Black Panthers, and shit. I didn't know anything about that shit. But who better to talk about it?

Then I got the idea I could write. For a time, I holed up in my house and wrote. Fueled by coke, coffee, cigarettes, and alcohol, I cranked out page after page of stories containing ideas and opinions that I thought were important.

"I'm a serious motherfucker," I told myself.

Finally, I got the guts to show my work to Reed. He sent it back with the note, "Man, dis ain't my language."

Well, that stopped my attempt at serious writing cold.

He could've said, "Motherfucker, you can't write."

But he made it hard. He was cold and, as I said, honest.

I heard that Shelley was hanging out with Miles. I don't think they were lovers. But just that they were spending time together messed me up.

Women get their heart broke, they cry.
Men don't do that. Men hold it in like it don't hurt. They walk around and get hit by trucks.
"Didn't he see that truck?"
"Man, he wouldn't have seen a 747. His heart was broke."

I was so pissed off about Shelley and Miles that I walked into a pawnshop, bought a trumpet, and blew it on a street corner outside an Italian restaurant. Only I didn't know how to play the trumpet. Not a fucking note. But I blew the motherfucker as if the shrill, discordant sounds that went screaming into the darkness would let everyone know how unhappy I felt inside.

Then Bill Cosby of all people walked out of the restaurant to see who was playing such shit. He had to have figured it was

someone real avant-garde or a terrorist. He looked stunned to see me.

"Man, what are you doing?" he asked.

"Playing the trumpet."

"No, you aren't," he said. "You're making everybody in the restaurant sick."

Bill invited me to join him inside, where he was eating with two of the tallest, prettiest white women I'd ever seen. I thought, Damn, wouldn't you know. But after a while, one of those amazon beauties gently stroked my leg underneath the table. I looked across the table at Bill and said to myself, "Sick, my ass. Man, that trumpet shit worked."

Berkeley was full of characters worse than me, and I seemed to get tangled up with all of them. I hung out with a coke dealer named Haywood who lived by the water in Sausalito. He once gave me a samurai sword.

"Here, man, cut off your head," he said encouragingly. "Do the honorable thing."

I also remember Geena, this hippie chick, whose entire self-worth centered around a pair of satin shoes Janis Joplin had given her. One night, in a fit of downright cruelty, I threw those shoes into the Bay.

Sweet Jesus was a pimp who controlled everything.

And I still shudder at the thought of Crazy Mary, a whore who had wooden teeth. I made a grave error with her once. I gave her money.

In her eyes that made us something.

She followed me around town. She showed up at clubs while I was on stage. She raised tons of hell.

"Where is he?" she screamed in a voice that ripped through even the noisiest nightclubs. "Where the hell is my Richard?"

One time she barged into the bathroom while I was inside doing my business. I kicked the door shut. She pushed it open

again with her shoulder. I smashed it shut again and told her to get the fuck away.

"Open this goddamn door right now!" she yelled.

"No."

"Why not? You're just shitting. Everybody shits."

Crazy Mary scared me. She wanted to fuck me up as much as she wanted to fuck me. Finally, I went to Sweet Jesus and told him about my situation. He promised to help, and from then on Crazy Mary with the wooden teeth didn't bother me anymore.

She didn't bother anyone. The really scary people like Huey Newton didn't bother me. Huey and I met at a party in Oakland and then did cocaine in my hotel room. As we got high, the Black Panthers' minister of defense got angry because his woman was coming on to me and I didn't tell her to stop.

The scene got very tense. It seemed certain something was going to happen. Either Huey was going to lose control and hurt me or I was going to provoke him into hurting me by saying something stupid. Both seemed likely.

We were talking about jail. He admitted to being worried about going to prison himself.

"Why you scared of jail?" I asked.

" 'Cuz if I go, everyone's going to want to fuck me," he said.

I didn't disagree.

"But if they put their dick in my mouth," he added, "I'm gonna bite it off."

"That's a plan," I said. "But right before you bite, you know, you're going to taste that dick in your mouth and wonder whether or not you like it."

Huey Newton shot up from his seat and punched me. The blow caught me on the side of the head.

"Fuck you."

It could've been messy. Both of us were high, we had guns, and we were out of our minds. Fortunately, I decided my best move was to watch as Huey grabbed his woman and marched out of my room.

I knew that I could stir up more shit on stage than in a revolution.

I could be a revolutionary, but I like white women. I have a white-women disease.

One night when I was snorting cocaine in Haywood's house in Sausalito, I met Casey de la Vega, a stewardess who I referred to as the Contessa for both her beauty and the sound of her last name. She fell in love with my sense of helplessness, treating me as if I was a doll or something. She cooked for me, dressed me, and even tried giving me her Porsche.

A few months later she followed me back to L.A. There was no single reason I left Berkeley and returned home. By the end of 1970 I just felt full. I knew it was time to go back and resume my career as Richard Pryor, comedian.

For the first time in my life, I had a sense of Richard Pryor the person. I understood myself. I knew what I stood for. I knew what I thought. I knew what I had to do.

I had to go back and tell the truth.

The truth.

People can't always handle it.

But I knew that if you tell the truth, it's going to be funny.

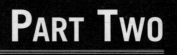

PART TWO

PART TWO

FASCINATIN'. That's what he is. Course the boy knew nothin' 'bout the shit he was talkin' 'bout, but knowin' shit ain't no prerequisite for achievin' great things. Lotta stupid people think they're smart and a lotta smart people know they're stupid. Everybody else, they just workst hard, try to get by, drink every now and then, and take a little pussy.

Ol' Rich was like that in some respects. He blew back into town too stupid to know better and too smart to care. The government was about to get all over his ass for not payin' taxes. Woman sued his ass for child support. And then his ex-wife was 'bout to get a divorce from him. If he'd taken the time to think 'bout things, he might not've come back to California.

Told me once, "My wife went to court, man, and she looked so young and pretty, like a little girl, and I said, 'Who is that bitch?' She told the judge this and that, and when I looked up, he was crying. The judge was crying.

"I looked at my lawyer and asked, 'What do I do now?' and he said, 'You're on your own, Rich.'

"Then the judge said, 'Nigger, we want everything. Do you have any dreams? 'Cuz we want them, too.'"

After the boy finished tellin' me that, I took a taste of wine and remarked that dreams is the blood of the soul and that he obviously possessed way too much soul for any judge to take away. That's what drugs do to ya. Leech the soul. Course, he

didn't listen to me 'bout that, either. Was too busy gettin' that cocaine in his nose. Reminded me of a dog lickin' his balls.

Called him every day for a week and asked, "Boy, whatch you doin'?"

"More," he said.

"Well, you wanna go do somethin' else?"

And each time he said, "Why?"

No one there to tell the motherfucker otherwise.

IT WAS DIFFERENT when I first went to Hollywood. See, after the Big One—World War Two—I tried to get into the motion picture business, too. Read about it in the papers. Said, "We want stars." Shit, in that respect, I was just like Rich. I knowed I was a star. Natural-born. 'Cause I couldn't do nothin' else.

Also, I figured Hollywood was gonna be like it'd been in France. Wall-to-wall pussy.

So I come out and went for this audition. Motherfucker said it was for King Kong. He gave me the script. I didn't know what the story was. King Kong. I said, "I don't mind being a king. Shit, that's a pretty good part. Change the motherfucker's last name, you know, to Williams or somebody. A little too Chinese for me, that Kong shit."

The director said, "I don't believe you understand. What I'm trying to say is that this is a movie about a gorilla."

I replied, "Well, you got the wrong nigger, motherfucker. I ain't no motherfucking gorilla. And I don't appreciate you calling me to this audition."

I took the script and threw the motherfucker down. Them motherfuckers had me out of there so fast, motherfucking dirt didn't even get on the rug. Snatched me right out like that. And I got on the freight train and went all the way back home.

Considerin' that experience, maybe I should've warned the boy. 'Cause I knew what was gonna happen to him. Could've

told him nobody in Hollywood give niggers no good parts. Oh, they'll smile at you, take you out to lunch, let you get some money in your pocket. But they still be lookin' at you like you were a gorilla.

Take what they did to the boy. They pretended to be there for him. Scratching his back. Hollering, "We gotcha, Rich. No worries, brother." 'Cept when he fell, you know what? They missed his skinny black ass.

They caught the monies.

No problems there.

But they missed his ass.

Fortunately, the boy's like one of them old-time niggers. In them days, niggers were too hungry to die. Nowadays, you shoot a nigger, he falls over. And sad to say, most of the niggers nowadays be shootin' themselves. Doin' the dirty work themselves. Shit. Ain't got no pride. Back in the old days, nigger'd live just to spite the motherfucker who wanted him dead. Didn't want to give up the wine or the pussy.

That's what Rich was like. Didn't want to give none of it up. In fact, he wanted more. More, more, more.

"Did you ever get it?" I asked.

"That's the thing about being an addict," he said. "You never know. Good or bad, you never know."

EIGHTEEN

Back in L.A., I started working out again at Redd Foxx's club. One night Redd gave me a fedora to wear. It was more than a friendly gesture. I saw it as the passing of a torch. The master had given me his blessing.

I took it seriously. My first concert film, *Smokin'*, filmed at the Improv in New York, in April 1971, contained new bits like "Black Cat with Neat Hair," "Colored Guys Have Big Ones," and "Dracula and the Brother." My second album, *Craps After Hours*, also explored race, sex, and drugs, but with even more shape and sting.

I knew routines dealing with getting high, fucking my wife's girlfriend, and rednecks looking for pussy were different from anyone else's. But I didn't want merely to shock people. I also wanted to be good. I wanted my stand-up to be like a night at the theater.

Mooney was the one who told me what people thought about me. I was hot in the black community long before I cracked the mainstream. But word spread. Clubs were packed whenever I played. My shows were events, sojourns into territory considered dangerous, taboo, and, as all of us know, true to life.

That's part of what made it so damn exciting. Me and the audience were breaking new ground.

People don't talk about nothing real. Like you talk about shit that's real. Like jackin' off.

A lot of people say they don't jack off.
I did.
I used to jack off so much I knew pussy couldn't be as good
as my hand.

I didn't see why that shit I talked about was considered controversial. It didn't make sense.

You can't talk about fucking in America. People say you're
dirty. But if you talk about killing somebody, that's cool.

My personal life had no brilliances either. I lived with Casey
in a house overlooking the Sunset Strip. It was not a scene that
could be described as loving or tranquil.

We had a birthday party at a fancy restaurant once. Invited a
lot of people. Got dressed up.

But Casey and I arrived fighting and continued yelling
through dinner. Finally, the waiter served the cake. I blew out
the candles and then smashed the cake in Casey's face.

As I got up to leave, the waiter offered her a towel. In a deliberate, ladylike fashion, she cleaned herself up and then to the
waiter said, "I'll have my coffee now."

That was tame compared to the other shenanigans that went
on when the Contessa wasn't around. Sometimes I spent days
at a time hanging out, snorting cocaine, and bullshitting with
Mooney (the only one who never got high), Dirty Dick, and
Prophet, an artist friend who resembled Miles Davis. When the
air cleared, we ventured down the hill to the Candy Store or the
Daisy, exclusive private clubs in Beverly Hills.

I wasn't a star, but they still let us rub elbows with a crowd
that included Elizabeth Taylor, Peter Lawford, and Sal Mineo.
Once, I saw a drunk Richard Harris chase Bobby Darin out of
the Daisy. At the Candy Store, I followed Kim Novak around
like a dog hoping for a sniff. Another time, Mooney and I arrived just as Steve McQueen was leaving. He shoved his face

straight into mine and asked, "Is that Dick Pryor? Is that him?" I looked him right back and said, "No."

As I walked by, I heard him say to Mooney, "The guy looks just like him."

"And you look just like Steve McQueen," Mooney said.

If that was a put-on, I was once the victim of an even better act than mine. I spotted her standing beside the dance floor at the Candy Store. She told me her name was Mitrasha, and she was as beautiful and exotic as her name, a dead ringer for Josephine Baker. After a night of drinking, flirting, kissing, and dancing, I took Mitrasha home, where we did blow and got down to business.

The next time we were together, Mitrasha forgot to do the tuck and fold. When I reached down, I discovered that she was actually a he. For some reason, I didn't care. Either I wanted the nut too badly, I was too high to object, or I was as sexually confused as Mitrasha. It was probably a combination of all three reasons.

Mitrasha and I carried on for several weeks. We even went out dancing at the Daisy. I never kept him a secret. Mooney, for instance, knew I was fucking a dude, and a drop-dead gorgeous one at that. I even admitted doing something different was exciting. But after two weeks of being gay, enough was enough and I went back to life as a horny heterosexual.

I was the only dude in the neighborhood who'd fuck this faggot. A lot of dudes won't play that shit.
In the daytime.
But at night, they be knockin' on the door.
Then I saw him like ten years later. He be, "Hi, Rich."

A while later Mooney delivered a message from Mitrasha. He'd realized a lifelong dream and undergone a sex-change operation. Now biologically a woman, she wanted to get back together.

I passed.

By then, I had more than enough to handle.

Given the word on the street, I wasn't surprised Motown founder Berry Gordy and director Sidney Furie assumed a lot of shit about me when I auditioned for *Lady Sings the Blues*. From the questions they asked, I realized they thought I was a junkie. They thought I shot up heroin. I never had.

But if it was going to get me a job, I didn't mind, you know.

"What would you say to Billie Holliday if you caught her doing drugs?" asked Sidney.

I closed my eyes for a moment. I'd grown up around people like Billie Holliday. I knew women like her. I knew that if I was her friend and caught her doing drugs, I wouldn't be surprised. I wouldn't get angry. I might not like it, but I'd understand, I'd be sympathetic to her need.

So I pretended to fix up some shit as I talked to her. Said, "Baby, how could you be doin', you know . . . Don't be thinkin' you're hidin' it . . ."

They gave me the role of Piano Man right there. They said I did great.

I was very excited. I talked about becoming a movie star all the time. Not because I saw myself as a star. I just had all this juice inside me, this swirl of emotions and ideas that I felt could be brought out on the big screen.

"You're the greatest actor I ever seen," Mooney once said. "You know why? Cause you can't act."

"I can't?"

"No, but you sure can lie. You convince yourself of somethin' and then you tell it like it was true."

And so it was in *Lady Sings the Blues*. I modeled myself after a piano player I knew from Collins' Corner in Peoria, named Jimmy Brinkley, and I tried not to get high as we shot the movie. It seemed to let me hold my own. Diana Ross was great,

mysterious, gorgeous. Billy Dee's self-assurance in front of the camera made me jealous, though I thought he took himself way too seriously. At the end, I felt like I'd opened a new door.

Suddenly, people wanted to meet me. One night Warren Beatty and Julie Christie came to my place. We talked about movies and sheep. Julie owned sheep in England; Warren wanted me to do a movie with him. But I worried that if we worked together I wouldn't like him as much.

I accepted another offer instead. Mel Brooks called and asked if I was interested in working with him on a script for a western. Mel and I had never met, but I knew of his brilliant reputation starting with Sid Caesar. I was excited just to talk to him. After the script arrived, I read it quickly, and Mel and I talked again.

"So this is a comedy?" I asked.

"Yes," he said.

"Then why don't you make it one?"

I joined Mel in New York, where he had set up shop in a hotel with writers Andrew Bergman, Norman Steinberg, and Alan Unger. We tossed out lines and acted out ideas each day for eight or nine hours. Mel acted as ringleader, saying stuff like, "Great, Richard, we'll make this guy black," and laughing when I came up with the fart scene.

I knew *Blazing Saddles* was going to be one of the funniest scripts ever, and before we even finished writing it Mel was talking about me starring as the black sheriff. But when it came time to make the movie I think people at the studio more powerful than Mel didn't want me.

They were scared of my reputation. Yes, I was funny, nobody could deny that. But they also saw me as a volatile, vulgar, profane black man who wisecracked about getting high and screwing white women. It scared the shit out of their Brooks Brothers sensibilities to think about risking millions of dollars on a movie starring a person like me.

I think Mel liked me, and I think he could've fought to keep me as his star. I think Cleavon Little did a good job. However, I

know what kind of job I could've done. But Mel, bless his heart, had a decision to make, and he chose to get his movie made.

It might've been different had *Lady Sings the Blues* come out before *Blazing Saddles*. The reviews I got for playing Piano Man surely would've changed some of those tight-assed minds. But both films were shot at the same time.

Some ten years later I saw Mel in a bathroom at a nightclub in London and he tried to make amends.

"If it wasn't for you, I wouldn't have been able to do it," he said.

"Don't tell me that here," I said. "Tell them that on television."

And then we both laughed.

Carefully.

Following the release of *Lady Sings the Blues*, I should've been one of the hottest young actors in Hollywood. There was talk of an Oscar nomination in the press. People knew that I'd cowritten *Blazing Saddles,* one of the funniest pictures ever. I had ideas and talent. I deserved the type of multipicture deal that film-makers Spike Lee and Robert Townsend would get from studios fifteen years later.

But that wasn't happening then. The only scripts that came my way were for low-budget, exploitation films. It was as if baseball player Barry Bonds had a great season and then was forced to begin the next one in the minors.

Still, I took what was available, including *Wattstax, Hit,* and *The Mack.*

It was frustrating not to be able to do serious work. I felt shackled, teased, and tortured by the system. But what were the options?

I went to see Logan's Run, *right. They had a movie of the future called* Logan's Run. *There ain't no niggers in it.*

I said, "Well, white folks ain't planning for us to be here. That's why we got to make movies. But we got to make some really hip movies. Not movies about pimps. We done made enough movies about pimps, because white folks already know about pimping. 'Cuz we the biggest whores they got."

I couldn't win. In 1973 I worked on the picture *Some Call It Loving*, which shot for several days at a church in South Central L.A. One afternoon the priest invited me into his office. An elderly black man sat in the corner. The priest, oblivious to the onlooker, informed me in a grave tone of voice that several girls who'd been watching the production claimed that I'd molested them. I was as high as a bubble band, but I still knew bullshit when I heard it.

"That's what they claim?" I asked.

"Yes," he said.

"Well, they're wrong," I snapped. "I didn't molest them. I fucked them. And their dogs, too."

Suddenly, the old black man perked up. As I stormed out, he asked me why I'd said that.

"They're talking bullshit," I said. "So I just added to it."

NINETEEN

In 1973 television, normally the most restrictive medium, turned into an unanticipated land of opportunity. Flip Wilson and Lily Tomlin were launching shows. As a rule, variety shows were as unhip as vanilla ice cream. But Flip and Lily wanted their shows to have an edge, and they saw me as the guy who could add that exotic spice.

For me, Flip's show was an opportunity to delve further into characters that I was developing in my stage act. During one sketch, Redd Foxx and I played a couple hustlers in a pool hall that reminded me of Pop's place in Peoria. Before we taped, Redd gave me an old overcoat that helped me get into character, but I did so good that he took the coat back as soon as we finished.

"Why do you want it back?" I asked.

"Because you were funny," he said.

"Do you like the coat?"

"I do now," he replied.

"Shit."

I was more inspired while working on Lily's two specials later that year. That was no doubt due to the way I felt about Lily herself. She turned me on. I went gaga over the way she dressed up in various outfits and became all those different people. I thought she was phenomenal and loved watching her work. She'd make me goofus from laughing so hard.

Then she'd switch gears and inject a poignancy that made

you think about the way you looked at the world. That shit was inspiring. It took comedy to a different level. I tried doing the same during a skit in which I played a junkie in a soul-food café, someone hoping to get both dignity and dinner. In another bit, Lily and I were a prejudiced aristocrat and a smelly wino who bridged their differences while stuck in an elevator.

"I may be a wino," my character, Lightnin' Bug Johnson, stated. "But I'm still a gentleman."

"Goodbye, Mr. Johnson," her Miss Audrey Earbore said. "Stay in touch."

Lily and I went to each other's house a few times. She was always inspiring. We got each other. We had conversations that spiraled into the ozone. In minutes, we'd create enough characters to populate entire neighborhoods. And the deeper and funnier it got, the more I wanted to get in her pants. But nothing ever happened, and we stayed friends and admirers.

The following year, Lily's second special won an Emmy award for comedy writing. I gave mine to Miss Whittaker and Carver Center. If not for her, I never would've gotten that award.

If not for her, I never would've gotten anywhere.

Not that everything was hunky-dory. In 1974, after *Blazing Saddles* finally reached theaters, my ignorance of the law, rejection of society's rules, and general lack of responsibility caught up with me. First, I was stopped by cops one night for outstanding traffic warrants while driving Mooney's 1952 Ford and, as was my custom, I didn't have any ID on me.

It wasn't a pretty picture as I tried to assure the peace officer I was who I said I was.

He preferred to throw my ass in jail.

Cops put a hurtin' on your ass, man. They really degrade you. White folks don't believe that shit. They don't believe cops degrade you.

"Oh, come on, those beatings," white folks say. "Those people are resisting arrest."

That's 'cuz the police live in your neighborhood. Niggers don't know 'em like that. See, white folks get a ticket, they pull over. "Hey, officer, glad to be of help."

Nigger got to be talking about, "I—am—reaching—into—my—pocket—for—my—license!" You know? 'Cuz I don't want to be no motherfucking accident.

As soon as that was cleaned up, the government kicked my ass by filing an indictment for failure to pay income taxes on $250,000 earned between 1967 and 1970. It looked to me like *The People* v. *Richard Pryor*, otherwise known as *David and Goliath, Part II: Screw the Nigger.*

I tried to explain, but "Oops" didn't cover it.

Neither did "Sorry" or "I'll try harder next year."

My lawyers plea-bargained four counts against me down to a $2,500 fine and ten days in jail.

I went to jail for income tax evasion. I didn't know a motherfucking thing about no taxes. I told the judge, "Your Honor, I forgot."

He said, "You'll remember next year, nigger."

With the release of my third album, *That Nigger's Crazy*, I hit the road. This was breakthrough time. The LP sold more than 1 million copies and became my first crossover success. I wish I had a dollar for every person who's told me how they hid that album from their parents and laughed all night when they finally dared play it.

But that's cool. That's how it was supposed to be.

This was new stuff. It was like listening to Lenny.

Everything was fair game. There was no turning back.

I had found my groove.

★　★　★

Not everyone approved. My grandmother told me not to use her anymore on records. Told me she didn't talk like that. I said, "Mama, you forgot."

Others couldn't help themselves. Backstage in Detroit, two black cops told me that they'd arrested a black guy who started spouting my line, "I—am—reaching—into—my—pocket." They nailed him for doing Richard Pryor and then finished the routine, saying, "Okay, spread them cheeks. Put your face on the ground." Then all of them laughed.

That was beautiful.

In Hollywood, I didn't have to say nothing to be popular. I walked into the Daisy one night and its owner, Jack Hansen, skewered me with his arm and proclaimed with a broad grin, "Richard, you're a movie star. Now we can fuck!" But that's how it went. I waved at women and they were mine.

If that was a joke, Deboragh McGuire, an exquisite black model in her early twenties, didn't get it. After spotting her on a few occasions at the Candy Store, she ignored my panto-mimed pickup attempts without so much as a smile or a wink in return. Nothing. Which made me want her even more. Each time I turned to my companions, usually Mooney or my friend David Banks, and whined how badly I wanted to leave with her.

I wanted it so badly it hurt. Truly hurt.

Finally, one Friday night David said, "Man, it might help your case if you talked to her."

"Why don't you do it for me?" I asked.

David, who's the definition of jive, squiggled up his face.

"I don't got nothin' to say to her."

"Don't fuck with me," I said. "Go over there and tell her I want to talk to her."

That was a mistake. It was like asking promoter Don King to be brief. David was overkill. She didn't like him. However, in order to get him away from the table, Debbie offered to com-promise.

"If he gets up off his ass," she said, "then maybe I'll talk to him."

After sending over a bottle of champagne, I walked over and let her talk to me like a dog. But I liked it, you know? Reluctantly, she agreed to drive with me back to my house for a party. I'd invited Lola Falana and some other friends. Later, Debbie confessed the only reason she had gone was to meet *Soul Train*'s host Don Cornelius.

Even though I was bedeviled by her, Deboragh didn't like me. She didn't need me. As a teenager, she had met this rich, older white man who helped her skip through the massacre. He taught her things, took her places, and she loved him.

That fact alone made me insanely jealous. I telephoned Debbie as if hers was the only number I knew. Day and night. The more attached she was to him, the more determined I was to take her away. It was sick, really it was.

I tried to get Debbie to hang out with me on the set of *Uptown Saturday Night,* but she wasn't ready to get involved with my craziness. I didn't blame her. One night I got so pissed at not being paid nearly $100,000 in royalties owed me for *That Nigger's Crazy,* I opened fire on my gold album—not to mention the wall—with a .345 Magnum. Another night Freddie Prinze and I, after getting nuts on coke, stood in the backyard and fired round after round into the sky.

The Contessa, who was still living with me, freaked out. She felt as if World War Three was breaking out in the Hollywood Hills. She called Mooney and asked him to come over and calm us down.

"He won't stop doing coke!" she wailed. "He's crazy!"

You can't tell nobody not to snort no cocaine. Mother-fucker's gonna snort it anyway. It took me a long time to learn that shit'll kill you. Once a big booger came out of my nose. A

motherfucking black one this long. Scared the shit out of me. I said, "Goddamn, please, I'll quit. Just let it stop."

The only thing that stopped was me and Casey. One night in early 1975, we went to a party up in the Hollywood Hills. Without telling me, Casey left with a friend of mine who had become a well-known actor. They got into my car, which was parked alongside the curb, and began some kind of funny business driving lesson.

Before long, we heard a loud crash. Everybody left the party and ran outside. The neighborhood was quiet and dark. However, we didn't have to look hard to see the source of all the noise. My car had crashed through a house down the hill. The tail end was sticking out. It looked like a stunt from a movie.

Casey and my friend were okay, but neither offered an explanation. But Mooney offered a guess:

"He must've been teaching her how to use a stick shift," he said.

It didn't matter to me.

I bought a new car, and Casey packed up her shit and made plans to get the hell out.

I don't mind women leaving me, see. But they tell you why. Fuck that. Just leave. You know? 'Cuz there ain't shit you can say while they're talking to you. 'Cuz you know it's true. All you can do is stand there and look silly.

But when the shit gets too thick, nigger's got a great answer.

"Well, fuck it then! Take your shit and get out. Yeah, motherfucker. Pack this. You packing shit. Pack this motherfucking shit. Goddamn it. I don't care where you put this shit. I don't give a fuck where you put this shit. Shit, I'm gonna find me some new pussy."

She didn't give a shit what I did or said. Somehow she made everything seem like my fault.

Women come back at your ass, though. *"If you had two more inches of dick, you'd find some new pussy here."*

Bullshit.

"I know the dick was good to ya. If it wasn't good, why was you hollerin'?"
"I was hollerin' to keep from laughing in your face."

Nothing was as terrifying as rejection.
Even when it worked for you.

TWENTY

By early 1975, I was a hot commodity, and if I wanted to grab a lucrative payday, one was there for the taking. TV series. Las Vegas casinos. Millions of dollars. But the money didn't interest me. I knew that if I was any good, it was going to be there regardless.

Instead, I went the opposite direction. Declined everything and continued pursuing my own thing. My manager at the time didn't understand. He knew the futility of asking me to tone down the shit I did on stage. But he pleaded with me to think sensibly. He wanted those monies.

"What I'm saying might be profane," I explained. "But it's also profound."

My belief in myself was unwavering. My job, as I saw it, was to throw light where there had been only darkness. I was John Wayne, taking up the fight for freedom and justice. Then Roberta Flack introduced me to Atlanta-based attorney David Franklin, the only black manager I knew of in the business, and I felt as if I'd found the guy who could help me become the hero I envisioned.

We couldn't have been more dissimilar. David was straight, upright, and uptight. I was a mess, short-fused, paranoid, unpredictible. However, we had a common interest—respect. Both of us wanted it. For ourselves and our people.

We were going to break down all the barriers.

As teammates.

He'd block, I'd toward the goal line.

The roll began during a five-week run at the Comedy Store—my gymnasium—where I began preparing new material for another album. One night between bits, I saw the likeness of an old man I'd seen somewhere else. Somewhere in my life, you know? It was as if he was standing beside me onstage. Right there, waiting for me to notice.

"Over here, Rich. Look at me."

Once I noticed him, inspiration took over. As with other characters I did, like the wino or Oilwell, I suddenly knew everything about this wise old man who I called Mudbone. Every black town had someone like him. Some old geezer who talked shit about his life's experiences. Fancied himself a philosopher. That first night I talked about Mudbone for two minutes. A month later I did a half hour on him alone.

I didn't know if he was any good as a character. But I liked him as a person.

I imagined myself at that age.

I was born in Peoria, Illinois—that's a city nigger. And when I was little, there was an old man. His name was Mudbone. And he dipped snuff. And he'd sit in front of the barbecue pit and he'd spit. See, that was his job.

I'm pretty sure that was his job, because that's all he did. But he'd tell fascinatin' stories . . .

My third album, *Is It Something I Said?*, was recorded over a week of performances at the Latin Casino in Cherry Hill, New Jersey.

The O'Jays opened the show. I'd never seen them. I stood backstage and listened. They were fantastic. The place was nuts. Then it was my turn and no one would settle down.

"Please take your seats," the emcee said over and over.

But no one listened.

Finally, I walked out, grabbed the mike, and said, "Will you niggers please sit down!"

And they did.

Then I went on and did a show that stands out as one of my best ever.

Good God, there are a whole lot of niggers here today. And some white folks too. You motherfuckers came in a bunch, didn't you! . . . Shortage of white folks lately. You all stop fucking? White folks into yoga. You can't get no nut doing yoga. You have to get the pus-say!

They stop fucking because some white man told them there were too many people on Earth. There's no room for him to ride his horsey.

There will be no shortage of niggers. Niggers are fucking.

We got to have somebody here to take over!

The comedy gods have many tentacles, you know. And they swoop down and touch you at different times. But when they do it's like salvation. Or deliverance. It's as close to flying as man gets.

The magic doesn't happen often, but when you're on and rolling nothing that I've ever touched comes close.

Not cocaine.

Not even pussy.

Afterward, David Banks went back to L.A. to edit the tapes, while I traveled to New York to host "Saturday Night Live." In only its first few weeks, the show had emerged like a gunshot blast as the hottest, hippest show on TV.

Even though "SNL" 's cast members John Belushi, Chevy Chase, and Dan Aykroyd pushed the envelope each weekend,

the show's producers were concerned that I might take it too far even for them. During rehearsals, writer Michael O'Donoghue came to my hotel room to discuss ideas, but my suggestions scared the hell out of him, and all he could say was, "You can't do that on television."

"See, that's what I'm talking about!" I protested, airing my frustration over the constraints of TV.

Aside from that, I never heard any discussion of censorship. No talk about holding back from anyone, including the cast, who gave me the impression they didn't listen to shit anyway. Behind the scenes, though, the network wrung their hands over the possibility that I might say "fuck," and producer Lorne Michaels, bowing to that concern, secretly installed a five-second delay to the live broadcast, giving NBC a chance to bleep it.

If I'd known, I never would've shown up.

In any event, I caught the cast's enthusiasm, and I think it was reflected in the show. Following an opening monologue—my *Exorcist* routine from "That Nigger's Crazy"—Belushi and I traded swipes as samurai bellboys who argued about which one of us got to carry a guest's luggage upstairs. It ended when I took my sword and cut the front desk in half, prompting Belushi—in the only sentence he'd ever utter in English as that character—to say, "I can see where you're coming from."

But we really stretched the rubber band of what was normally seen on television in a skit where Chevy Chase was a personnel executive giving me a job interview. Although we began innocuously with words like "dog" and "tree," the game quickly escalated to a tension-filled contest of racial epithets when Chevy said, "White."

"Black," I replied.

"Bean," he said.

"Pod," I responded.

"Negro."

"Whitie."

"Tarbaby."

"What'd you say?"

"Tarbaby."

"Ofay."

"Colored."

"Redneck."

"Jungle bunny."

"Peckerwood."

"Burrhead."

"Cracker."

"Spear-chucker."

"White trash."

"Jungle bunny."

"Honkey."

"Spade."

"Honkey-honkey."

"Nigger!"

"Deeeeeeead honkey!"

Movies were next. Although *The Bingo Long Traveling All-Stars and Motor Kings, Car Wash,* and *Silver Streak* were all box office winners, each one had its disappointments. I wasn't speaking to Billy Dee when we did *Bingo Long.* On the set of *Car Wash,* I was too coked out to know any better. And after *Silver Streak,* which began as a minor part but ended as a costarring role with Gene Wilder, I felt I could have done better.

Afterward, I was inundated with scripts, but I worried that my insurgent brand of humor didn't translate as well to the silver screen as I'd hoped. Although my funky, jive-talking characterizations gave credibility to otherwise poorly written cutouts, I still felt limited by the ideas other people had originally created.

And in that way I compromised what I wanted to stand for. But then maybe I was just fooling myself by thinking there

was more freedom in movies, since I was never going to find an outlet as unrestricted as the stage. Just me, the mike, and the audience.

You knew that, Rich.

Yes, I did.

So?

Well, there was still a little child inside me who wanted to go behind the screen as I'd done in Peoria and look for Little Beaver.

And?

The monies. I wanted the monies.

So what'd you expect?

More than I got.

You all know how black humor started? It started on slave ships. Cat was rowing and dude says, "What you laughin' about?"

He said, "Yesterday I was a king."

Deboragh and I went fishing in Hawaii. Since I was a child, I've loved to fish. We always argued about who was going to catch the biggest fish, and at the end of the day, we argued about who'd caught the biggest fish. However, on this particular day, we were out in deep water when she caught a motherfucker that had no intention of letting her pull him in. But she put up a fight that matched his and got him all the way up to the boat.

I took one look at the motherfucker and worried that he was going to get on board and say, "You caught the wrong fish, motherfuckers. Now everyone in the water. Let's see who filets who."

You know?

But this fish took a turn and then jumped straight up into the air. Broke Deboragh's line. You could hear it go.

Ping!

We looked at each other and laughed. We'd had so much

fun. We had fun just thinking about it later on. Hemingway wrote one of my favorite books about a monster fish that got away. On *Bicentennial Nigger*, my fourth and most political album, I tried explaining that sometimes the shit you don't get is as memorable as the shit that you do get, you know.

They'll have some nigger two hundred years old in blackface. Stars and stripes on his forehead. Little eyes and lips just jiving. And he'll have that lovely white-folks expression on his face. But he's happy. He's happy cause he's been here two hundred years.

He'll say, "I'm just so thrilled to be here. Over here in America. I'm so glad you all took me out of my home. I used to live to be a hundred fifty. Now I die of high blood pressure by the time I'm fifty-two. That thrills me to death. I'm just so pleased America's going to last.

"They brought me over here in a boat. There was four hundred of us come over here. Three hundred sixty of us died on the way over here. I love that. That just thrills me so.

"I don't know, you white folks are so good to us. Got over here and another twenty of us died from disease. Ah, but you didn't have no doctors to take care of us. I'm so sorry you didn't. Upset y'all, too, didn't it?

"Then you split us all up, yes, sir. Took my mama over that way. My wife that way. Took my kids over yonder. I'm just so happy. I don't know what to do. I don't know what to do if I get two hundred more years of this.

"Lordy, mercy. I don't know where my own mama is now. She up yonder, in that big white boat in the sky.

"Y'all probably done forgot about it. But I ain't gonna never forget."

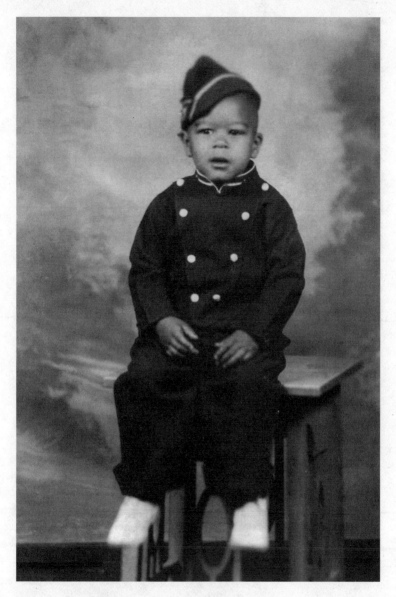

Here I am at two years and eleven months (1943).

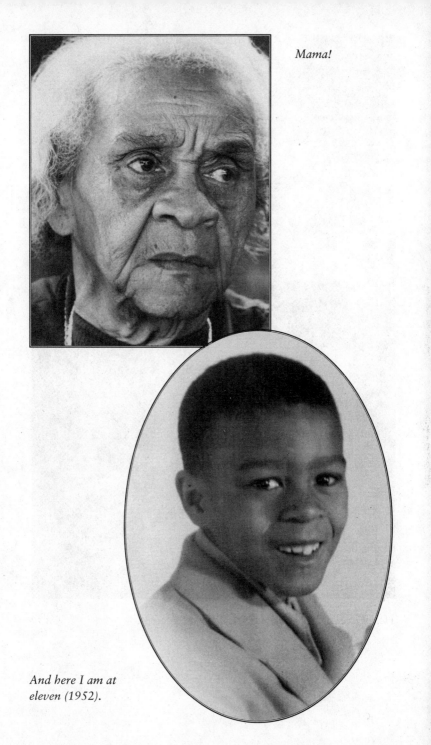

Mama!

And here I am at eleven (1952).

With a friend on board a ship bound for Germany, where I served in the army from 1958 to 1960.

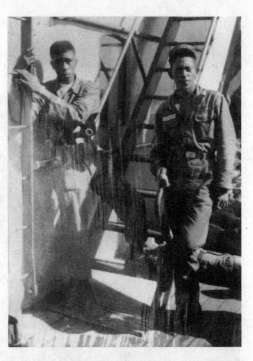

Uncle Dickie, with his daughter and two of his friends.

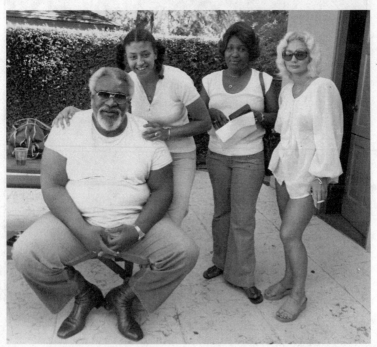

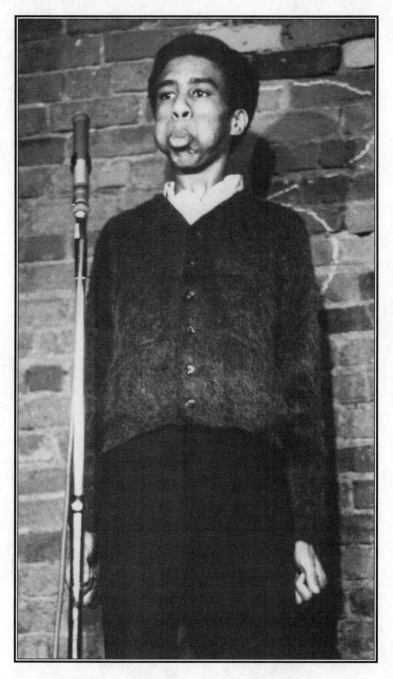

Performing in Greenwich Village, New York City (1964).

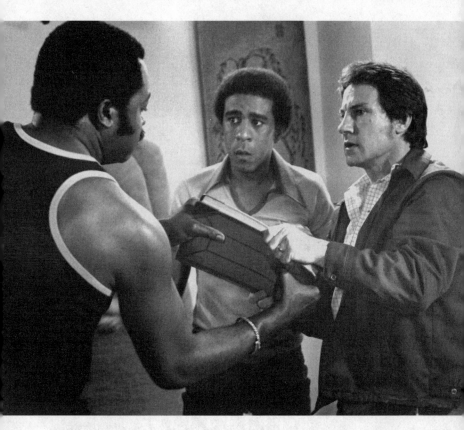

With Yaphet Kotto and Harvey Keitel in Blue Collar *(1977). (Copyright © Universal City Studios, Inc. Courtesy of MCA Publishing Rights, a Division of MCA Inc.)*

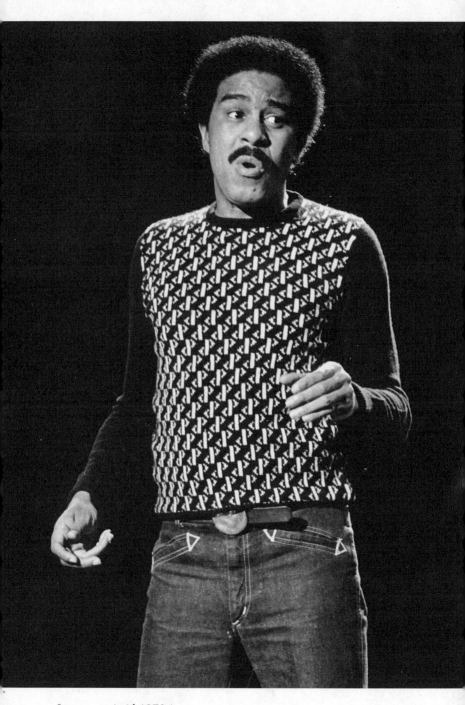

In concert (mid-1970s).

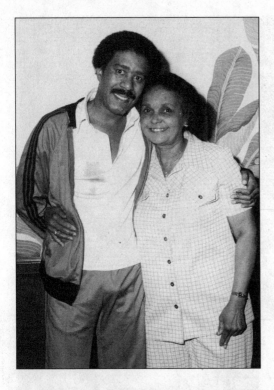

With Aunt Dee on the set of California Suite (1978).

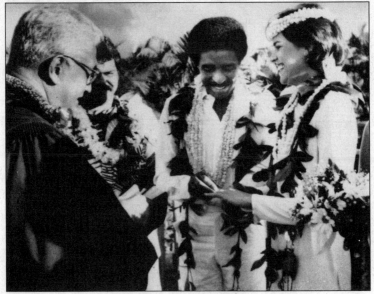

With Jennifer at our wedding in Hana, Maui, Hawaii (1978).

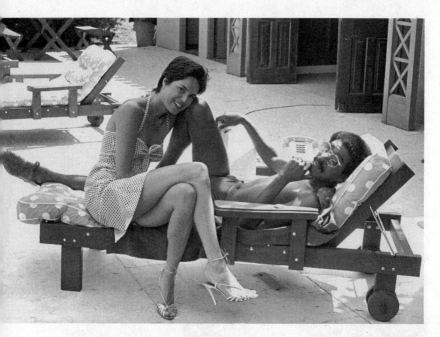

Poolside with Jennifer in Northridge, California (1978).

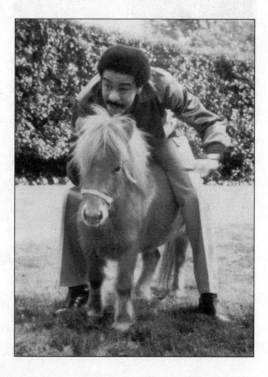

With my miniature horse, Ginger (1978).

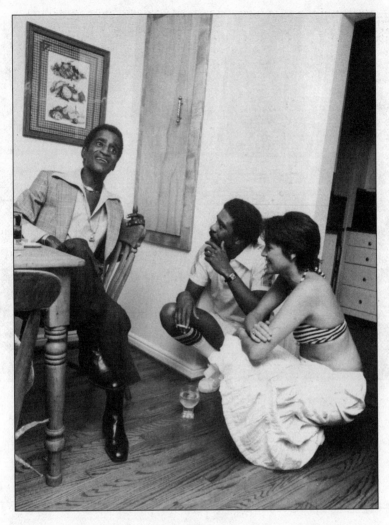

In the kitchen of our Northridge house with Jennifer and Sammy Davis, Jr. (1979).

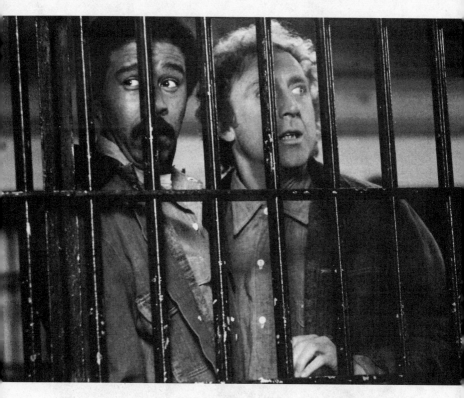

With Gene Wilder in Stir Crazy. (Copyright © 1980 Columbia
Pictures Industries, Inc. All rights reserved. Courtesy of Columbia
Pictures.)

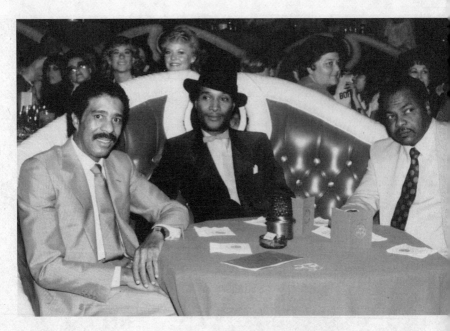

With Paul Mooney and David Banks in Las Vegas (1982).

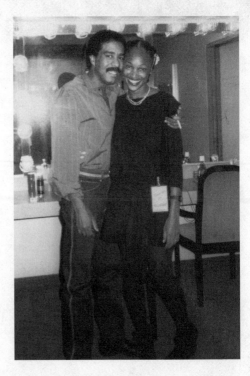

On tour, backstage, with Deboragh (1984).

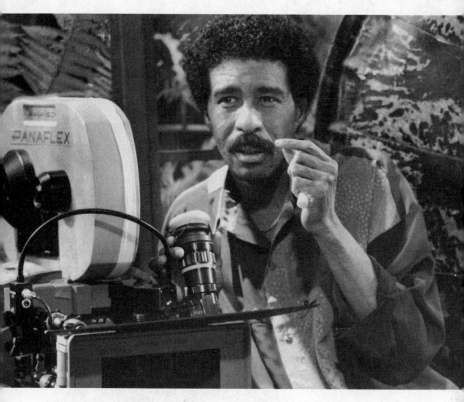

Making my directorial debut with Jo Jo Dancer, Your Life Is Calling. *(Copyright © 1986 Columbia Pictures Industries, Inc. All rights reserved. Courtesy of Columbia Pictures.)*

Above: With Flynn, wife No. 5 and No. 6 (1985).
Below: With Flynn and our son, Steven (1988).

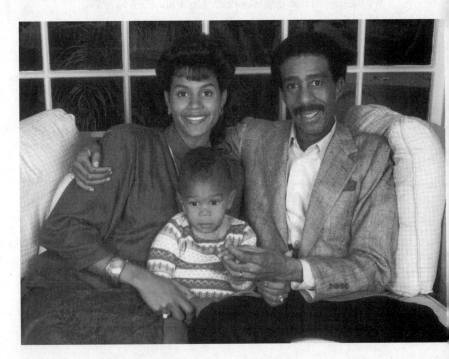

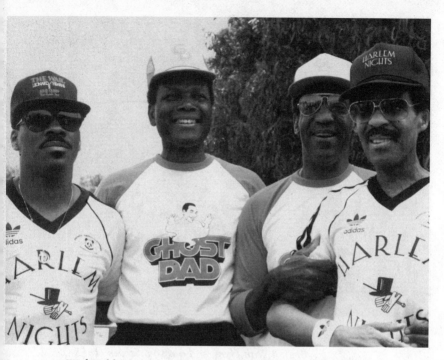

With Eddie Murphy, Sidney Poitier, and Bill Cosby (1989).

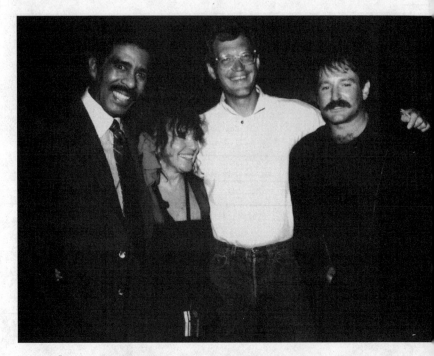

With Mitsy Shore, David Letterman, and Robin Williams (1989).

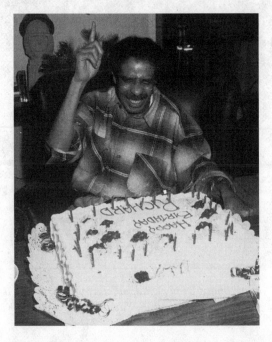

Celebrating my fifty-fourth birth-day, at home (1994).

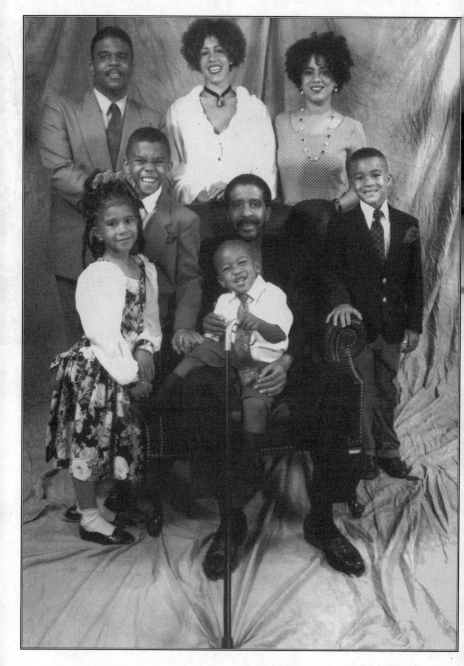

Surrounded by my children (clockwise from top left): Richard, Jr.; Rain; Elizabeth; Steven; Randis (my grandson); Kelsey; and Franklin (1993).

TWENTY-ONE

Women. Drugs. Movies.

It doesn't matter. One of the scariest things in life is to get what you wish for.

Toward the end of 1976 producer Hannah Weinstein asked me to go through the script for *Greased Lightning,* a film based on the life of black stock-car driver Wendell Scott. As I sat on her living-room floor, she ticked off the film's different characters as well as the actors she had in mind to play them, including Cleavon Little. I heard his name and assumed he was going to play Scott.

"Who do you want me to play?" I asked.

She looked at me as if I was stupid.

"The lead," she said. "You're going to play Wendell Scott."

Well, that fucked me up. Although I complained that the only reason I made stupid films like *Car Wash* and *Silver Streak* was because they were the only scripts offered, I was blown away when a movie that seemed to have substance came along and the producers wanted me to star. Was I ready to carry a film?

Said you were, motherfucker.

Yeah, but . . .

I was going to be cool for about four weeks (back when I was a kid), hanging with my man Matt. Matt was bad. Knockin' motherfuckers out. Bam! Bam! He was killer, Jack.

Henry Hanson, though, he'd knock a motherfucker through a brick wall. Matt backed off. Then I was standing there all alone. Henry say, "What you got to do with it, little nigger?"

"I was just—I come home with Matt. I wasn't doing nothin'. I was gonna play some basketball. Can I go now?"

The movie was shot in Madison, Georgia. It got off to a rocky start when the original director, Melvin Van Peebles, tried stirring up shit about there not being enough jobs for blacks on the production. His effort fizzled when I refused to support him.

I said, "Man, I got a job. What the fuck are you talking about?" He was replaced by Michael Schultz, who'd directed *Car Wash*.

It was a nod toward keeping me in line. Though I hadn't been involved, the studio worried about my volatile reputation. I was more concerned about doing a good job, and to that end I vowed to stay clean throughout the entire movie. I rented a farmhouse on some of the prettiest property I'd ever seen, and flew my grandmother out from Peoria to take care of things.

Through thick and thin, Mama was like a security blanket for me. She knew the real Richard Pryor. There was no need to pretend around her. I don't know how she felt about hanging around a movie set, but she liked fishing, and we spent a lot of time together casting our lines in a beautiful freshwater lake out in the field. One day she caught the biggest bass of her life. Started to scream as if she wanted to tell Jesus himself.

That was nice, Mama, wasn't it?

Meantime, I hooked my costar Pam Grier. The first scene we shot was a romantic one with both of us in the bathtub. I tried to be truly amazing. The director yelled "Action." Pam sang "Amazing Grace" in my ear. It was quite a scene.

Pam and I stayed together for about six months. After the movie, we went on a romantic getaway to Barbados, where she got deathly ill after eating shellfish. Back home, we enjoyed a

much healthier life. We shopped, played tennis, watched TV, and hung out.

Unfortunately, our relationship wasn't able to survive Hollywood. Of the two of us, I became the star, but I was put off by how much I thought Pam believed that stardom belonged to her. In my head there was only one Numero Uno, and it wasn't her.

White women take more shit. You be home and shit and you be ready to go out. You say, "I'm going out, baby. Take it easy."

She say, "Okay, toodle-loo."

You say that to a black woman, the bitch starts dressing, too. Says, "Yeah, nigger, me too. Shit. What the fuck. You can't go out without me."

After *Greased Lightning,* the pieces fell together. Everyone in town wanted to be in business with me. David Franklin negotiated separate multimillion-dollar deals with Warner Brothers and Universal, where I set up offices in a bungalow next door to Telly Savalas. I also had projects going with Paramount and Columbia.

As befitted my new stature, I spent $500,000 on a Spanish-style hacienda on three and a half acres in Northridge, a rural suburb outside of L.A. An electronic gate kept unwanted visitors out, while its guesthouse, tennis court, pool, orange groves, and a stable—home to a miniature pony—made it seem as if I never had to leave.

On the downside, the estate was in utter disrepair inside and out. The rambling grounds were overgrown and forlorn. The interior was shabby and old. In a way, the house was very much like me. It looked good. It had tremendous possibilities. But it needed work.

I got some money and finally bought a house. First house I ever had. And them motherfuckers who come to fix it, boy, they

*can kill you. Everything's five hundred dollars when they come
to your house.*

"What do you want? It's five hundred dollars."

I said, "I ain't told you what I want."

"I don't give a fuck. It's five hundred dollars."

I hired Lucy Saroyan, the daughter of writer William
Saroyan and Carol Matthau (she'd remarried Walter Matthau),
to redecorate from top to bottom. Some blond actress introduced us. Lucy was smart, energetic, and friendly with everybody in Hollywood. She played with life as if it was a toy. I
think she thought working for me was going to be a continua-
tion of the party.

But by the time I finished *Which Way Is Up?* in February,
Pam and I were sailing on rocky seas. I was pursuing Deboragh
again, obsessed with prying her from her older lover. And then
I started up with Lucy.

It was a circus. Pam was telling people that we were getting
married. I was fantasizing about marrying Debbie, and in the
meantime I was fucking Lucy.

One time when my grandmother was visiting, all three
women came by to see her at the same time. They sat in the den,
talking as if they were friends. Pam, Debbie, and Lucy. Unable
to deal with this, I hid in the bedroom and listened to them
make small talk.

Finally, I called my grandmother in to see how things were
going.

"Mama, which one of them should I marry?" I asked.

She looked at me as if I'd lost my mind.

"I wouldn't give a nickel for any of those bitches," she said.

My grandmother refused to see me as anything but the little
boy she helped raise. That same visit she tossed the housekeeper
Mercy and the cook and all their helpers out of the kitchen and
made dinner. Afterward, she washed dishes and then called me
over to help dry. I shook my head as if she'd told a joke. I was
watching TV.

"Mama," I laughed.

"You didn't get too big for that, did you?" she asked.

"Mama, I don't want you doing that. I got ladies who do that stuff for me. I pay four people, you know?"

"Does that mean you ain't gonna help?"

A moment later, she stood over me, and I swear to God I never saw the skillet that was in her hand. But I felt it, that's for damn sure. She whacked me good, right over my head like in one of those cartoons. I might as well have been nine years old as she grabbed my collar and led me into the kitchen. I dried everything, too—dishes, counters, floors, chairs, tears.

The press said many things about me being the new black superstar; only one thing was certain: it wasn't easy being Richard Pryor. After the movie *Blue Collar,* which Paul Schrader wrote in about two days especially for me and Harvey Keitel, I went straight into preproduction on my own weekly comedy-variety series on NBC.

When I committed to do a ten-week comedy-variety series, I thought I could do something significant. I saw only the possibilities of TV as a way of communicating. I mean, one week of truth on TV would blow people's minds. You got 20 to 50 million people listening to the real shit every week, there's going to be a revolution in the way everybody thinks.

But the reality of what the network censors allowed on prime time undercut all my enthusiasm. Because I didn't want to sell out completely, I walked into one of the earliest meetings with the show's writers—headed up by Mooney and David Banks—and quit the show. I had no heart for the censors, I explained.

"You want to see me with my brains blown out?" I ranted. "I'm gonna have to be ruthless here because of what it does to my life. I'm not stable enough."

I wasn't stable, but it had nothing to do with the censors. In August, Lucy hired her friend Jennifer Lee to assist her while

decorating my house. Jennifer was a dark-haired flower who blossomed right in front of my eyes one night as she sat on the edge of a bed and played the guitar and sang.

I encouraged her to hang out more often. She had depth and intelligence. She seemed to understand me more profoundly than anyone I'd ever met. I'd catch her watching me, our eyes would lock, and I knew that she knew the shit I was thinking.

She was in the guest room the night Lucy and I broke up following a deranged night of cocaine and violence. The next morning, Lucy tried to persuade Jenny to leave, too—which would've fucked me over since my house was completely torn apart—but something possessed Jenny to stay. Maybe she knew the trouble had been coke-related. Maybe she wanted me. Maybe she thought she could help me. Or maybe she simply felt safe in the morning light.

In any event, I realized that she could handle herself when our first date—an Andrew Young fund-raiser at the Beverly Wilshire Hotel—ended in potential disaster. We'd gone with a friend and his girlfriend. In the limo on the way back, the girl-friend laid into Jenny about being white and dating a black man.

Sisters look at you like you killed your mama when you're out with a white woman. Why should you be happy?

Outside the door to Jenny's quaint bungalow in West Holly-wood, I took her hand and gave her a gentle kiss.

"I'm sorry for what she said in the car," I said. "I don't know what you've heard or read about me. But I don't see colors. I don't believe in prejudice. We're all people, you know? That's hard enough."

And that's the truth.

TWENTY-TWO

I t was weakness. The day after a plane flew over my house towing a sign that said SURRENDER RICHARD, I let myself be swayed into going ahead with the TV series, though I got NBC to agree to reduce the number of shows from ten to four. The less the better.

I should have just taped my personal life and sold it as a weekly drama. Episode one: Although Richard is in love with Jennifer, he proposes to Deboragh.

"I thought Pam Grier said she was marrying you," Deboragh said.

"She did," I replied. "But that's not true. Don't worry about it."

I still don't know whether I wanted to marry Debbie because I loved her or because I figured it was the only way to bring my obsession with her to the point of do or die.

"Well, I first have to talk to *him*," she said, referring to the older man who'd virtually raised her.

"Okay," I said, putting the phone down.

I sounded like a reasonable man. But I wasn't close.

After hanging up, I numbed myself with vodka and cocaine. The demons began hammering my brain. Putting in overtime. Before I knew it, I drove to Deboragh's house and was pounding on her door. No one answered. I screamed.

Suddenly, it opened just a crack—enough for her to look out and tell me that she wasn't going to let me in.

"I'll call you," she promised.

A few days later, she did.

"Okay," she said.

"Okay, what?"

"Okay, you win. I'll marry you."

Episode two: On September 18, Lily Tomlin invited me to appear at a star-studded gay rights' benefit at the Hollywood Bowl. By the time I walked on stage, I was out of control. I was drunk, stoned, and incensed at what I perceived to be the mistreatment of a black singing group compared to some of the white acts on the bill. When I got to the mike, I asked 17,000 of the richest, most powerful and influential motherfuckers in Hollywood where they were when Watts burned.

Then I added, "You Hollywood faggots can kiss my rich, happy, black ass."

I was the talk of Hollywood the next day. I'd pissed off everyone from studio heads to headwaiters. Lily tried excusing my behavior, or at least explaining it by saying, "When you hire Richard Pryor, you get Richard."

In the aftermath, I was sorry and ashamed. I regretted the incident. But when you're fucked up and try to make a point, something gets screwed up as the words travel between your brain and mouth.

Your brain says, "You want to say something, Rich? Great. But first come on into the lion's den."

"Oh, okay."

So then you want to tell your wife that you love her, but you end up saying, "Hey, bitch, get off my back."

Episode three: The night before Richard marries Deboragh, he pulls Jennifer into the bathroom and starts kissing and groping her.

"You're getting married, right?" Jenny asked, confused but not resisting and in fact already in love with me.

"Supposed to be," I replied, lifting her dress.

"So how come you're kissing me like this?"

It was a good question. I wanted to possess Deboragh, but I wanted to *know* Jennifer. She knew famous actors and musicians. She'd seen things. She'd been there, you know? And I envied that.

"I guess I want it all," I finally answered.

Before we got any further, Deboragh came home. Right away she smelled trouble. Sniffed the funny business before she got upstairs. She wanted to fire Jenny, but I played it smooth, saying that was fine with me, but then she'd have to take over the redecorating. Knowing Deboragh was a grandiose bitch who never did a day's work in her life, I prayed that she would react in character—which she did.

"Well, maybe we should keep her around just to finish up," she said.

"Uh, good idea," I replied. "Okay."

The wedding, if you can call such a spectacle that, took place the next day—barely. I was drunk. My daughter Elizabeth wore black. Pam Grier showed up uninvited. And Deboragh, the bride, who was an hour late and had to be revived after taking too many Quaaludes, said, "Thank God you were drunk when I got there, because if you'd seen what I looked like . . ."

The following morning I showed up on the set of "The Richard Pryor Show" still wearing my wedding tux, ready to tape the third of four shows.

By then, I was already resigned to failure. Not only were we pitted against "Happy Days" and "Laverne and Shirley," the two top-rated shows, but the network censors thwarted me from the git-go. On the very first show, they refused to air the

opening bit, a close-up of me reporting how delighted I was to have my own show.

"There's been a lot of things written about me," I said with a straight face. "People ask, 'How can you have a show?' You'll have to compromise."

At that point, the camera panned back and showed me standing naked (I was in a body stocking), with my balls cut off.

"Well, look at me," I continued. "I've given up absolutely nothing."

With a supporting cast that included Robin Williams, Sandra Bernhard, and Marsha Warfield, we still managed to deliver an exciting, surprising, and provocative show. In one skit, I played the first black president of the United States, who's asked at a press conference if he planned on continuing to see white women. After revealing the strain of such a delicate subject, he replied, "As long as I can keep it up."

Then he added, "Why do you think it's called the White House?"

The show was no vanilla milkshake. It was poignant: In one sketch, a wino returned home to his wife, who was played by writer Maya Angelou. She used her Pulitzer Prize–winning genius to elevate this takeoff on my "Nigger with a Seizure" routine into a monologue about the woeful self-destruction by black males.

The show also had its share of punch lines: As a slick black evangelist with a global-sized Afro, I groused about not having the "crossover buck, the Billy Graham dollars."

I'm proud of the effort. But the medium's limitations were as frustrating as low ratings. The show also took a tremendous toll on my health. My drugging, drinking, and relationship excesses were lethal when combined with the pressure of being a perfectionist and putting on a weekly series.

I imagined resting when Debbie and I finally honeymooned in Maui, but it was nothing to put on a postcard home. I spent the first night drunk and covered with vomit in a shower while she complained about the awful condition of the bungalow we had reserved. It was old, there were bugs, and the hotel didn't provide room service.

"Are we going to eat cornflakes for a week?" Debbie asked.

I attempted to redeem myself the next evening by going to the grocery store and cooking fried chicken, mashed potatoes, and corn on the cob. But it was a temporary reprieve.

At the end of October the craziness began all over again when I went to work on *The Wiz* in New York. I couldn't help myself. I caroused with sleazy, doped-up nogoodniks all night. I was as lit as the white suit I wore playing the Wiz himself. I answered my wake-up calls by saying, "Oh, shit, I made it again."

I didn't realize the extent to which I was wreaking havoc on my system and jeopardizing my health until I went to Peoria in early November for my grandmother's seventy-eighth birthday. The fall weather was brisk and energizing. But I was wiped out. Too many drugs, too little sleep, too much work, too many problems.

Still, I fell immediately back into my old habits, much to Deboragh's chagrin. One afternoon she and I, Uncle Dickie, and my grandmother went fishing, and in the middle of the outing Uncle Dickie and I disappeared with what Debbie described as the "two most unattractive white women ever—dogs."

She was packing to go back to L.A. when the phone rang. "Deboragh," Uncle Dickie said, "Richard's had a heart attack."

To be sure, I'd almost gone the way of my dad. Bit the bullet with an ugly whore. My heart had begun palpitating. I'd gotten sick and had trouble breathing. But even then I didn't give it much attention.

"Hi, Rich."

Then the pain arrived.

It was late getting to the party.

If the other shit didn't get my attention, that did.

"Oh, fuck!"

Never mind that I'd been on the cover of *Newsweek* or hailed by *Time* as the new black superstar. Never mind my latest picture, *Which Way Is Up?*, opened that week. Never mind I had money, a mansion, women, and cars.

I got my ass home and hollered like a kid: "Mama! Mama! Help me, Mama!"

Them motherfuckers hurt. I don't care what nobody tells your ass. I was walking in the yard and someone say, "Don't breathe no more."

I said, "Huh?"

He said, "Don't breathe no motherfucking more. You heard me."

"Okay, I won't breathe. I won't breathe."

I tried to ease a little air inside my mouth. Then I heard, "Say, motherfucker, didn't I tell you not to breathe?"

"You told me not to breathe."

"Well, why you walking? Stand still, motherfucker."

"Okay."

"Get your ass down."

"Okay, I'm down. I'm down. Don't hurt me."

"Shut the fuck up. You thinkin' 'bout dyin', huh?"

"Yeah, yeah. Dyin'."

"Why didn't you think about that when you was eatin' that pork, motherfucker? Drinking that whiskey and snortin' that cocaine, motherfucker?"

My family worried themselves sick. They were probably closer to death than I was. They saw their money supply gasping for air, moaning, and writhing in pain. They probably wondered if this wasn't some sick joke. Me coming home to die in

front of them. They weren't going to have none of that shit. Not about to lose my fame and money.

They called an ambulance. Told them to get into the ghetto quick. Told them a white woman had been shot.

I woke up in the ambulance and I was looking at nothing but white people staring down at me. I said, "Oh, God, I fucked around and wound up in the wrong motherfucking heaven. Now I got to listen to Lawrence Welk the rest of my days."

I spent four days at the hospital in ICU, where doctors determined I'd had a "scare" rather than an attack. My grandmother gave all sorts of explanations to the press, ranging from too much smothered steak and cabbage to a heart scare. No one mentioned a family history of heart disease or the chance that my ticker didn't enjoy the "white lady"—cocaine—as much as I did.

No one mentioned anything.

The doctors simply told me to take it easy.

"Remember, Mr. Pryor, moderation."

"Right. No problem."

TWENTY-THREE

Our New Year's party started out like everyone else's. Debbie and I invited a bunch of friends over to celebrate as the clock ticked past midnight. We drank and snorted cocaine and kissed as the calendar changed to 1978. But none of us anticipated starting the new year with a blast.

By morning, though, I was plastered. Debbie and I were also fighting like cats and dogs. Then she threatened to take off with her girlfriends, all of whom sat on one side of the living room snickering at me. Being someone who didn't take kindly to insults on my manhood, I went for the ultimate fuck-you:

My .357 Magnum.

I grabbed it from my nightstand table. Then I waved it in her face. Didn't bother Debbie one bit. She refused to flinch. Stayed right in front of me. I said to myself, "This bitch is crazy, you know?"

"You gonna shoot something, shoot me," Debbie said.

I took most challenges, but not this one. I pointed the gun away from her. She moved in front of it.

"Deboragh, stop!" I said.

"Then put the gun down now," she demanded.

"Fuck you."

I ordered Deboragh and her friends outside. Not that anything changed. We just yelled at each other in the driveway. A moment later, they decided enough was enough and made a bee-

line for my Mercedes, obviously planning a speedy getaway. But I stopped that by jumping between them and opening fire on my car.

I thought it was fair myself. My wife was going to leave me. I said, "Not in this motherfucker, you ain't. You may be leaving, but you gonna be walking away from this motherfucker because I'm gonna kill this here. So go get them Hush Puppies and get your ass down the road.

Then I opened fire.

I shot one of them tires. Boom! That tire said, "Ahhhhh." Sounded good to me. I shot another one. "Ohhhhhhh."

The vodka I was drinking said, "Go ahead, shoot something else."

I shot the motor. But the motor fell out. The motor said, "Fuck it."

I was the last one who could explain why I did such a stupid thing, but apparently "I'm sorry" wasn't enough. One of the womens called the police. If you want to get a cop to respond quickly, all you have to say is, "Hello, Officer, I want to report a black man with a gun." It's like announcing the start of hunting season at an NRA convention. The cops arrived so fast I barely had time to run inside and smoke all my dope.

Then the police came. I went into the house. 'Cuz they got Magnums, too. And they don't kill cars.

They kill nig-gars.

They arrested me for assault with a deadly weapon. I went to jail and was freed on bail later that day. The charges were dropped in February.

Within six months, Deboragh and I were officially divorced

and back to being friends. I probably should've given my love life a vacation. Maybe taken a decade or two off. Instead I grabbed hold of Jenny and lulled her into the calm center of my hurricane.

"What's wrong?" she said. "Are you trying to catch a train?"

It was the first time we made love.

"What do you mean?" I asked.

"Slow down," she said. "Slow down."

I wish it had been possible.

From the beginning, Jennifer and I were mismatched lovers who couldn't get over thinking how lucky we were to have found each other. She came into the picture knowing exactly what to say and do to inspire my mind and excite the rest of me. To her, I was one in a million, a prince who didn't see his royal standing.

And I felt elevated around Jenny. In this well-bred, college-educated beauty, I thought I might've found somebody who could love me so hard and passionately that I'd finally be able to love myself. But our relationship was marred by a tragic weakness that would nearly destroy both of us.

Jenny was almost as big a dope dummy as me. In a test of wills, she was as strong and stubborn as me. She drank with me. She snorted coke with me. But the worst of our secrets was shared the first time I slapped her.

When a man hits a woman one of two things happens: either she hauls ass in the opposite direction or she becomes yours.

Violence is like voodoo. The sting is like a hex. You become possessed by each other. Locked in a diabolic dance.

I lived in that dark place you go when you grow up with people telling you that you aren't worth shit, and Jennifer, bless her heart, followed me down that destructive path. Whether we were vacationing in Maui, locked behind the gates at my house,

or on the road, we never left that faraway place where passion met brutality.

It gripped us both equally. I broke furniture. She threw bottles. We ripped each other's clothes. Even the lighter, innocent moments were tinged with red. One night we were in my study when I leaned across the desk and told her that I wanted to suck her pussy.

"Say that again and I'll hit you in the nose," she said.

I scooted closer.

I spoke slower.

"I—want—to—suck—your—pussy."

Suddenly she popped me in the face.

Boom!

I smothered the sting with my hand and saw that it was covered with blood. Jenny ran downstairs and roused all 350 pounds of my Uncle Dickie from in front of the TV in the kitchen.

"Help me! Help me!" she screamed. "I hit Richard and he's bleeding!"

Uncle Dickie hadn't budged when I entered the scene.

"Where is she? I'm gonna kill the bitch!"

Moments later it was like nothing happened. I apologized. I promised it wouldn't happen again.

"Just stay with me, baby," I said. "Don't leave."

And she didn't.

I didn't excuse such behavior. In all honesty, I didn't even think about it. From as far back as I can remember, I saw men handle their women with a certain roughness. One time as a child I followed my father and stepmother up the stairs of our house, watching as my dad beat the crap out of Viola. It was very upsetting. It wasn't a fair fight. I knew he shouldn't have been beating her.

"Daddy, don't hit her," I pleaded. "Don't hit her no more."

He turned around.

"This is my woman," he snapped. "Now you get your ass back down those steps and mind your own business."

I remember my mother and father was fighting once and I was going to jump in, Jack. Not my mother, motherfucker!
But he beat the shit out of me.
"Nigger, what the fuck?"
"That's my mama!"
"That's my woman, motherfucker!"

I never understood. I always wondered if maybe she liked him kicking her ass. Or maybe it was a man thing to do.

It wasn't until later I realized that letting them go is the man thing to do.

But it's hard to be that strong.

When I took Jenny to Peoria, it was to show her all the sights and people of my youth, the places where I'd grown up and hung out. I wanted her to see what I couldn't describe, the smells and details, the colors and the sounds. But whether or not I realized it, I was also putting her in the midst of my long-time struggle to break free from a past that was often more powerful than I was able to admit.

From their visits to L.A., I already knew most of my family weren't too fond of Jenny. They sensed she had the grit and determination to help me pull away from them, and they feared that more than anything. Mine was a family of survivors. They enjoyed my fame and fortune. They were extremely happy that I'd made a better life for myself. But at the same time they felt that my success also entitled them to a better life.

So when Jenny and I settled into Mama's, they made sure that I knew my place. Mama served soul food. Uncle Dickie started a poker game. Cousins, aunts and uncles, and friends of theirs appeared from out of nowhere. The hours passed. Jenny

went to bed. Dickie arranged for womens to come by. The sun rose and they started the same shit all over again.

"Never forget where you came from, Rich."

" 'Member your roots, son."

"Where would ya be if not for all the material we've been givin' you? Shit, I feel like I wrote half your act."

I could only take so much. Then I burst.

I looked at Mama. At the others. I was famous. The *New York Times* loved me. I lived in a mansion with a swimming pool and tennis court. I'd bought some of these people their homes, paid their mortgages, given them cars.

None of it mattered.

Suddenly I was crying like a baby.

"You never loved me. Ever since I was a little boy you wanted me to be a pimp. I couldn't do it."

At thirty-eight years old, I was crying the tears they never let me. The tears I never let myself cry.

"Let me be who I am, goddamn it. You want me to be like all of you, stuck here in Peoria, doing nothing with your lives."

Mama tried calming me down.

"And you took me away from my mother," I continued. "I loved her. Didn't you know that, Mama?"

A few hours later Mama got me one of her whores and I left Jenny alone with her guitar, to sing the blues.

Our blues.

That was the drill. The tug of war. I apologized and we went back home to L.A. Then something happened inside me. One summer night Jennifer and I were driving home from a dinner party at a friend's house when I abruptly turned the car around and drove to the Comedy Store. I hadn't been there for months, but when we arrived there I waited my turn and then climbed

on stage and ended a long drought between standup performances.

Bonded by a great sense of purpose—me delivering the best
comedy of my career—Jenny and I became inseparable. Even
dependent on each other. Jenny picked out my clothes. She
dressed me in Armani suits and made sure to stick a gardenia in
my jacket lapel before I went on stage. She sat in the back of the
Comedy Store and took notes. In the morning we ate breakfast
by the pool and critiqued and honed routines that became the
heart of my concert movie *Wanted: Richard Pryor Live in Concert* to comedy perfection.

Jenny praised me for telling the truth, for being able to take
my life and turn it into a funny theater of the absurd. However,
it wasn't only me. My life worked for me. For instance, before
Jenny and I went on vacation in Hana, she fired the housekeeper
and replaced her with the weekend maid. A few days later the
maid telephoned us in Hawaii, sobbing and hysterical. She'd left
my cousin's Great Dane in the backyard with my miniature
horse, Ginger.

"Oh, Mr. Pryor," she cried. "Ginger was eaten. The dog ate
her."

*I remember the first time the dogs saw the horse. They
thought it was another dog. My cousin had a Great Dane stay-
ing with us. They ran over to see the horse and then that smell
hit their ass.*

"Hey, that ain't no goddamn dog."

*"You smell that shit? Ain't no dog in the world shit like that,
Jack."*

*Great Dane say, "I don't know what it is, but I'm gonna
fuck it."*

Come back and say, "Can't fuck it."

Other one say, "Well, let's eat the bitch."

One night Jenny and I made love. First, I had an orgasm and
she didn't. I pounded my chest. She called me Macho Man.

I don't give a damn if you come or not, 'cause I'm Macho Man.

Then she had an orgasm.

And you can tell when you made good love to your woman, right? 'Cause she will go to sleep.
That's when you really are Macho Man.

One day Jenny demanded credit for that bit.
I said, "Go register it at the Writers Guild. Then we'll talk."

After working all summer at the Comedy Store, I set out on a large tour that fall. The halls sold out. The reviews were worshipful. There was nothing better than spending an hour and a half on stage, making people laugh. With the comedy gods smiling down on me, I was in heaven.

But the feeling was short-lived. The time I spent by myself between shows was hellish. I hated being alone. I was my own worst company. After one show, David Banks and I were hustled by bodyguards to a waiting limo. A moment later, I ordered the driver to turn around and the bodyguards to relax.

"You did too good of a job," I said to them. "Now we're gonna go back and this time let a few womens through, okay?"

Fortunately, Jenny was with me most of the time. She prompted me to read books, visit museums, and see shows. She kept me fully engaged in real life rather than allowing me to indulge my inclination to sit in a darkened room, doing dope and entertaining lowlifes.

Sometimes her task was easy. Other times we fought without remorse.

The year closed on a dark note. At the end of December, my grandmother suffered a severe stroke. Gravely ill, she didn't appear long for the world. Jenny and I flew to Peoria so I could be by her bedside.

Even then I was conflicted between past and present, between my family and my future. Knowing my grandmother didn't like Jennifer, I nonetheless escorted her into the hospital room to sit with me. Seeing my grandmother dying was difficult for me to face. I needed Jenny's support, and I said so.

"Mama," I said, motioning toward Jenny, "this is the woman I love."

Rather than respond, she reached out and touched my overcoat, which she had bought me. She rubbed it with two brittle, bent fingers.

"Are you cold, Mama?" I asked.

Her lips moved, but I couldn't hear what she was saying. Then Jenny filled me in on what was really going on.

"She's not cold, Richard," she whispered. "She just wants to be loving. She's trying to love you."

That was nice, Mama.

"It feels like blue azure," Mama managed to say.

"Yes, Mama. And it's warm. Very warm. Thank you."

Though sick and inches from death, she was still a formidable woman in her own way. Her doctors were trying to put a tube up inside her, but she wasn't letting them. Desperate to help, I stood in the doorway, tears running down my face, and told her that if she didn't let them work on her, I'd do it myself.

Before I left, I saw her relax.

I guess she knew.

I never saw anyone deal with death like that. I mean, serene and shit, you know? Me, I'd be screaming, "Death, get the fuck away from me!" But Marie, she took it calmly. A few hours after I left her room, she died.

Yes, she did. She died.

And that was something.

TWENTY-FOUR

Five years earlier I had looked out from the cover of a record album with a funny face and a wry look in my eyes and said, "That nigger's crazy." It had been a joke. But after Mama died, nothing struck me as funny.

The world was mine. My concert movie *Wanted* was an instant smash after opening in October. Reviewers seemed grateful that, after so many big-screen misfires, my brand of humor had finally been successfully captured on film. Then Hollywood, which loves a hit movie, also seemed to rediscover me.

Surely I wasn't white.

Suddenly I wasn't black either.

I was green.

But as Kermit the Frog said, "It's not easy being green."

Projects were heaped at my feet. A sequel to *The Sting* with Lily Tomlin. Neil Simon wanted to write *Macho Man* for his wife Marsha Mason and me. Producer Ray Stark brought me *The Toy* and *Family Dreams*. Through my own deals with studios, I talked about developing a movie based on George Orwell's *Animal Farm* and remaking *Arsenic and Old Lace*. I was also offered the lead in a film based on the life of jazz great Charlie Parker.

But it seemed too much to handle. Instead of taking advantage of being a hot commodity, I was awash in a depression which had crashed over me following Mama's death. I truly felt as if I was flailing underwater, stuck in a surreal nightmare.

Despite whatever problems I had dealing with my grandmother, she had always been my anchor, my tether to some sense of reality, and with her gone I began drifting and floating over the landscape without any course.

It was like the word game I'd played with Chevy Chase on *Saturday Night Live*.

"Mama."

"Dead."

"Life."

"Death."

"Richard."

No one dared think about how I might respond to that suggestion, except for Jennifer. The flow of hookers and my frequent, all-night, sometimes weeklong disappearances into the squalid home of a strung-out female drug dealer who plied me with my life's two essentials told her I was in trouble. These flights occurred every night rather than every now and then. Yet she stayed at my side. Put up with me. Berated me. And dragged my ass home.

Any doubt that I was on a path to self-destruction was erased the day I emerged from the bath with half my mustache shaved off, then dressed in a red jogging suit, silver shoes, and a top hat, and announced that I was going out.

"Oh, really," she said. "Where ya' goin'?"

"Shuffling off to Buffalo," I grinned madly.

After that, she checked my ass into a hospital. It was clear the egg had cracked.

In the hospital, I spent a few days detoxing while under the thumb of some good sedatives—a contradiction in terms if you want my opinion, though I wasn't complaining. Once my eyes cleared, I began talking to a psychiatrist, a scholarly-looking black man who made me realize how affected I was by my grandmother's death. I'd told myself it didn't bother me, but it did.

"Everybody's dying around me," I said. "It makes me scared."

Ironically, I had a hard time in the therapist's office. All I had to do was talk about myself, but I found that painfully difficult. I figured it was too personal. But God bless him, the man tried.

"What exactly about cocaine do you like?" he asked.

"It fucks me up good. I like that ping it puts in my head."

"Do you see how it removes you from reality? Mentally as well as physically? You spend days and even weeks isolated in your house, alone in your bedroom, getting high."

"Yeah, but that's okay."

"Why's that? Why's it okay?"

"I don't see any need to be in reality because I've seen how ugly the world is."

He didn't buy that shit. Not for an instant. Wanted to know how I was so confident of the world's ugliness when I wouldn't venture into it and check things out. He started asking me where I'd been, the places I thought were ugly, places I thought were nice, and finally, as if setting me up, he asked how I could make such extreme statements about the world when I'd never been to the origin of the world's beauty.

Okay, I bit.

"Where's that?" I asked.

"Africa."

Excited after reading Richard Leakey's and Roger Lewin's *Origins*, Jennifer and I left for Kenya on Easter Sunday, 1979. From the moment we touched down at the small airport in Mombasa, I sensed something extraordinary. Through the jet lag, I knew something was different but couldn't articulate it. Couldn't get good reception. I strained to hear a beat that was too far away. However, I realized the shrink had been right. The place really was beautiful.

My eyes were full.

It was so beautiful. It was black. Blue black. Original black. The kind of place where you go, "Black."

And landing at the airport in Nairobi, it just fills your heart up. You see everybody's black. And you realize that people are the same all over the world. Because people in Africa fuck over your luggage just like people in New York.

The next day we went to Nairobi, where the sensation of being in Africa grew even stronger. Something was indeed different, exciting, alive, but radically so. We took a tour of the National Museum, and that completely rearranged the cells in my brain. Did a whole rewiring trip on me. By the time I sat my ass down in the hotel lobby, I knew what I was feeling.

"Jennifer," I said. "You know what? There are no niggers here."

She glanced around the hotel lobby. It was full of gorgeous black people, like everyplace else we'd been. The only people you saw were black. At the hotel, on television, in stores, on the street, in the newspapers, at restaurants, running the government, on advertisements. Everywhere.

"There are no niggers here," I repeated. "The people here, they still have their self-respect, their pride."

Over the next week, we traveled into the bush. Settled into a lodge in the middle of Masai territory. I loved their attractiveness, their ancient yet timeless tribal look, their ornate beads, their twisted, elongated earlobes, their pride and grandeur, and the way they stood guard over an earth that belonged to them before it belonged to any other humans.

The animals were a different story. We went on a safari. Not to shoot, only to look. But we still went deep into the jungle, driving until it felt as if we had driven to a different planet. It was so pretty, and there were no people. Just monkeys, giraffes, elephants, hippos, jackals, and lions. Moving in packs, kicking up dust, looking for food.

I couldn't take my eyes off a lion who was tearing into a Cape buffalo. Motherfucker ate like my dad.

"Oh, goddamn, this is good. Shit. Goddamn."

It wasn't no zoo.

We all go to the zoo and fuck with the lions, cause the lion can't get out. You say, "Hey, lion! Hey, motherfucker!"

But when you see a pride of lions, about twenty of them motherfuckers, hanging out, they have a different attitude. They see you and say, "Yeah, get your ass out of the car. Bring the camera, too. 'Cause we gonna eat all of that shit."

After three weeks, I had no doubt that being in Africa had had a profound effect on me. It seemed especially so when it came time to return to the United States. The land had been timeless, the people majestic. I had seen and felt things impossible to experience any place else on Earth. I left enlightened.

I also left regretting ever having uttered the word "nigger" on a stage or off it. It was a wretched word. Its connotations weren't funny, even when people laughed. To this day I wish I'd never said the word. I felt its lameness. It was misunderstood by people. They didn't get what I was talking about.

Neither did I.

I wished that I'd kept my mouth shut.

But that was a hard thing to do. An impossible thing to do.

It wasn't too late, though.

And so I vowed never to say it again.

One thing that happened to me that was magic was that I was leaving, sitting in the hotel lobby, and a voice said, "What do you see? Look around." And I looked around, and I looked around, and I saw people of all colors and shapes, and the voice said, "You see any niggers?"

I said, "No."

It said, "You know why? 'Cause there aren't any."

'Cause I'd been there three weeks and hadn't said it. And it started making me cry, man. All that shit. All the acts I've been doing. As an artist and comedian. Speaking and trying to say something. And I been saying that. That's a devastating fucking word. That has nothing to do with us. We are from a place where they first started people.

In Africa.

In Kenya.

Dr. Leakey, a white anthropologist—which I have to say so white people will believe me—he found remains of a man that stood up and walked on the earth 5 million years ago. You know that motherfucker didn't speak French.

I mean, black people—we are the first motherfuckers on the planet.

My epiphany was highly personal. I would do what I could to make my feelings known at home. It was a vision that extended beyond black people and included people of all colors. My comedy was colorblind. None of it would've ever worked if the world was all one color.

I mean, even black ain't beautiful if it's the only color you look at every day. Life's richness, its beauty and excitement, come from the diversity of things. The multitude of colors that greet you when you step outside the door each day.

I no longer wanted to be someone who pointed out the differences—especially racial ones.

I wanted to help people see how similar all of us are.

I came back home and thought of Malcolm's turnaround at the end and how beautiful it was and how people considered him a traitor for it, and it made me teary-eyed all over again because he had been right.

We're all just people.

We're all the same.

What else I found out in Africa is the fact that aside from us being from the original people, so are the white people.

We all family.

That's it, Jack. And fuck all that other shit. 'Cause it don't mean nothing except about some cash.

TWENTY-FIVE

Holy shit.

I didn't expect the reaction I got when I disavowed the word "nigger." Mooney and David Banks told me that people thought I'd gone soft, sold out, turned my back on the cause, and all that political, militant shit. I received death threats. Kooks showed up at my house, threw shit over the gate. I got letters. And comments from people who thought they owned me and didn't want me to stray.

It was the same as the struggle I had with my family when they said, "Don't forget where you came from."

They wanted my voice to be theirs.

And they didn't want mine to change.

But I wasn't Malcolm, Martin, or anybody else. I was a drug-addicted, paranoid, frightened, lonely, sad, and frustrated co-median who had gotten too big for his britches. I'd wanted laughs, not racial struggles. I'd wanted to be liked, not hated. Overburdened, I'd walked too far out onto the wing, lifted too much weight, and finally I buckled under the pressure.

I was terrified of the jacket.

Confused, I squandered away the summer, working two days for $50,000 on the lame comedy *In God We Trust* and preparing for a major role costarring with Cicely Tyson in *Family Dreams* (later retitled *Bustin' Loose*). But neither picture, when it came to facing facts, was of the caliber I should've been doing if my head hadn't been lost in a haze of vodka, coke, and anger.

As it was, my finest performances were at home. Jenny and I acted like schizophrenic lovebirds: passionate one moment, attempting to murder each other the next. Calling the cops, then persuading them nothing was wrong. This woman turned out to be just as tough and crazed as me. My Uncle Dickie used to say, "You know why? 'Cuz the Irish are niggers turned inside out."

Seemingly destined for the Domestic Violence Hall of Fame, we nearly rewrote the record book the night I stood in the living room, cranked to the gills, and grabbed my .357 revolver. I fired three rounds, then turned and pointed the gun at Jenny, and ordered, "Get out, bitch." Thirty minutes later, when we made up, I said, "I'm glad you didn't make me kill you."

It was classic.

I was the victim.

Nothing was my fault.

I offered no apologies. Take my behavior on the set of *Family Dreams* in Seattle that October. Erratic and ornery from dope, I must've worn out Cicely to the point where she spoke to her husband, who called me one afternoon in my trailer and in his own way asked me to shape up.

"Rich," he said.

Only one man in the world had that voice.

"Miles!"

"Rich. That's my woman."

Then he hung up.

Even so, I knew what he meant. But I was too far into the shit.

Sorry, brother.

Needless to say, going to Dirty Dick's meant I had one thing on my mind, and it was no secret to anybody, because I was so goddamn open about using cocaine that it had become a cornerstone of my act, such as it was. When I walked into his place

one afternoon in November 1979, I saw him going through this complicated process to fix up a tiny rock of 100 percent pure coke and then smoke it.

It transfixed me. My feet might as well have been in cement blocks. I stared and tried to comprehend the nuances of the ritual. It was like watching someone do a new dance step. It looked cool, the expression on his face, total bliss, real out there, and when the motherfucker came down from that rocket blast, he looked at me like he'd just come.

"Oh, man," he said.

"Yeah?"

"Yeah, Rich. You know, I just seen God."

"God?"

"Motherfucking God."

When I first did it, I knew it was going to fuck me up, but I had to do it. Had to be hip. Motherfucker said, "You ever try this?"

I thought, He's going to string me out. He's a dope dealer who needs me to get hooked so he can get some freebase. This dude used to snort a little coke. But I saw him and said, "What's wrong with you?"

He said, "Have you ever freebased?"

"Say what?"

"Freebased?"

He told me he saw Jesus.

Dirty Dick didn't have to ask if I wanted to try it. From the look in my eye, he just started to cook the rock.

"I'll do everything," he said. "You just suck on the pipe. Like it was a chick's dick."

Honest to God, I was scared that first time. I thought it was going to be something else. But it was nice.

That was the worst part.

That it was nice.

★　★　★

In a terribly ominous, ironic forewarning of the calamity that lay ahead, I started a fire the first time I freebased at home. The rambling house was still, dark, and quiet. I was by myself, behind closed doors in my bedroom, seated at a little table, chasing that first high. Rock, lighter, rum, pipe. I thought that I was in touch with the Lord.

"Oh, Jesus," I muttered. "Oh, God."

I should've sensed right then the magic pipe was more than I could handle. But you don't have any sense when you smoke that shit.

Jenny told me that when she came home the place had the feel of a haunted house. If it wasn't ugly before, it was then. Strange. Spooky. Menace in the air. I heard her call me, but I didn't respond. When she walked into the bedroom, I was standing beside the bed, pipe in hand, and staring at the pink comforter, which was on fire. The room was filled with smoke. Flames danced at my feet as if grasping for me.

"Richard!" she screamed.

My assistant, Rashon, ran in, grabbed the burning blanket, and took it outside. From numbsville, I tried to explain.

"I don't know what happened. I was just trying to light the pipe the way you're supposed to. But the rum on the cotton tip must've dropped on the blanket and . . ."

As I dove deeper into the gloom, I corrupted those around me, missed a $100,000, one-day cameo in the biblical spoof *Wholly Moses,* and barely noticed Christmas and New Year's. In less than a year, I'd gone from my artistic peak to personal pits.

I didn't give a fuck.

Didn't even notice.

It started out innocently enough. Every now and then. A little bit. "Naw, not now. No base. Fuck it." Pretty soon, I noticed I wasn't walking as far away from the pipe as I used to. I used

to put the pipe down and go, "I'll be in here." Then mother-fuckers you used to share with come by and you say, "Hey, ain't you got some of your own shit."

If you're unlucky, you sit and wait for someone to fix your rocks, and that's all you think about—when am I going to get my turn? The person who cooks has got all the power. I was fortunate. I had money. I cooked it myself. I was fascinated with shaking up the shit, cooking it, watching it bubble down, you know?

I was like a kid watching magic.

Performing it myself.

Spellbound by the power of turning powder to rock.

You put it on the paper end and—*dink*—it would be a rock, you know?

I was out one night and we was doing it and a woman says, "The fire don't last long enough." We kept trying to get it, and I said, "What kind of fire do you want?"

The dude says, "The kind that lasts forever."

You want to know the difference between sniffing and smoking?

Snorting you get high.

With base, you hope you don't die.

Bill Cosby had once said of me that the line between comedy and tragedy was a thin one. From where I stood on the eve of filming *Stir Crazy* in Tucson in early March, there was no line. My mind was somewhere other than on this crazy caper about two truck drivers who bust out of prison after being mistakenly convicted of robbery.

I immediately set myself apart from costar Gene Wilder and director Sidney Poitier. Rather than stay in the luxury hotel

where they were encamped, I rented a ramshackle home in the hills that was as isolated as I was trying to make myself. My unwillingness to play team ball created tension as thick as the smoke in the pipe that prevented me from showing up for work until noon or later. Another fuckup.

If unprofessionalism had been my only indiscretion, I might not have made so many enemies. But I lived up to my badass reputation by trying to make friends with the prisoners at the Arizona State Penitentiary, showing them that I was cool by getting them water and even sneaking them drugs.

Shit, Rich, what were you trying to prove?

I always said the black man had been fucked over in the revolution. We're nice people. We just got a bad break. But I was there six weeks and I talked to some of the brothers there. Thank God we got penitentiaries.

I said to one, "Why'd you kill everybody in the house?"

He said, "They was home."

Although I was lucky to make it through the movie, I was even luckier not to have landed in jail alongside the murderers, thieves, and drug addicts like myself when I started buying coke through a connection with some motorcycle gangbangers. Unbeknownst to me, they were being monitored by state police and federal agents, including their visits to and from my trailer and my hillside house.

We became targets, too. One night Jennifer smelled cigarette smoke. Then we heard the crunch of gravel outside my house. It wasn't merely my paranoia. Jennifer had been sober for months. We definitely were being watched. The next day, agents and cops were all over the set. For the first time that I knew of, I was in danger of getting busted.

My dumb-ass solution?

Confrontation.

Show them who was hip.

"I hear you guys are mad at me," I said to one of the federal narcs. "Sorry."

They didn't give a shit about my sorry ass.

"We suggest you don't buy any more dope while you're here," he said. "And if you try to leave the state with any, we'll arrest you."

Fair warning. But I couldn't help but do whatever stash was left before returning to L.A. I even got to the airport, then ordered the driver to turn around so I could go back and dig up the emergency stuff I'd buried in the yard.

Nobody can talk you out of doing shit when you've made up your mind to hurt yourself, right?

As the movie finished in L.A., Jenny left me. To her, it was a life-and-death decision. She feared the base was going to kill her if she didn't escape.

My bitch left me and I went crazy.

I was convinced that Jennifer was cheating on me. That's why she left. That's what was really driving me crazy. At first, I hired various dealer lackeys to tail her. Then one night I decided to punish her myself. I trapped her in the bedroom and nearly strangled her to death while repeating, "Jenny Lee, today you're going to die."

But I fell in love with this pipe. The pipe controlled my very being. This motherfucker say, "Don't answer the phone. We have smoking to do." Or the pipe's talking about "Now come on, don't put me down anyplace where I might fall. Because it's two in the morning and it's hard to get one of me."

I had the same suspicions about people who worked for me. I feared they were stealing money from me, making business

deals I didn't understand. I didn't know whether I was paranoid or not. In my state of mind it didn't matter. But just to be safe, I began withdrawing large sums of money from the bank and hiding it in lock boxes at home.

I was high around-the-clock.

I was paranoid.

I was sad.

I cooked up base in the kitchen and ran to my bedroom where I smoked it.

I had conversations in my mind with everybody. Entertainers. Presidents. All of them.

That was a strange place.

I was doing so much I embarrassed cocaine dealers. They said, "Richard, man, goddamn. Come on. Shit. Why don't you just snort the shit?" "Okay, yeah, I'll just snort it." "How much you want?" "A kilo. Just for the weekend."

Football Hall of Famer Jim Brown tried to intervene.

Jim Brown asked, "What are you doing?"
"Freebase."
"What's free about it?"

After cooking up a fresh batch of rocks one night, I walked from the kitchen toward the bedroom. To get there, though, I needed to walk down a long hallway. About halfway through, I was confronted by an apparition. At first, it was too far in front, dancing through the walls too quickly for me to get a long, clear look.

As I took another step, it sprang out from the wall right in front of me and I saw that it was me. Skinny, orange-skinned, wearing black underwear. I was the devil. I pranced around myself in fiery circles, playing, laughing, closing in, weirded-out.

Eight months before, when Dirty Dick had started me freebasing, he promised I'd see God.

Motherfucker. Look who showed up instead.

The devil.

"Are you really me?" I asked.

"Yes, I am you," the devil incarnate said.

Then he—rather, I—disappeared inside the wall again. In the instant, I sprinted into the bedroom and locked the door. I fought the urge to open it a crack and look back, certain that if I did, I would die.

The motherfucker.

And I knew why he was there, too.

He wanted to kill me. Put my ass out of its misery.

TWENTY-SIX

After freebasing without interruption for several days in a row, I wasn't able to discern one from the next. Night and day became different shades of gray. Nor did I care about such details as time. But after waking from a short, unrefreshing, troubled sleep late on the morning of June 9, I drove into Hollywood, where I entered my bank and demanded all the cash from several large accounts I had there.

My brain was strung out. That morning's smoke-a-thon rekindled my paranoia that people were stealing from me.

I wanted my money.

While I was ineffectually arguing with the bank manager, who explained that he needed prior notice for such a transaction, Jennifer called my house and pleaded with my Aunt Dee to get me help. She'd never seen me so wasted and sickly. When Aunt Dee reassured her that I was fine, Jenny made a beeline out to Northridge in order to confront me herself. But the sight of me in the dark, clutching my pipe, told her it was useless.

"I know what I have to do," I mumbled. "I've brought shame to my family. I've hurt you. I've destroyed my career. I know what I have to do."

Shortly after she frustrated herself out the door, Deboragh phoned me. We hadn't spoken for almost a year, but she felt compelled to check in and see how I was doing. It was as if she

and Jenny, the two people who didn't give a damn about my power trips or being cut off, sensed it might be time to say goodbye. They knew it was a scary time.

"You're the only one I trust," I told her. "They're trying to get my money."

"Who is?" she asked.

"It's not fun anymore," I mumbled.

"What's not fun, Richard?"

"I don't think I can get out of here, you know?"

The house was full. From Rashon to my cousin and Aunt Dee, not to mention the housekeepers and cook, people were doing their thing. They were trained to leave me alone. Oh, Mr. Pryor, he's in his bedroom. They didn't mention that the door was locked. By late afternoon, the only reason to suspect I was present was the continuous smell of acrid smoke and the foreboding vibes that sent into the rest of the house.

Nothing changed as darkness took the heat out of the beautiful spring day. Hovered over my rocks, pipe, cognac, and Bic lighter, I smoked and soared and crashed and smoked again, repeating the deadly cycle over and over again as if I was chain-smoking Marlboros. But I didn't allow time even for cigarettes. I'd never felt more paranoid, depressed, or hopeless.

Hopeless.

As if I was drowning.

Voices swirled in my head so that I wasn't able to tell which came from me and which were hallucinations. My conversations became animated, like those crazy people on the street. I heard people who had worked for me talking outside the bedroom window. They were loud, rude, laughing, angry. They made fun of my helplessness. I yelled at them, louder and louder, and still they refused to answer.

"What the fuck are you doing out there?"

As that craziness went on, I continued to smoke until I ran out of cocaine. By then, I was experiencing serious dementia. Stuck in a surreal landscape of constantly shifting emotions. No

weight. Floating at the distant end of a tunnel. Miserably alone. Frightened. Voices growing louder, closing in. Wave after wave of depression. Needing to get high. Real high.

No more dope.

Unsure what to do, I panicked.

"God, what do you want me to do?" I cried. "What do you want me to do?"

I didn't wait for a response.

"I'll show you," I said with the giddiness and relief of a certified madman. "I'll show you."

More laughter mixed with tears.

"I'm going to set myself on fire."

Hysteria.

"Then I'll be safe. Yeah, then I'll be okay."

Now here's how I really burned up. Usually, before I go to bed I have a little milk and cookies. One night I had that low-fat milk, that pasteurized shit, and I dipped my cookie in it and the shit blew up. And it scared the shit out of me. Not the blowing up, but the catching on fire.

Imagining relief was nearby, I reached for the cognac bottle on the table in front of me and poured it all over me. Real natural, methodical. As the liquid soiled my body and clothing, I wasn't scared. Neither did I feel inner peace.

I was in a place called There.

Suddenly, my isolation was interrupted by a knock on the door. A bang, really. My cousin opened it and looked inside at the moment I picked up my Bic lighter. I saw him trying to figure out what I was doing.

"Come on in," I said.

He zeroed in on the lighter in my hand.

"Oh no!" he exclaimed.

"Don't be afraid."

Then I flicked it. The lighter didn't work. I tried it again and nothing. Then I did it a third time.

WHOOSH!

I was engulfed in flame.

Have you ever burned up? It's weird. Because you go, "Hey, I'm not in the fireplace. I am fucking burning up!"

Instinctively, I jumped on the bed, thinking that I'd grab the comforter, wrap myself up, and smother the flames. But God's wonderful. That comforter was just laying on the bed, not tucked in or anything. But the damn comforter wouldn't come loose. Wouldn't let me pick it up or wrap it around. It wouldn't move an inch. It was just stuck.

"*Ahhhhhhhhhhhhhhhhhhhhhhhhhh!*" I screamed.

I was in a place that wasn't heaven or earth. I must've gone into shock because I didn't feel anything.

I sat on the floor when my Aunt Dee rushed in. She peeked in the room as if she was scared at what she'd see. I motioned her to come in.

"Smother him!" she yelled to my cousin.

"What the fuck you talking about, smother him?" I said, though I don't know if any sound came out.

In my mind, I thought that "smother him" meant something bad. Like, "Put the sorry motherfucker out of his misery."

Still on fire—though unaware that I'd turned into a human barbecue—I rubbed the back of my head and looked at my hand. Flames rose from my skin. Scared the shit out of me. I screamed, "What the fuck is that?"

"You're on fire," my auntie exclaimed, and then to my cousin she barked, "Put a sheet over him."

Again, in my delirium, I thought that they wanted to kill me. Taking advantage of their confusion and horror, I leaped up and jumped out the window. That really took them by surprise.

Sprinting down the driveway, I went out the gates, and ran down the street.

"Come back here, honey!" my auntie called.

But I kept going. Running, running down Parthenia. I was out of my mind.

Catching on fire is inspiring. They should use it for the Olympics. 'Cause I did the hundred-yard dash in about 4.6 in the underbrush.

There was a lot of traffic on Parthenia. I saw people looking at me, you know, and I couldn't understand what they were looking at. It felt like a parade. I wondered if I was missing something good. But they were looking at a man burning up.

And you know something I noticed? When you run down the street on fire, people will move out of your way. They don't fuck around. They get the fuck out of your way. Except for one old drunk who's sitting there going, "Hey, buddy, can I get a light? Come on, pal. A little off the sleeve?"

By the time I hit Hayvenhurst, my pace had slowed to a walk. A police car pulled up. Two cops tried to help me. I tried reaching for one of their guns. They could've blown my fucking head off. I wanted them to shoot me. Hoped they'd finish what I'd already started.

But I had no fight in me. My hands and face were already swollen. My clothes in burnt tatters. And my smoldering chest smelled like a burned piece of meat. They held me as an ambulance pulled up and helped get me inside.

"Oh, Lord, you got me now," I muttered.

Then my Aunt Dee, out of breath, bless her heart, got there. She climbed in and started talking to the ambulance attendant. More conversation I couldn't understand as they began treatment for my burns by covering me with a fluid-treated sheet.

The siren wailed.

"Is there?" I asked.

"Is there what?" someone asked.

"Oh, Lord, there is no help for a poor widow's son, is there?"

TWENTY-SEVEN

A t the Sherman Oaks Community Hospital Burn Center:
"Do you know who I am?" the man in the white coat
asked me. "I said, 'Do you know who I am?'"

"Yeah," I said. "You're the doctor."

In the background, I heard people whispering that I'd fucked
up. That I'd fucked up royally.

You can really tell when you've fucked up because the doc-
tor goes, "Holy shit! Why don't we just get some cole slaw and
serve this up?"

They wrapped me up in cloth shit. I complained that it felt
tight. The pain was so bad I turned numb.

"You're going to touch me first. Then I'm going to die?"

The Burn Center's waiting room turned into a circus of the
most concerned. My family filled the place. Aunt Dee, Uncle
Dickie, Maxine, and Shelley. My kids also came in case they
needed to pay their last respects.

Some in the group couldn't wait for the outcome. They simply went back to Northridge and picked the house clean of jew-
elry, televisions, and shit.

But that family shit was kid's stuff compared to the way God
was torturing me for having transformed myself into a human
torch. Physically, I was scarred from the tip of my ears down to
my thighs. The most severe damage was concentrated on my up-

per body, where third-degree burns turned what was once smooth, unmarked, brown skin into a raw, fleshy paste that oozed brown pus and left the nerves exposed.

Emotionally, I didn't know which way was up. I have only vague images of: calling my agent and asking him to get me the hell out. An orderly asking for an autograph. Not permitting Jennifer to visit—my way of punishing her for God only knew what. Probably for getting clean. Jim Brown guarding the door. Deborah wincing at the sight of me.

To be sure, I had the look of something created by a Hollywood special effects department. Wrapped in gauze. Slimy stuff dripping down my face. Moans coming out of my mouth.

But little registered with me other than the sheer, ceaseless pain. The intensity was punishing. It drove me in and out of consciousness. I conversed with God, pleading, cajoling, trying my best to get his attention.

Finally, I heard him respond: "Richard, this fire is too much. I'm going to relieve you for now. I'll call you later."

He kept his word, too. One day the male nurse who cared for me—a big black man with incredible patience and kindness—entered my room holding a sponge for me to see. He showed me both sides—one soft, the other full of little bristles. Didn't look like much. And the way he described it to me, in a real slow, even voice, made me feel like a kindergartner.

This guy Larry Murphy would come in and he kept talking to me every day. He said, "Now we gonna wash you pretty soon and put you in the tub."

I said, "Yeah, man, goddamn."

And he said, "And we gonna wash you."

"This—is—a—sponge, and—I—am—going—to—wash—your—back," he said.

"Okay," I said.

"And—it's—going—to—hurt."

"Ain't going to hurt me, man," I said.

One day I said, "Motherfucker, put me in the tub. I don't want to hear this shit anymore. Just wash my ass, please."

So they put me in this tub and he said, "How do you feel?"

After some preparation, he ran it across my back and I swear to God I screamed like a baby. Can't even describe that pain. Shitfuckmotherfuckerohgoddamnshitohfuckgodhelpmefuck-fuckfuckfuck doesn't even come close.

"Don't touch another motherfucking thing on me! I'm get-ting out and walking out. I don't care if I die, but you ain't gonna touch me with that motherfucking sponge. Please, don't touch me with that stuff."

After receiving this treatment twice a day for four weeks, a nurse mentioned that they weren't authorized to give me painkillers, but if I asked for them—

"I've been here all this time and you're just now telling me that all I have to do is ask?" I said incredulously.

"Yes, Mr. Pryor."

I went right back to my room, buzzed my doctor, and told him that I wanted painkillers. I watched as the nurse injected Demerol in my IV. Moments later, the most throbbing pain I'd ever felt melted into thin air. It was like a pleasant little hum overtook my entire being, brain and body, and I understood the nod of heroin addicts. They go for that hum.

Between the scrubbing and the skin grafts that initiated the long, painful healing process, I had no doubt of the horror story I created. Toward the end of my hospital stay, I also began talk-ing with a therapist, who tried addressing the problems and feelings that led to my suicide attempt. This psychiatrist got right to business. Made me talk about my ma, my grandmother, my father, the neighborhood where I grew up.

I cried like a baby and I wasn't even being scrubbed.

★   ★   ★

The toxicity level of my blood was so high from the amount of drugs I'd done prior to the accident that doctors erroneously thought I must've been sneaking coke into the hospital. They questioned me daily. During that time, though, the only drug I had—other than what was prescribed by doctors—was television. Every Sunday, I watched the religious shows. Those televangelists became my new addiction.

They were so obviously full of shit, hustling the poor in the name of God, that I started imagining what would happen if Jesus himself surprised one of those charlatans by walking into the picture and tapping him on the shoulder, you know?

"Well, hi, Jesus. I was just talking about what you said in—"

"Said what? In where? Man, what are you talking about? I can't even write. Don't know how to spell. What are you talking about?"

"Well, you know that you said you were so and so—"

"Man, I didn't say none of it. I didn't say any of that stuff in that book. But here I am."

"Hallelujah."

"Yeah, thought I'd visit the United States. I hear and see so much. You all say so much about me. Put so many things in my mouth. Make me out to be different, like I give special concessions for special people and so forth. But my law is my law, no exceptions."

"Amen."

"Don't know what you're so happy about, brother. In any case, as long as I'm here, there're just a few people I'd like to say hello to. Like I remember there was a guy who had this dream that one day people of all colors . . . Ring a bell?"

"Martin Luther King, Jr."

"Yeah. Good guy. I'd like to say hello."

"He was killed. Assassinated."

"What? I don't believe it."

"God bless his soul."

"You leave my Father out of this. Now how about this leader you people used to have. Man said something about not what the country could do for you but what you could do for . . . I'd just like to have a quick word with him."

"He was also assassinated."

"I don't believe you people. I also know of some children, little children, who said their prayers every night. I loved hearing them pray. Such good kids. Little voices sounded like music. I'd just like to say goodbye to them."

"I'm sorry."

"Them, too? Just because they were different colors?"

"I'm afraid so."

"I'll give you something to be afraid of, Jack. I mean, how can you mess up so badly. How can you just destroy love? My Father gave you this world, and I gave you love. If you mess that up, too, I hope somebody will have mercy on you because I certainly won't."

"Thank you, Jesus. Now people, how can you resist a heartfelt plea like that? Please, send in whatever you can—ten dollars, twenty dollars, fifty dollars. We have payment plans . . ."

Going home was a relief. Buoyed by 25,000 letters from well-wishers and an army of visitors, I settled into the slow, painstaking, and painful routine of recovery. Basically, that consisted of taking baths and rubbing salves into my skin. At night I slept in a corset that was supposed to prevent my grafts from shrinking. I was also supposed to try not to scratch, but my fingernails scraped the soft, itchy skin until I drew blood.

In my state, pleasure and pain were the same. I was fortunate to have survived my fiery accident, but after the doctors, treatments, and pills were all done, I was still afflicted with the same old problems, fears, and pains that had caused me to drink a bottle of vodka a day, spend upward of $250,000 a year on cocaine, beat women, and then work to make them love me again.

The scars I now had on the outside only mirrored the ones I'd had on the inside my entire life.

Naturally, I got hung up on the superficial. I didn't think I could ever let a woman see me again, you know? That was something basic. Something immediate. For a while there, I flashed on the Great Pussy Drought of the 1980s and, brother, it was a frightening thought.

If I couldn't fuck no more, then what, you know?

I was wrong, though. Deboragh, bless her heart, was my first woman after the accident.

After the fire, a lot of people said, "God was punishing you." No, if God wanted to punish my ass, he would've burned my dick. When the fire hit, my dick went to work. "Emergency! Piss, come—do something! Don't let the fire get to the balls!"

And my chest was hollering, "Help!"

My dick said, "Fuck you. Every man for himself. Spit! I'm protecting the balls."

With Deboragh, it was like I'd never done it before. But then oh, God, did I do it, you know? It was beautiful.

I felt myself fall in love.

With Deboragh. Always with Deboragh.

But also with life.

I saw it all—the brightness that starts the day, makes the flowers, causes a hobo to smile, and inspires a woman to sing. It was right there, man.

Life.

As bright as the fucking sun.

I rubbed it all over my damn face.

And for that moment, it was mine and I was glad to be alive.

TWENTY-EIGHT

'd never been higher than I was in Hawaii one day toward the end of 1980. After ten hours' worth of flying lessons, I took over the controls of my single-engine Grumman Tiger and piloted the plane myself from Oahu to Maui. It was a transcendental moment. My whole life I'd wanted to fly. As a kid, I'd told one of my teachers about my dream and he'd laughed at me. I could still hear him say, "Richard, you can't do that."

Yet at age forty, I was doing just that. Likewise, plenty of people doubted whether I'd be able to refrain from my self-destructive ways. Privately, I was among them. But as I soared above the lush, emerald green island, banking to the right, then to the left, and then slowly circling the island's crystal blue perimeter, I was overwhelmed by the freedom of being above it all, and I felt as if I could prove them wrong, too.

Any doubts I had about how the public would react following the accident were quickly erased. After its December release, *Stir Crazy* went on a tear at the box office, grossing more than $100 million. In April, the Hollywood community showed their support with a standing ovation when I presented an Oscar at the Academy Awards. Then *Bustin' Loose,* which I finished after recovering from my burns, continued my winning streak that summer.

In Hawaii, the high life was replaced by a healthy, isolated

life in Hana. I retreated into the slow lane of my newly completed, modern, Japanese-style home, which was situated on a hill overlooking five plush, gorgeously landscaped acres of flowers and trees. Every room had its own deck. I looked outside, into the gardens and then out beyond, to the ocean, and one word came to mind:

Yes.

But fruit juices, jogging, and shoji doors didn't ensure life would be as sweet as the orchids in my garden. The affection I craved was still damn elusive. I tried Deboragh. I dallied with a Korean actress. I coerced my cute Japanese maid in Hawaii. I pretty-pleased Jennifer back into my life. I tried all thirty-one flavors, whatever I felt like at the time, but when it came to womens, relationships, trying to satisfy the urge to get loved, I couldn't find the right prescription.

It's not that I lacked for love, but what I was able to feel was as momentary as the high I got sucking on the pipe. My therapist plumbed my childhood for reasons. Motherfucker made some points that were hard to accept. But true.

"That's why life stinks," I said.

"What do you mean?"

"To me, this life stinks because all we want is love," I went on. "That's all anybody wants. Black, white, orange. Race, nationality, none of that shit matters. We're all human beings and we all want love. That's all."

"I think you're right," he said. "How does that make life stink?"

"Because the motherfucker's fleeting, you know? It won't stay put."

Was that the problem, Rich?

Or was it that you didn't love yourself?

★   ★   ★

In February 1981, I returned to the mainland to prepare for work on *Some Kind of Hero*. Drug-free until then, my Northridge house was filled with the ghosts of when I wasn't clean. They'd waited around like ghoulish fans for my homecoming, but instead of wanting my autograph, they asked, "When we gonna smoke, Rich? When we gonna get high, man?"

The big house had been vacuumed and cleaned of all my old drug paraphernalia eight months earlier. The day of my accident the stuff had been thrown out. Not on account of me. No, nobody wanted the police to find it. But as soon as I walked inside that place, I knew there was some shit around. I sensed it. Sniffed it like a bloodhound.

After waiting till the house was quiet and I was alone, I went to where I kept my supersecret stash. A little drawer. Lo and behold, I had the exhilarating rush of a prospector who pans the river, sifts through the silt, looks down, and sees a golden nugget sparkling in the sunlight.

Eureka!

There was a little rock.

One perfect little rock.

I picked it up and marveled at its whiteness. Brightness. A star in the night sky.

Make a wish, Rich.

A few minutes later, I found a glass pipe.

Locked in the bedroom, I flicked my Bic for the first time since the fire.

"Oh, Jesus," I sighed as the rush began. "Oh, God."

Though I appeared to be in fine form as *Some Kind of Hero* filmed that summer, I'd climbed aboard the old self-destructive roller coaster without anybody knowing it. I wanted so badly to prove that I was the same old Richard Pryor that I actually became him. I kept a tiny pipe in my trailer and got loaded whenever I could get my hands on some coke. By August, I was back in the same rut.

So was my personal life. My six-month affair with *Hero* costar Margot Kidder ended just before the movie did, when she discovered that I was cheating on her. She didn't get mad— much. But she got even by coming over to the hotel where I'd taken up permanent residence and scissoring the Armani wardrobe hanging in my closet.

Thank God that's all she cut.

In the meantime, I repaired old ties. Before *Hero* ended, I'd proposed to Jennifer. It took three tries, including a final proposal at a pool party in Hana where I smoked some Maui Wowie pot that was as powerful as an LSD trip, before she finally accepted.

Our marriage took place in a backyard ceremony on August 16, 1981, and Jenny looked resplendent in white and flowers, but the event was short on celebration. As for a reception, Margot sent an angry telegram. My pretty Japanese maid, who'd taken to keeping a bottle of vodka by the Mr. Clean—using one to mop and the other to mope—got sloppy drunk and cried that she was losing me. And in the morning, having sobered up, I called my attorney in L.A. and asked him to get the damn marriage annulled.

"I woke up and realized what I'd done," I explained. "I said, 'Shit, I don't want to be married.'"

By October, I had initiated preliminary divorce proceedings, slept with other women, and physically pummeled Jennifer, but something in me couldn't let go completely. Pressured into making another concert film, which I wasn't ready to do, I knew instinctively that I had to hang on to Jenny in some way, shape, or form. She'd gone through it with me before.

"You aren't ready," she counseled. "Don't do it."

"But they're telling me that I have to cash in," I countered. "They say now's my time. Now's my time."

But December came and I knew it wasn't time. Rather than work out for weeks and then tour, honing each routine to a razor sharpness, as I did before the first concert picture in 1979, I

went up to Oakland the week before we filmed and fucked up. Too much booze, too much coke. I was little better when I got in front of the camera the first night at the Hollywood Palladium.

In a scene reminiscent of my breakdown in Las Vegas fifteen years earlier, I asked myself, "What the fuck am I doing here?"

Then I walked off stage.

Over the next couple days, I delivered the goods, enough so that producer Ray Stark, agent Guy McElwaine, and other powers behind the movie were mostly satisfied, but all of them knew they'd need to reshoot parts. As for me, I split for Hawaii. Told Jennifer, "They made the gentle mistake of giving me the money in advance. Bye-bye."

"They didn't give you all the money," she said.

"Yes they did," I said, flashing an evil smile.

Eventually, I finished the live-concert film by performing at what was essentially an invitation-only party, but after the footage was spliced with the Palladium bits, it still played as inspired, cutting-edge theater. Even so, *Live on the Sunset Strip* wasn't as great an overall performance as the first concert picture, but with routines like "Mafia Club," "Africa," and "Freebase," it had its moments.

And, fortunately, so did I.

It's nice to be able to laugh later.
I thank you all for the love you sent me, and I mean that sincerely.

Offstage, I was not nearly as sentimental. In January 1982, I embarked on Jennifer's and my belated honeymoon, a cruise through the Caribbean. If we hadn't been fighting at the time of departure, she would also have been on board the *Silver Trident,* the luxury yacht I'd leased for the occasion. In her place I found other female amusement when I wasn't too fucked up.

But I missed her terribly, and after ten days of ship-to-

shore, me sweet talking and pleading from such appropriately romantic-sounding locales as Teardrop Cove, she succumbed to the lure of our mad addiction to each other.

It may not have been a traditional honeymoon, but there was no mistaking it as anything but ours. Wild and woolly, we were George and Martha sailing across the high seas of love. Passionate lovemaking spoiled by drinking and fighting. After less than two weeks, she jumped ship and got a divorce lawyer, and I finished up the vacation with another woman.

As always, Dr. Jekyll's good intentions were fucked up by Mr. Hyde. The shit was beyond my control. I couldn't escape the darkness.

Late on the night of March 4, 1982, John Belushi, Robin Williams, and Robert DeNiro had come by the Comedy Store looking for me to participate in their wee-hours carousing. Luckily, I happened not to be there. Otherwise I might have—and to my mind, probably would have—ended up going back to the Chateau Marmont and doing cocaine with Belushi, who died early on March 5.

It could have easily been me.

I was just as lucky in cheating death a month and a half later when I worked on *The Toy* with Jackie Gleason in Baton Rouge, Louisiana. I didn't much care for the picture. Like the others, I did it for the monies. But Jackie and I hit it off famously, like kindred souls.

The shit Jackie talked between setups was funnier than anything we got in the movie. He knew about gangsters, gamblers, comics, vaudeville, strippers, and sharks. He'd start talking about something that happened in the 1970s and then suddenly he'd be swirling around the 1920s and '30s, describing people and joints so good I could smell them.

One day he asked me to get him some grass. I found some and gave it to him on the bench where we used to sit and talk.

It overlooked a lake that had no fish in it. But Jackie didn't like the way I handed it to him. He showed me a sneaky way of handling the exchange, and then he winked.

"That's called a switch," he said.

We laughed. Two stars. Getting paid a few million dollars. And we were practicing dope deals.

Goddamn, that was funny to me.

Then things got serious. One day I felt my heart pound in rebellion to my secret dalliances with the evil white lady. An ambulance rushed me to a New Orleans hospital. I really thought I might actually die right then, and the only thing that really bothered me about it was being in the South. Down there, people didn't care if a black man died. Or else the Klan would be so glad they'd declare a holiday.

Otherwise, I figured the rest of my family had gone. Maybe it was my time, you know?

But it turned out to be a warning. According to the doctors, it was my Wolff-Parkinson-White syndrome acting up, a sudden arrhythmia, which they could treat. I explained that the palpitations had come during a scene I shot in a swamp opposite a live alligator. The gator had said, "Ah, blackened catfish." With that, my heart began sprinting for shore.

It didn't know the rest of me couldn't swim.

Deep down, I knew the truth. Lying in my hospital bed, I let my mind wander back to the time when I'd asked Redd Foxx why I always wanted more, more, more cocaine, and how he'd looked at my ignorant face and told me it was because I was an addict.

An addict.

I didn't tell anyone.

As if it was a secret. As if it wasn't true.

But who were you fooling, Rich?

Even then you wanted more.

TWENTY-NINE

Yes, I was unrepentant, even with that scare, as I went off to London to play the villain in *Superman III*. And yes, the movie was a piece of shit. But even before I read the script, the producers offered me $4 million, more than any black actor had ever been paid.

"For a piece of shit," I'd told my agent when I finally read the script, "it smells great."

But the money couldn't buy what I needed. One night Margot Kidder stopped by my room to see if I'd go out with her. She observed me sitting in the middle of the floor of a vast, luxurious suite, sucking on a crack pipe. I was surrounded by empty vials.

She muttered something about me being such a sad sight.

So fucking sad.

What could I say?

"What did you say, Rich?"

"Nothing. I just kept smoking."

There were moments when I dreamed of escaping my misery just as I had before I'd set myself on fire. I just couldn't find an escape that suited me. I took my kids to Hana for Christmas, making a big show of it though in truth it was nothing more than an empty gesture. I wasn't capable of anything else.

Remember when Rain stood in the doorway. She and the others were going to the beach.

"Daddy, come with us," she said. "Come on."

I was grouchy and hungover. I looked out at the beautiful Hawaiian afternoon, sunny and warm. The blue Pacific glistened in the distance like a sapphire I might've given a woman after having the guilties for cheating on her. None of it registered with me.

I wanted the kids to go already.

But they wanted their dad.

So?

That's what I thought.

I just wanted to do my base.

Then the strangest thing happened. Left alone, I asked myself what I was doing. You know? In a moment of clarity, I glimpsed the absolute pitifulness of my situation. Got a clear view through the window of hopelessness and despair.

You go through changes in your life and you just fucking change. Something happened in my life just fucking changed my mind about all the shit. I used to think I knew everything, man. I'd be fucked up and I knew it. I knew all the shit.

And all of a sudden I didn't know shit.

I was one of the dumbest motherfuckers that ever lived. If you catch me on the wrong day and ask me my name, you're gonna get trouble.

"How'd you end up like that again, Rich?"

Although the answer was in my heart, I dealt with what was in my hands. Trembling but determined, I tossed the shit in the garbage. For real. No hiding the pipe in one drawer and the rock in another and tiptoeing away for a few minutes. I chucked it. Grabbing my cigarettes, I walked to the beach. As I shuffled onto the sand, my kids looked as if they saw an alien.

In a way, they did.

"Daddy!"

Even I was tempted to turn around and look at who they were talking about.

"Daddy!"

But then it was great. Rain taught me how to float. Bobbing in the salty water, I got into the sensation of buoyancy, the feeling of levitating off the ground. I imagined drifting away from my addiction, away from the dark rooms where I was prisoner to the pipe. Staring up at the sky, I saw the immensity of the spinning world. The gulls squawked. My kids squawked. The water slapped the shore.

Like music.

And I was in the middle of it.

Alive.

And grateful to be there, you know?

Several weeks later, I got a call from a friend. Coincidentally, she'd checked herself into rehab and wanted me to help her in recovery by participating in therapy. Ordinarily, I would've told her no. In my neighborhood, the administration of affection had always been a one-way street. However, in my newfound sobriety I asked where and when and hopped on a plane.

Although there was no bigger skeptic than me, the therapy sessions had an unanticipated effect on me. I listened in the group meetings, where people stood up and told harrowing stories caused by their addictions. I thought back to when I was seven and my grandmother took me to an evangelist in Springfield and pleaded with him to rid me of the devil.

Even then I thought that shit was funny.

But now I heard things that sounded too familiar to laugh off. Gradually, I recognized the picture being assembled by these confessions was of me.

I had to quit drinking. I got tired of waking up in my car driving ninety. You know? Trying to talk to the police when your mouth don't work.

One day, caught in the fervor, I stood up and admitted that I, too, was a drug addict and alcoholic.

It wasn't anything I didn't know already.

Amen.

Or hadn't known for many years.

Sing it, brother.

But to say it out loud, in front of strangers, without adding a punch line, man, that was like saying adios to the greatest, funniest character I'd ever created.

My best work, you know. And it scared the hell out of me.

Hallelujah!

"I know you, motherfucker," I said. "We ran for a long time. But I'm tired of you hurting me. Let's declare a truce. Leave each other alone. See how it goes, you know?"

No response.

"Okay?"

No response.

"Please?"

"We'll see. If you just shut up."

Even sober, I couldn't control my addiction to the womens. Deboragh started out by my side when I began a lengthy spring tour in preparation for another live-concert film. But after a performance in Washington, D.C., I met twenty-year-old Flynn Be-Laine. Within two days, I shuffled Debbie off to Buffalo, so to speak, and cozied up to Flynn.

By any standards, Flynn was drop-dead fine. Strong legs, nice breasts, and sweet smile.

I was like a mouse sniffing around a trap.

But it was good, you know?

There were other womens, too. A Julie in New Orleans, where I filmed most of *Here and Now.*

But when I added the finishing touches to the film in New York I had Flynn meet me there. Then I set her up in L.A. By

August, though, I lost interest in her and went back to Jennifer. Naughty me. I couldn't help myself, and neither could she.

Flynn, bless her, was tough. She didn't give up. I wanted nothing to do with her, but she had other ideas. One day Jennifer slipped into my Rolls and saw a pair of baby booties hanging from the rearview mirror. Her eyes rolled.

"Flynn sent 'em," I said.

"You know what she's telling you, right?" Jenny asked.

Indeed. In February 1984, right before I received the Black Filmmaker's Hall of Fame Award, Flynn broke the news: She was pregnant. Clearly, I was a productive motherfucker, deserving of some Hall of Fame. But instead of celebrating Flynn's announcement, I ran to Deboragh, seeking consolation, advice, excuses. Seeking something. She knew as well as I did that my own need for parenting far exceeded my ability to be one.

My life's sentence, you know?

But that poor-pitiful-me shit didn't play in Peoria, and it sure didn't play on Debbie's doorstep.

"Well, what am I supposed to do about it?" Debbie asked. "I didn't get her pregnant."

"I've got to do the right thing," I said.

For some reason, I thought I saw the pieces of my life falling into place much like a puzzle. Events took on a pattern and meaning. Such nonsense began making a certain amount of sense. I don't know why.

Following my accident, I had tried to write my autobiography but never quite got a grip on the three-hundred-pound alligator that was my life. Still too close to the fire. Didn't have perspective. I kept at it, though. Thinking about shit. Writing down bits and pieces, thoughts and shit.

Finally, I asked Mooney and Rocco Urbisci, a writer friend, to help me stitch it all together, and the result was *Jo Jo Dancer, Your Life Is Calling*. Originally, I intended it to be a straight-out

comedy, but I couldn't keep the sadness and emotion from spilling onto the page. It was beyond me, you know? Like therapy. I went with it.

Maybe a documentary would've played better. It would've had the edge of my standup. More dick, less heart. Or maybe more heart and less dick. I don't know.

I never will, either.

Jo Jo was the latest and biggest project my company, Indigo Productions, produced as part of a $40 million deal with Columbia Pictures. For my money—which it was—Indigo was a fiasco, something much bigger than I could handle. I didn't know how to run a company, and, come to think of it, I didn't even want a company, you know?

Jim Brown did, though.

I made my friend Jim president.

At the end of 1983 I fired him and all hell came down on top of me.

Jim, a complex man, liked running that company more than I liked having it. He hired lots of people. He made lots of noise. He commissioned numerous scripts. Started up all sorts of projects.

However, I wasn't happy about where the company was going. The only thing I cared about was the work, and when I sat down to read the scripts that had been developed, I couldn't find one that stood out as special. Not one screamed to be made, you know? I had to ask myself a serious question, something I tried my damnedest to avoid.

"Rich, do you want the company?"

"No."

And that's basically what I decided to tell Jim when I fired him.

I caught shit, though. The black film community was outraged. The NAACP turned on me. Everybody, it seemed to me, acted like it was my obligation to employ people just because of their skin color. They didn't understand. I didn't want to employ anybody—black, white, or purple.

I didn't give a shit anymore.

Jo Jo was the exception. The project was my own creation, my own madness. Certainly, it takes a degree of madness to produce, direct, co-write, and star in a movie. By the time I took all that damn film in the editing bay, I felt like a snake charmer slowly being strangled by his own charming pet viper. I just wanted to know how I might've fucked up. Not that I could see anything wrong. I was too close, and everyone around me only said how brilliant it was.

"Genius, Rich, that's what it is."

All that shit.

But goddamn it, I knew better. I just wanted someone to tell me where the holes were, you know?

"Right there," the doctor said. "Look there."

Flynn's legs were apart. My eyes were riveted to that amazing sight: my son Steven entering the world. On November 16, 1984, I actually stood in the delivery room and watched him being born, and now I can finally say it:

I'm glad I was sober.

If you've never seen a baby born, you ain't seen shit. I know if men had to push babies out their asshole, there'd be no question about abortion. Not even a smither of a question.

I saw this woman who I loved lying on a table with her legs open, a baby coming out of her pussy, and she had a smile on her face. Right then I knew she was crazy. That was proof.

I was just praying to God that the baby didn't come out and grab her hemorrhoids.

Then he came out, and that made me realize women have been bullshitting us. You know when you're fucking, really working, doing some serious damage, and she says, "It hurts." Well, if your dick is not as big around as my thigh, you ain't hurting shit, okay? I saw a baby, a whole entire human being, come out of this lady's pussy.

The doctor let me help pull him out. It was my baby boy, you know? And you hold it in your arms and do the stupidest shit. While she was recovering from the pain and the blood and shit, I took that little guy and held him up in the air. Like, "Behold the only man greater than myself!"

Then the doctor says, "Can you give him back to the mother so she can feed him?"

"No, motherfucker, I'm not finished beholding yet."

I still refused to marry Flynn, and it cost me. I came back from a gambling binge in Las Vegas. Had my winnings in a briefcase. Some $600,000 I'd won at the blackjack table. Flynn's lawyer was the first to congratulate me.

"That's about how much she'll need to take care of the boy," he said.

But that's life sometimes.

A simple, unpredictable roll of the dice.

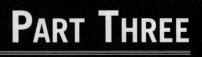

PART THREE

MUDBONE, PART THREE

NOW somethin's obvious to me. These here times we live in are tryin' times. But ya know what? Ain't never been no time when folks didn't have to try.

Shit, ya gotta try.

Every day ya gotta try'n get your lazy ass out of bed in the mornin'. Ya gotta try'n get somethin' to eat. Somethin' to drink. Try'n get a little pussy now and then.

Now Rich, he had spunk. He had a heart attack and then went on TV and said he could still make love nine or ten times a day. Absolutely knew he could. All he had to do was meet a woman and then he'd prove it.

'Cept it was a cover-up.

Boy was suffering.

Worn out. I know'd he was tired.

Loss of nerve. Maybe.

Bad breaks. For sure.

Not long after his movie came out, people were talking 'bout how he'd changed. Looked skinny and sickly.

People started talkin' it was AIDS 'n' shit. Thought never crossed my mind.

'Cause I know human nature.

Truth is, you lock yourself in a dark room and breathe that devil's snot every day, you gonna miss all the sunshine. Naturally, you gonna be miserable, quit tryin', give the sickness

space to rent. Flower don't get sunshine, it ain't gonna grow. People don't get enough sunshine, they ain't gonna see any reason to try'n bloom, either.

Reminds me of a fella I knew named Black-Eye Titus.

Shit, you probably never heard of old Black-Eye. But I knew him well. Heard of him long before I met him, but that's 'cause Black-Eye was famous. Famous the same way ol' Josh Gibson and Buck O'Neil were famous baseball players. White folks ignored them 'cause they were black, but Josh and Buck knew they were among the greatest who ever played the game.

Same with Black-Eye. He was the greatest entertainer I ever saw, and that includes a lady I once knew in Paris. She could whistle Dixie without using her mouth, if you get my drift. But that's besides the point.

A great dancer 'n' singer, Black-Eye came along at a time, way back in the 1910s and '20s, when not much notice was given to black performers like him. People too busy payin' attention to Al Jolson, who was okay if you liked schizophrenics. But I never much understood that blackface shit.

Course, Black-Eye noticed what was goin' on with Jolson and got the notion of rubbing white shit over his face. Only thing you'd be able to see were his black eyes—the reason for his name. Black folks loved his ass, though. Paid him just for walkin' down 125th Street, and that was after his show. And those white folks who saw him left dazzled.

He had a chance to go as big as Jolson.

Maybe bigger. But that's what scared folks.

One night when he was asleep in his car—had to sleep in his car 'cause no hotel'd give him a room—some motherfucking Klansmen snuck up and cut off his legs. Laughed that he was no man no more. He was half a man. Exactly how they considered black people in general.

I was supposed to see Black-Eye perform that next night. Had a pretty little girl. But the curtain went up and a kid named Callaway came on. Nothin' was ever said 'bout Black-Eye and no one heard of him again.

★ ★ ★

'BOUT forty-somethin' years later, I was passin' through Peoria, Illinois, and wandered into Collins' Corner, a little black
'n' tan joint in town, where I was supposed to see a young per-
former. There happened to be an old man at the piano, playin'
'n' singin' and smilin' at some of the ladies. The fat ones. And I
didn't think nothin' much of it, 'cept that I liked the way
he sang.

Then I got up to meet a pretty thing. That's when I noticed
the old man was in a wheelchair.

Upon closer inspection, I saw he didn't have no legs.

Well, I put one and one together, and sure enough it was
two. Black-Eye Titus was still alive and kickin', so to speak.

"Was down 'n' out for a spell," he explained.

"You was the greatest," I said. "What happened?"

"It's this way," he said. "I never much noticed my legs was
gone as much as I did my spirit. If I couldn't dance—because
that's what I did best—then I figured I couldn't do nothing.
'Sides, when I didn't have on my face, nobody knew I was
Black-Eye, including me."

"You mean without the cream . . ."

"Yep. Without the cream, there was no coffee."

We probably would've kept talkin' if Bris Collins, the club's
owner, hadn't told us to shut up or get out. As happened, he introduced a young singer-comedian named Richard Pryor, which
was the whole reason I was there anyway. Passing through
town just to give him some advice.

I wished I woulda told him 'bout Black-Eye. 'Cause before
we quit talkin', ol' Black-Eye told me how he spent years tryin'
to drink himself to death. One night he figured he was on his
way to doin' just that. And when he opened his eyes in the
mornin', it was because he felt something warm on his face, and
it felt mighty good.

"Turned out it was just the sun," he chuckled.

"And that was enough?" I asked.

"Well, the thought dawned on me that it could be. A little pussy, a little warmth. Same thing. It's like God's up there playin' craps, and all of us peoples is just one roll of the dice. You ain't gonna be a seven every day, but you can hope, and most times that's enough for me."

THIRTY

As a reward for *Jo Jo,* I decided to sprint across the country in my Ferrari. People asked why. Simply because I had a Testarossa, you know. That was reason enough. Going 130 miles an hour, I wanted to blaze my own path into the future. Slip in and out of time as it applied to people. Flee the past. Escape Hollywood, a town I didn't like in the first place.

But where were you going, Rich?

I didn't know.

I was just going. Going fast, too.

But where?

Maybe nowhere. Maybe just away.

Or maybe I was trapped.

Trapped in a cosmic joke, you know?

If so, I wasn't alone. Geraldine Mason, a pretty actress who'd auditioned for *Jo Jo,* sat beside me. She had stars for eyes, a smile as bright as a sign in front of the hotel in Las Vegas where we partied for a few days, and, as far as I knew, she really wanted to be with me.

We sped through Las Vegas, intent on getting to Peoria in record time. Somewhere along the way, Geraldine mentioned she might be pregnant. I didn't know there was such a condition as "might be pregnant."

"Maybe we'll get lucky," she said softly. "Maybe nothing will happen."

In my entire life nothing was something that never happened to me, and that didn't change in 1986.

That summer the first signs of a serious problem surfaced. It snuck up on me while I finished shooting *Critical Condition* in L.A. I remember being tired by that time, feeling drained of my normal energy. Then one day the floor caved in. I had been resting in a chair between setups and camera changes when director Michael Apted finally asked me to take my place.

I heard him loud and clear.

No problem.

"Okay, Michael," I said.

The message was relayed to my brain.

My brain said, You have to get the fuck up, Rich.

But nothing moved.

Raise your ass up off the chair, my brain continued.

I tried. But nothing moved.

"Come on, Richard," the director said. "Quit fooling around."

I wasn't fooling around. That's what scared me.

"I'm not joking," I called. "I'm trying to get there."

And I was. Real hard. But my body wasn't buying that shit. It was fucking with me. Like ha-ha-ha, you know?

I saw my legs. Told them to get up and go. But the job order got lost around my waist. My legs were on vacation.

Numb and dumb.

I didn't panic. Probably because I didn't know what the fuck was going on. I had to believe it was just a strange muscle twitch. Something that was going to pass. After massaging my legs, I shuffled my feet in place, a tentative start up, and then, just as strangely as the motherfuckers had quit, they started back up again.

My brain was going nuts: You're under your own power. Good, Rich. But what the fuck is going on? Don't matter. Just don't fall.

I walked funny, but at least I made it to where I was supposed to be and did my scene without incident.

Afterward, I didn't know what to make of the problem. I hoped I could forget about it. Tried to, anyway.

But it sure tripped up my sanity, you know?

After I guested on "The Tonight Show" a short time later, people noticed a dramatic change in my appearance. I'd suffered a noticeable loss of weight. My body was spindly and my face looked thin and tired. Suddenly, the rumor mill overflowed with speculation that I had AIDS. I didn't know what the fuck was wrong with me, but blood tests proved it wasn't AIDS.

I tried ignoring the symptoms, but that became impossible. At a charity basketball game, I fell down while dribbling the ball. Nobody was around me. My legs just took a time-out. I went splat. I looked like a motherfucking clown, though it obviously wasn't funny. After resting, I finished the game. But the incident shook me up.

Frightened by the way my eyesight and balance came and went without informing me of its schedule, I finally saw my longtime physician. After he asked a ton of questions and performed numerous tests, I asked him what he thought might be the problem. He looked at me as if I'd just walked through the door.

"I'm not sure," he said.

Well, I knew that much. Motherfucker did everything but make lemonade from my piss and didn't know more than I did. That infuriated me, you know?

Because something was wrong.

"I don't believe you," I said.

My intuition told me that he suspected the problem, but didn't want to tell me. Conservative doctor shit.

"We need more information," he counseled. "I really think you should go to the Mayo Clinic for more tests."

It took until August for him to finally persuade me it was in my best interests to stop ignoring the problem and go for an examination. Childlike in my fear of what they might discover, I

asked Debbie to accompany me. Though we hadn't spoken for a while, she agreed. In spite of all the reasons we couldn't live together, we still loved each other.

For the next week, I went through a series of intensive, often frightening and exhausting tests. Embarrassed when my eyes' inability to focus prevented me from describing pictures on large cards, I shifted into unrestrained terror when I saw the needle they were going to use during my spinal tap. At least the pretty nurse was nice.

"Now, Mr. Pryor, don't move," she said.

"I won't," I replied. "I'm looking at your titties."

The brief glimpse might've been the lone bright spot. Unable to handle the fear of what the doctors were going to find, I secretly turned to the only relief I'd ever known. One night Debbie, worried by the unusually long time I stayed in the bathroom, opened the door and caught me fumbling with a tourniquet and syringe as I shot up with Demerol.

Oh, Mama.

I stared at her, helpless and frightened and silent.

Mama.

She didn't say a word. She took in the scene and backed out of the room, shutting the door.

In the movies, I would've heard crying coming from the other side. But there was nothing.

Just the sound of my heart beating and the silent cry in my head for my mother to make it all better.

At the end of the week, Debbie and I finally met with the doc. For five days, I'd been asking what they thought and getting mystified shrugs in return. Now they had a diagnosis. In a plain, emotionless voice, the doctor told me that I had multiple sclerosis. Debbie and I turned and exchanged blank, worried looks.

Multiple sclerosis.

Those two words hit me like a ball on a backboard.

Bounce.

"Oh, I got it?" I said. "What is it?"

The doctor's face was all funny and shit. I'd never heard a doctor just say, "Ahhhhhhhhh."

"So what is it, doc?"

"Ahhhhhhhhhhhh."

"That means you don't know anything about this shit, right?"

"Ahhhhhhhhhhhh."

He told me that the MS was still in its infancy. That I was fortunate.

"Your prognosis is good," he said. "Many people with MS can live for a long, long time. But . . ."

I told the doctor: "You don't know how the fuck I got it and you don't know when it's going away. So don't be bringing up theories about my cocaine. You didn't even know I did no cocaine."

He still said. "Maybe it was those two ounces you did that time."

I said, "Man, what do you mean, 'that time'? I did two ounces every time."

"Well, slow down."

I flew back to L.A. in shock. Neither Debbie nor I mentioned a word about MS the entire flight. I didn't know what to think. Living life so large, bigger than life, you tend to believe you have some sort of superhuman power. I'd left the ghetto behind. The whorehouses of my youth were like postcards from past journeys. I'd walked through fire. Seen my own motherfucking flesh regenerate. I wanted to see myself as a blessed motherfucker. But suddenly I felt the floor start wobbling. Like in an earthquake, my footing was unsure. All my different incarnations

stared at me. Child, comedian, asshole, addict, man, father, husband, actor, victim, superstar, patient, child.

They all wanted to know the same thing.

"What now, motherfucker?"

It occurred to me then that at the outset of life God gives you a certain number of angels. They hover above you, protecting your ass from danger. But if you cross a certain line too many times, they get the hell away. Say, "Hey, motherfucker, you've abused us too many times. From here on, you're on your own."

That's what scared me—the prospect of being alone. One option was to marry Flynn. Despite all my philandering, she remained as determined as ever to become the next Mrs. Richard Pryor. She'd become a devout Jehovah's Witness, once even trying to convert me while sitting on the edge of my bed. But I didn't hold that against her any more than I did other shit.

Worn out and in deep denial, I caved in to fears of being alone, and on October 10, 1986, we married in a civil ceremony performed in a judge's chambers. She brought a girlfriend to witness the occasion; I didn't bring nothing but misgivings.

In the weeks following the wedding, I started working out new material at the Comedy Store. Some people talk to psychiatrists, but my biggest insights had always come onstage, so for me it was therapeutic. About the AIDS rumors, I said, "That was funny the first time I cleared out an elevator." Flynn's and my twenty-two-year age difference also proved fruitful. "My wife is young," I said. "The school bus had her back on time today."

But it just wasn't the same as before. My performance lacked the passion that had always given my performances an incendiary edge. After leaving the Mayo Clinic, the only constant was the level of chaos in my life. It reached the danger zone when Geraldine gave birth to my son Franklin. The news pissed off Flynn, who wanted to be the mother of the youngest Pryor offspring.

What could I do, you know?

Try—to—get—a-way!

If only I'd been able. Separated in early December—after less than two months of marriage—our divorce was finalized in January. As we left for court, Flynn sashayed out of the house wearing a fur coat with nothing on underneath.

The upshot?

Roughly ten months later, Kelsey was born.

She was my sixth child. Her mother was my fifth ex-wife.

I wondered if I was ever going to roll a seven. Probably not. Better not. Later on, I got a vasectomy to make sure I damn well didn't.

But God love us all anyway, you know?

THIRTY-ONE

In the dream, I was standing opposite my father in the middle of a big field, throwing a baseball back and forth. For a long time, we played in silence, enjoying the warmth of the afternoon and the rhythm of the game. Then I started asking questions about my life. Mostly about my womens. Stupid shit. Like what he thought about Deboragh's ashtray. Did he like what Jennifer wore a particular night we went out. Shit like that.

As my arm tired, I asked if he knew that I'd gone to the Mayo Clinic and been diagnosed with MS. He caught the ball and threw it back. Suddenly, it seemed like a test.

"How do you feel, son?" he asked.

"Eh," I said with a shrug. "Sometimes better. Sometimes a little worse."

I threw the ball back and the game resumed. A while later, he interrupted the silence again.

"How do you feel, son?" he asked.

"Dad, if only I'd have known."

But the future doesn't let you know it's there until it bites you in the ass, particularly, as I discovered, when it includes multiple sclerosis. Chronic, disabling, and hard to detect, the disease attacks the central nervous system, destroying the protective casing that surrounds nerve fibers. Although rarely fatal, it produces symptoms that range from loss of coordination and muscle strength to mood shifts and depression—with some

bladder weakness, memory loss, spasms, and even paralysis thrown in for good measure.

It was as if God had all this shit left over from the other afflictions he created and decided to throw it all into one disease. Kinda like a Saturday Surprise. It was a motherfucker. It ate you up from the inside out.

Instead of denial, I went into depression. By early 1988, I was hitting booze and pills pretty hard, spending a lot of time isolated in Hawaii. On a rare outing, I took Deboragh on a shopping spree to New York. While holed up at the Plaza Athénée, I snuck in a visit with Jennifer, who heard me ramble semicoherently about life and death and left thinking I was suicidal, though she never heard me reveal the reason why.

In August, I returned to Gotham City to star in *See No Evil, Hear No Evil,* another lackluster comedy reteaming me with Gene Wilder. My excuse was the money. I don't know what everybody else had in mind. Physically and emotionally, it was difficult to involve myself in the work. The picture also reunited me with Jennifer, who pestered me with questions about my distant, sullen, and markedly slower demeanor.

"Why are you walking like an old man?" she asked.

For weeks, I refused to answer. Why she didn't tire of such shit is testimony of our strange, twisted, and enduring love affair. Then one morning before I left for work, Jenny caught me unrolling my Comme des Garçons shirtsleeve over a thin stream of blood as I exited the bathroom. I'd just shot up.

"It's bunk," I said.

"Why, Richard?" she asked. "Why are you fucking with this shit again?"

The room was disturbingly silent for a long time before I was able to summon the courage to admit the last secret of my complicated life. But I don't think I could've said anything that would've shocked Jenny. We'd been through it all.

"I went to the Mayo Clinic for some tests," I said. "I've been twice now."

"And?"

"I have multiple sclerosis."

"So that's the reason you're walking funny?"

"Yeah."

"And the bunk?"

No reply.

I had limits to what I thought needed explanations. I had my limits.

Even in the early stages, the disease was unpredictable. It came without warning, like a relative showing up unannounced at my doorstep. I'd get up to walk across the room, and while my mind would picture me striding as always, I'd actually be splattered on the floor, a fucked-up tangle of surprised arms and legs. I had no control. I'd look up and say, "God, it's in your hands."

I got a taste of things to come shortly after I moved from my longtime Northridge residence—it was more like fleeing the ghosts—into a two-story, Spanish-style house in Bel Air. Once I was walking up the long driveway when I lost control and fell down. Frightened, I called for help. The people who worked for me thought I was inside the house and ran up and down the stairs. About the time my fear turned into frustration, one of them finally poked her head out the front door and saw me waving like a castaway on a deserted island.

"There you are!" she exclaimed.

"Right," I said. "But you don't get no prize because of it."

It was like that, you know?

At the end of 1988, I worked on *Harlem Nights,* Eddie Murphy's pet movie project. At the time, no one was bigger. Exercising his clout, he was the picture's writer, director, and star. He was trying to scale the same mountain that I climbed making *Jo Jo.* I should've warned the motherfucker.

I never connected with Eddie. People talked about how my

work had influenced Eddie, and perhaps it did. But I always thought Eddie's comedy was mean. I used to say, "Eddie, be a little nice," and that would piss him off.

But Eddie can act. I don't care what people say, the mother-fucker is a great actor.

So throwing me and Eddie together, after so much dreaming by agents and studio executives, sounded exciting as hell. The potential had guys in Hollywood putting money down on new Porsches and vacation homes. Then Redd Foxx joined the mix and Eddie's movie took on the air of history. Three generations of black comics looked like the middle of the 1927 New York Yankees batting order.

Only *Harlem Nights* wasn't a comedy, you know?

It was Eddie's movie—that's what it was. I just wish that I'd been in peak form. For obvious reasons, I never felt obliged to inform anyone about the disease, but the fact was, the MS shit gave me a difficult time. It was my secret, and it put me in a dark place moodwise through most of the movie. I finished thinking that Eddie didn't like me.

It wasn't true. But thoughts don't care about truth and shit. They sit up in your mind and fuck with you whenever.

"Hey, Rich?"

"What?"

"I didn't say anything."

Of course, even paranoids have reason to be scared. In March 1990, after cleaning up at the Betty Ford Center, I treated myself to a long-overdue deep-sea fishing expedition in Australia. However, before I even had the chance to set off from my Brisbane hotel, I got sick. Like severe lethargy and shit. Chills, weakness, weird pain. Despite my objections—I really wanted to go fishing—the hotel doctor checked me into a local hospital, where other doctors hooked me up to all this shit and told me that I'd had a heart attack.

"I'm glad you told me," I said. "Because I didn't know that. For real."

"We'll want to keep you here for a month," they said. "You shouldn't travel so far so soon."

"I thought the heart attack was a joke," I replied. "But what you said is really funny."

I liked Australia, but if I was going to die, it was going to be in my own motherfucking house, you know? Following an emergency call, my personal physician arrived from L.A., put me through treadmill and electrocardiograph tests, and then accompanied me back home, explaining I'd incurred a mild infarction.

Maybe. But the effects weren't mild. Afraid that I might die alone, without anyone around to love me, I remarried Flynn on April 1. It wasn't hard. Flynn was there. She had my kids. She liked being married to me.

Smart Rich.

How much did that foolish decision cost you?

Can't remember? Does it matter anymore?

No, because we divorced a few months later and then I was just as alone as before, you know?

But I didn't want to be dead without a wife. Honest. If I was going to die, I wanted a bitch there to cry.

I never considered how much I could stand. No doubt the fire, the MS, and now the heart attack had caught up with me, though I didn't really acknowledge it until shortly before I partnered with Gene Wilder in *Another You*. One morning I woke up and tried getting out of bed, but my legs wouldn't move. Not a fucking kick or twitch. Not only could I not stand, I couldn't even fall, and it fucked me up because I didn't feel bad, you know?

"I don't know what's wrong," I yelled at my doctor. "It just won't work!"

"Things like that happen," he said. "It comes and goes. Some days might not be as bad. Other days can be worse."

Rather than dwell on what could possibly be worse, I spent two intensely hard, exhausting, painful weeks learning how to walk again. By the time the cameras rolled, I was on my feet—fragile, wobbly, and obviously not in fighting shape—but I was on my feet. It took regular cortisone shots and steroid treatments from my doctor to keep me going, but I was determined to finish the picture.

Yet toward the end even that seemed iffy. The picture, which was strife-ridden after a change of directors, ran about eight hundred weeks over schedule. By that time, I was exhausted. I never had a conversation with Gene or anyone about my struggle with MS, but it was pretty clear my body was mostly beyond my control. They started keeping a wheelchair on the set.

Finally, my stuff said, "I put up with you this long. But no more, motherfucker."

Gene and I were doing a scene in which we went hunting and I was supposed to kill him after a run-in with a great big bear. They used a real live bear, who was trained, but a big motherfucker nonetheless. With claws and teeth. He stood behind Gene, and before I fired at Gene, I was supposed to talk shit to the bear. Now I don't know if the bear knew he frightened people, but he scared the shit out of me.

If he acted up, I couldn't run.

I was dinner, you know.

Even worse, when the director yelled "Action," I didn't move so hot. I tried hobbling around a bit, but my legs weren't operating like my brain was telling them to. Finally, the director must've overheard me arguing with myself.

"Run, Rich, run!"

"No, motherfucker. Just shut the fuck up!"

Realizing Richard couldn't move, he came over and in a private whisper asked if I would be more comfortable having a stunt man substitute for me. Momentarily relieved, I said, "Yes, that would be fine." But then the reality hit me. The only comparison that comes to mind is when New York Yankee great

Lou Gehrig was taken out of the game. Only there was no ceremony. I didn't have a stadium full of people cheering for me. Just a film set with a lot of folks anxious to get on with their work.

Yet that was the beginning of me not being able to do the shit anymore.

Whether I wanted to admit it or not.

The MS took over.

THIRTY-TWO

One morning at the end of May 1991, I pleaded with Deboragh to let me stay in bed and skip my scheduled doctor's appointment. At the time, she worked as my personal assistant. With our history of heartbreak, that was less a job than an excuse to be together rather than alone. She knew that I loved her dearly even though I'd been a perfect asshole in the past.

Ornery, depressed, and weakened by a general malaise that had turned my body into a lead weight, I begged and begged to be left by myself, propped up in bed, smoking, and staring at the television as if it was a Valium. Ordinarily, I got my way acting like a child, but that day Debbie didn't buy my shit.

"You don't look so good, Richie," she kept saying. "I really think you need to go."

Both of us knew how much I hated going to the hospital, even when it was for a routine checkup. But I have a suspicion that sometimes I get together with women for a reason other than just the quest of pussy. Though they mostly behave like bitches, they can also be like angels who watch out for Richard.

"Okay, I'll go," I said finally. "Only if you stay with me."

A few hours later, the doctor saw a funny blip on my EKG and checked me into the hospital for observation. If I'd been observing some foxy nurses sucking my dick, it might've been all right. But about four in the morning, I was awakened by a

sharp, horrible pain that made my body contort and writhe as if someone was trying to pull my nipple through my asshole. Then the shit all centralized in my heart, and I knew what was going down.

"Richard."

"Who's that?"

"God."

"Go away, motherfucker."

"Let's wrap it up."

"But I got more material."

The hallway flew by. Lights on the ceiling looked like steps leading to heaven (I hoped) or perhaps a Michael Jackson video. People rushed around me. Doctors hurried to explain the whats and hows of a quadruple bypass operation. I asked Debbie to sign papers that would prevent the vultures from eating up all the money. But there was no time. That was the biggest impression I had. Everything was moving fast.

Was I scared? Scared of dying? Shit, I don't know. A nurse sticking a giant needle into my arm. Another, she explained, was going into my heart. Okay, you know? I wasn't there to argue. But whatever drug they give you before an operation, you don't have to worry. It takes away all your pain and fears.

One minute I was dying. The next I imagined that Sammy Davis, Jr., was in the room, snapping his fingers and doing Sammy shit while Frank Sinatra sang a classic. Comedian Jan Murray stood in the hallway. Not wanting my life to turn into a fucking lounge act, I told Sammy to go and get Frank. I wanted him to help me get back in the main showroom.

I mean, if not Frank, then who?

"Okay, Bub," Sammy said. "I'll get him."

Groggy, confused, dulled, and numbed by drugs, I came out of the operation believing that some kind doctors and nurses had gotten together and arranged for my hospital bed to be placed

in the middle of a blue trout stream. When my eyes opened, I was gazing out on a beautiful scene in the woods instead of a cold and stark hospital room loaded with heart-monitoring equipment. I worked my fishing rod with as much ease as ever, getting some bites but never the big one.

The nurse who wandered in struck me as a nun. She was Sister Rosie. And I spoke with an Irish accent.

"Sister Rosie, don't stand in the trout stream," I warned.

The same thing happened when the shift changed and a guy nurse wandered in, checking shit. I thought he was an Irish priest and told him to get on out of the trout stream. He looked at me as if I should've known better.

"The Bulls are going to win," he said.

I didn't understand at first, but then something must've fused together in my brain, like a missing piece of railroad track, because suddenly I realized that I was in the hospital and that he was talking about the basketball play-offs.

"You mean the Bulls are going to beat the Lakers?" I asked.

Quick cut. I bet him $30 the Lakers would win. L.A. beat the shit out of Chicago. It was the only game they won the entire series. I was happy, man. But the motherfucker never came into my room again. To this day, I've yet to be paid.

At least I was around to collect, you know. I'd entered the hospital for a routine checkup but left with my heart having been removed, flipped over, and attached to new veins that had been relocated from around my legs and ankles. A long, Frankenstein scar ran down the center of my chest like a receipt from the grocery store. I'd been prepared to die. Expected it. But then I realized God chooses the checkout time.

"Hey, Rich, I changed my mind," He said. "You were right. You do have some more material. Get your ass back out there.

"Just don't smoke," my doctor said as I left.

I'd already gone through a pack of Marlboros in the hospital.

"What about the pussy?" I asked.

"Why not?" he answered.

That's what I said, too.

Why not?

Why the fuck not?

THIRTY-THREE

Enough was enough. In September, I decided to take my battle with MS public. The nudge came when producer George Schlatter asked if he could organize a special CBS tribute to me, and I agreed. The show brought together Arsenio Hall, Eddie Murphy, Patti LaBelle, and dozens of friends and performers in an emotional look at my entire career.

Until then, MS had been a private matter. My problem. I was too proud to want to be seen as debilitated. Nor did I want sympathy. Nor did I want to discuss any of the shit. I had more than enough problems trying to figure out why the fuck God had decided to give me MS. I asked the question daily. Sometimes hourly. It echoed in my head like a fucking church bell. Why me? Why did you give this shit to me?

But there were no answers.

So either I could drive myself crazy, which wouldn't have been too long a trip, or I could, as had been my practice since my first misstep in dog poo, milk the entertainment value, sail down the uncharted river of my life, and check out where in the hell the current took me.

After all, I told myself, "Fuck it, you know. This is my life. I've got MS, not death."

Some people found reason to joke otherwise. George had put on a similar event for Sammy Davis, Jr., not long before he passed away. The irony prompted Eddie Murphy, the show's emcee, to wonder how scared I was when George called.

Going into the Beverly Hilton Hotel that evening, I'd worried how people would react when they saw that I needed a cane to stand, that I had trouble walking, speaking, and even doing little things like eating. But at the end of the evening, I was relieved to finally put all the rumors to rest. No more hiding, pretending, or shit, and my bruised pride was mighty grateful.

But it didn't make coping with MS any easier. Each day, it seemed, I was forced to confront the disease. It was like being held captive by a truly nasty motherfucker. One day I would be able to get around using a cane. The next day I wouldn't have the strength to even hobble and would have to use my motorized cart, or "Mobie," as I called it. I spilled drinks, had difficulty eating, and, even more frightening, I once fell in the shower.

Although impossible to cure, I fought the MS by devoting part of every day to some kind of treatment. In addition to the cortisone injections and intravenous steroids that I'd been taking for nearly two years, I saw a therapist, took antidepressants for my mood swings, and worked with physical therapists. I also watched my diet and alcohol consumption.

My doctors said, "You're doing great. You could go on like this for a long, long time."

"Is that a reward?" I asked.

Considering the alternative, I supposed it was.

But even my best efforts only slowed the degenerative disease. That's when I unbaffled this baffling disease. Saw the big picture. Saw it as clear as the first day I got cable TV. It was a message from God.

"Hey, Rich, you ever heard the phrase 'delayed gratification'?"

"Yeah."

"Good. 'Cause you've done had a lot of gratification."

"So."

"Well, now comes the delay."

In some ways, it was more like a total stoppage. Despite two

Rolls-Royces and a Ferrari parked in the garage, I couldn't drive a car anymore. I couldn't climb stairs. I couldn't even have an orgasm. But my dick would get hard, you know? Rise to the occasion. Visit me like a friend or something. "Hey, Rich, how're ya doin', brother? Just wanted to say hi."

The motherfucker always caught me off guard.

"Come again?" I asked.

"Shit, motherfucker, I ain't even come a first time."

That's what it all boils down to, right? Can you or can't you? I tried, Mama, I tried. There were times when my dick got hard and I got so excited that I called people just to tell them about it. And the people I called weren't always womens, you know? It was whoever answered their phone.

"Hey, Herbie, guess what? My dick's hard and it's looking at me."

I never prayed in my life, but MS made me pray. I'd be in bed with a woman and I'd start praying, "Please, God, I know you're an extremely busy man. But if you could find it in your heart to grant me a tiny little favor. Not world peace. Not a cure for MS. No miracles, man. I just need my prick hard, okay?"

Eventually, I realized that I should deal with the basics rather than the luxury items—like my bladder. Before MS, I dialogued with my bladder, you know? Like I'd have to piss, but I wouldn't be near a toilet. So I'd ask my bladder, "Hey, there's not a bathroom nearby. You think you can wait till home? Only fifteen minutes or so."

"Yeah, no problem, Rich."

But MS ended all communication. I'd be on the street, talking with some womens, and suddenly I'd start pissing. Feel piss streaming down my leg, squirming into my socks and landing in my boots. It was no different than the other problems I had with, say, my legs. You know, I'd want to walk across the room, but they wouldn't go.

Then the womens, they said, "Don't worry. It's all right."

Clearly, though, it's not all right. I don't like to see nobody

piss. So why's it okay for people to watch me piss? And in the middle of the street? But people always say shit like that is okay so long as it isn't them.

Once all the shit ganged up on me at the same time. I was on the freeway, being driven back from someplace, and I was feeling cocky. Somewhere up ahead, a truck jackknifed, causing a monstrous traffic jam. It seemed every car in the world was on the freeway that day. Cars from as far away as Denver came just to clog up the damn road.

As we sat, I saw one of the prettiest bitches I'd ever seen in my life, and she was waving at me. I waved back and the bitch opened her car door, got out, and walked across the freeway to meet me. She kept waving as she weaved a path through the cars. Cute little friendly waves that told me she thought I was cute. Suddenly, my arm started twitching and doing shit, some wild shit, and I tried to get my arm down but it wouldn't go.

"Come on, arm. Quit that shit."

"No."

"Please."

"No."

Just as she got to the car, my bladder decided it was time to go, too. The floodgates opened, the tender of the pump house yelled, "Now!" and I prayed I didn't slide off the seat. She said something about how I was so funny but I could stop waving, you know. I didn't bother to explain. I couldn't. I was too preoccupied. Because while my brain thought about how much I wanted to fuck her, my dick was saying, "Go ahead and try. Ha-ha-ha."

I did what I could. One night I came home and pissed outside because I couldn't get to the door. Right in the flowers. I thought that was okay. In fact, I was grateful to have made it that far and been able to get my dick out. But you know what? The dog was pissed off. He ran across the yard, snarling.

"Rich, man, that's my spot. I been pissing on that geranium for two years. What the hell are you doing?"

"I had to go."

"But that's my geranium. There's a whole yard here."

I gave that damn dog an abbreviated look—ASPCA.

"Shut up, motherfucker," I said. "I may not be able to kick your ass anymore. But I still got my gun."

By the fall of 1992, I was resigned to a life in the slow lane and hopefully few surprises. If I went crazy, it was with my remote control, flipping through 120 channels with the speed I used to drive. But then one day I got my ass kicked. The phone rang. My assistant told me that my accountant was on the line, and he was very worried.

"He says that he heard you were dead."

"Tell him that I was," I said. "But I came back to check the books."

Rumors of my death spread as far as New York newspapers. It's a bitch to be watching the nightly news and see the mother-fuckers talking about you in the past tense. Friends called. The weirdest shit was when people who worked for me started to believe that I could go at any time. Like my housekeeper. She'd walk into the bedroom while I was sleeping and start making a lot of noise. When I didn't stir, she squeezed my toe.

"Oh, shit! What're you doing?" I screamed, waking up in a panic of discomfort.

"Sorry, sorry, Mr. Pryor. But I thought you were, maybe, well, maybe you were no longer living."

"Why the hell would you think that?"

"You were lying on the bed. With your eyes closed. Not hardly moving."

"That's how I sleep. How do you do it?"

"But the news on the TV in the kitchen. I heard you died."

"Well, they were lying."

There were probably countless ways I could've dispelled the reports of my premature demise, but the one I chose certainly

wasn't the easiest. On October 31, after weeks of working out new material at the Comedy Store, I performed before a sold-out audience at the Circle Star Theater outside San Francisco, my first concert in nearly six years.

Didn't matter how many times I done this before, I was scared, man. I truly was.

First of all, they call it standup comedy, but I found myself having to adapt the format with a big easy chair placed in the center of the stage. Swallowing more fear than I'd known my entire life, I gingerly made my way across the stage with the assistance of a silver-handled cane. Then I sat down.

It wasn't easy. The crowd thought they were there to laugh, but my physical condition also gave them some major drama.

Gave me some, too.

You know?

Afterward, I thought I had kicked ass. The reviews were mostly in agreement.

Encouraged, I hit the road. Although it wasn't anywhere near the same as it had been in the past—none of the drug-induced craziness, the spur-of-the-moment insanity with womens—the outpouring of love I felt was overly generous.

But after a few gigs, I realized that I had more heart than energy, more courage than strength. Just turning in a decent forty minutes exhausted me way too much. The mind was willing. But my feets couldn't carry me to the end zone.

Knowing I was unable to continue through the early months of 1993, I canceled the rest of the tour.

What a bitch, you know?

It destroyed me emotionally. All the shit that I wanted to say was in my head with nowhere to go. I could hear the applause. I imagined the rejuvenating effect of laughter. There was nothing like it in the world.

THIRTY-FOUR

had my first encounter with death when I was a kid visiting my grandfather's farm in Springfield. One night he took me for a walk. On the property next door we came across a dead cow. Enormous motherfucker lying on its side. For a moment we thought it was asleep, but it was dead. No question.

Don't know why, but my grandfather handed me a gunnysack and instructed me to kneel down and open it up by the cow's asshole. Then he kicked the cow in the belly. A second later, a possum ran out of the cow's ass. Straight into the gunnysack I held.

"Hold the sack, boy!" my grandfather yelled.

"Holy shit, Pop!" I exclaimed.

You know?

It was a fucking possum! Come out of that cow's asshole!

In any case, my grandfather grabbed the bag out of my hands and swung it over his shoulder, holding it there, despite the possum's squirming, until we came to a big rock. Then he slammed it against the rock, killing the possum.

Okay.

Then I started wondering what we were going to do with that dead rodent.

You know what we did with it? We took it home and my grandma cooked it. We ate the motherfucker. To this day, I don't eat anything with barbecue sauce, because I had to drown the

motherfucker in that shit in order to get it into my stomach. But it taught me about death all right.

Life is all there is.

When you kick, that's about it. Show's over.

I'm sorry whatever others may think. But ain't shit happening when you're dead.

A friend once said to me, "Life's a bitch. Then you die. And you don't get change."

You don't get change.

You know that's the truth. The shit they do to people in the funeral parlor, getting you ready for the funeral. If you don't wake up from that, you have to know that being dead means that you are dead. Fade to black, you know?

When my body shuffles off to Buffalo, I want to be cremated. I don't want nobody fucking with me again. Because there are people who like to fuck with dead people. Twist their toes around and shit. I don't want nobody fucking with my toes.

Or my nuts!

On the off chance that I'm wrong about death, I want to make sure that I can still fuck. If there's pussy in heaven, I'll be chasing it. Imagine that: chasing pussy for eternity. Sounds an awful lot like life, doesn't it?

Although death has occupied a lot of my idle thoughts the past few years, I look at it like a report of bad weather. Dark and stormy clouds today. Maybe clearing up later in the week. The truth is—has been and, near as I can figure, will continue to be until the last gasp—that MS may have kicked my ass into the blackness, but I have too much to live for to give up on basking in the light again.

Throughout the illness, the womens in my life have made sure of that. I hear from my first wife, Pat, from Shelley and Maxine. Geraldine's picture rests on my bedroom table. Flynn comes by, reminding me to exercise. Deboragh, who's remained

so understanding, has never left the spot closest to my heart. And Jennifer, bless her lovely soul, kicks my ass from treatment to treatment and makes sure I get a dose of laughter every day.

Then there are my children. Somehow they've managed to make it in life and turn out magnificently. Richard Jr. continues to keep the Pryor name alive in Peoria while Rain continues to prove herself in Hollywood. Elizabeth is in graduate school. And Steven, Kelsey, and Franklin have their work cut out just trying to grow up in this world.

At this stage of my life, I'm more amazed by their presence than ever. When I look at them, I see so much. I see all my debauchery, but I also see the goodness and the long road of hope and possibility ahead of them.

It makes me love them very much.

Do I have regrets? I think about what might've happened if I'd done things differently. But I can't go back and redo them. So why, you know? What is, is.

I'm glad I'm in show business. As crazy as it sounds, I don't think there are any people like us on earth.

I plan on doing more work—acting, writing, producing. The ideas swirl in my head.

I'm also proud of the work that I've already done. I'm glad I was alive at a time in history when it was possible to record what I had to say, because I think I had something to say. It sounds presumptuous, maybe, a guy from the whorehouses in Peoria. But why not? I came with perspective.

Looking up.

Looking out.

The view was clear. People are nice to each other and they're also mean to each other. That's the way it's always been and probably always will be. The fact that we're different colors is basically just an excuse for doing all that shit. But if people understand the differences a little better, learn to blend the colors, which was my job as a comedian, it's possible to see we're all the same.

Same needs and wants.

A little money, a little wine, a little pussy.

Lately, I've been thinking about something. Back when I was in the Army stationed in Germany, I was in charge of repairing utilities. I was always on the phone, calling different offices. One day I picked up the phone and started talking to this lady who had a nice voice that intrigued me.

A short time later, I got to meet her, and she turned out to be one of the nicest ladies I'd ever met. Although she was married, we used to make love all the time. Mornings, afternoons, nights. Her husband eventually found out. He knew she liked me. But for some reason, he didn't bother as long as I kept away while he was there.

Shortly before I shipped back home, we made love one more time, and afterward she said, "I will come and visit you in Peoria."

Sure.

That's what I thought, anyway.

Then one day, long after I'd been back to Peoria, I was in a bar, and who came in? This lady. She looked wonderful. No different. But I wasn't the same soldier, you know, and it panicked me. I knew she couldn't withstand all the shit in my life. So while her husband waited, I made love with her one more time at the Holiday Inn, and then we said our goodbyes and that was it, the last time we saw each other.

That's been in my mind lately.

Why, Rich?

Well, I've been thinking about where both of us were at that moment in our lives. The future was so unclear. Not bright or dark. Just the future. And our hearts were so strong. I hope that she's all right. I really do. I hope that she found whatever she was looking for.

Life can seem so complicated at times. Yet when you look

back what is it besides the accumulation of such encounters with people?

You never know.

As for me, I's amazed that I didn't OD on heroin, get stuffed with coke, or die from AIDS. I think it's remarkable that I'm still here, thinking these silly thoughts. Some people have said it's pure luck. Others say it's testimony to the human spirit. I think it has more to do with something else.

Through an old friend of mine I once said, "There ain't but two pieces of pussy you're gonna get in your life. That's your first and your last, and all that shit in between don't matter. That's just the extra gravy. But you never forget your first and you damn sure won't forget your last. And if you live that long, you're in big trouble."

I'd rather die of cancer than fuck around and remember my last piece of pussy, you know?

I got some this morning, and right now that's as far back as I want to remember.

Oh yeah, one more thing.

I always remember to keep some sunshine on my face.

INDEX